DEMENTIA:
NON-PHARMACOLOGICAL THERAPIES

NEUROSCIENCE RESEARCH PROGRESS

Additional books in this series can be found on Nova's website
under the Series tab.

Additional E-books in this series can be found on Nova's website
under the E-book tab.

NEUROSCIENCE RESEARCH PROGRESS

DEMENTIA:
NON-PHARMACOLOGICAL THERAPIES

ELISABETTA FARINA
EDITOR

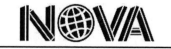

Nova Science Publishers, Inc.

New York

Library of Congress Cataloging-in-Publication Data

Dementia : non-pharmacological therapies / editor, Elisabetta Farina.
       p. ; cm.
  Includes bibliographical references and index.
  ISBN 978-1-61470-736-3 (hardcover)
  1. Dementia--Treatment. 2. Dementia--Psychological aspects. I. Farina, Elisabetta.
  [DNLM: 1. Dementia--therapy. 2. Dementia--psychology. 3. Rehabilitation. 4. Sensory Art Therapies. WM 220]
  RC521.D45565 2011
  616.8'3--dc23   2011024889

Published by Nova Science Publishers, Inc. † *New York*

CONTENTS

PREFACE

This book presents current research in the study of non-pharmacological treatment proposed in dementia care. Topics discussed include music therapy in dementia; predictors of effective support for carers of persons with dementia; computer-assisted spaced retrieval training of faces and names for persons with dementia; physical and mental exercises plus work therapy for Alzheimer's patients; recreational therapy interventions and Cognitive Stimulation Therapy.

Article 1- The use of music and sonorous-music elements in the field of dementia has been, for some years, much widespread, although the application experiences are very different in relation to the purposes and contents of the proposals. The contexts in which musical activities are proposed to people with dementia are numerous. Their main goal is to create a situation of wellbeing and socialization through various music proposals (rhythmic use of instruments, singing, movement associated with music, etc.). There are also the experiences of listening to music: music is potentially evocative, stimulates memories or states of mind through moments of verbalization after listening to music; further, music is used in order to facilitate the recognition of environments or structured moments of the day; finally, listening to music (classical music, favourite music, etc.) is used in the belief that it can effectively reduce behavioral disorders and enhance mood or socialization (Raglio, 2008a).

Article 2- As the number of patients diagnosed with a dementia increases, so does the need for managing cognitive impairment, behavioural and psychological symptoms. During the past 20 years, a significant amount of knowledge, new theoretical and practical approaches have been developed. Multiple therapeutic trials have led to the marketing of symptomatic drugs, including cholinesterase inhibitors for patients with mild-to-moderate Alzheimer's Disease. At the same time, and complementary to drug therapies, various non-drug, individual or group interventions, have been designed for patients and/or caregivers (Doody et al. 2001, Brodaty et al. 2003, Seux 2008).

Article 3- Apathy is defined as the loss of motivation not attributable to cognitive impairment, emotional distress, or reduced level of consciousness (Marin, 1991). Apathy occurs in approximately 71% of individuals with Alzheimer's disease (AD) within five years of diagnosis (Boyle and Malloy, 2004). Individuals living with AD with apathy require more management and support, given their reliance on others to schedule their activities and initiate tasks even when they are still physically capable of performing them. Studies examining the relationship of apathy to neuropsychological measures showed apathy was consistently associated with more severe functional impairments, more severe cognitive deficits, higher levels of burden and distress in caregivers, along with increased resource utilization (Landes, Sperry, Strauss, and Geldmacher, 2008; Starkstein, Ingram, Garau, and Mizrahi, 2005). Apathy is a negative symptom in AD that is often overlooked by healthcare providers, yet one that if left untreated, leads to more rapid than expected functional decline (Starkstein, Jorge, Mizrahi, and Robinson, 2006). The causes of apathy are described as complex and related to underlying pathology, atrophy of the frontal lobes, and their connections to the temporal lobes (Levy and Dubois, 2006). Damage to these areas of the brain reduces the individual's the ability to initiate, sequence, and complete tasks without assistance.

Article 4- In recent years there has been a growing interest in reminiscence work with older adults. There appears to be a general assumption that reminiscence work has a positive impact on those who participate, including people with dementia (e.g. Woods and McKiernan, 1995; Gibson, 2004). However, the evidence to date with older adults with dementia has been very limited and offers little insight into these approaches. Only five studies could be included in the revised Cochrane review of reminiscence work in dementia (Woods et al., 2005), each evaluating a different modality of reminiscence work, and the results from these did not allow firm conclusions to be drawn. In light of the widespread application of these techniques, the effects of clearly specified reminiscence approaches need to be carefully evaluated.

Article 5- Improving the quality of care for people with dementia is a key priority of the National Dementia Strategy (DoH, 2008), and staff training is essential to the development of good standards of care (Innes, 2001). However, a review of training in dementia (McCabe et al, 2007) showed mixed results, with half of the studies finding no effect of staff training on the resident they provided care for, even when increases in the knowledge and skills of staff were demonstrated. The authors suggested that training can bring secondary benefits including increasing job satisfaction; reducing staff stress levels and turnover rates, possibly through an increased sense of competence, morale, and self- worth. Moniz-Cook et al. (1998) found that following a training programme, staff often went back to prior ways of working. As the title of one report suggests, 'Training is not enough to change care practice' (Lintern, Woods, and Phair, 2000).

Article 6- One of the great challenges of the 21st century will be the provision of adequate care to the growing number of elderly people, and in particular, those with dementia. With an estimated 24 million people world-wide suffering from dementia at present [1], a number expected to double every twenty years, and the parallel decrease in the number of persons of the working population who are potentially available to offer formal and informal care [2], health care systems require significant adaptation to meet the future demands of persons with dementia. Because of the expected disproportional grow of institutionalized care, relatively more people with dementia will need to be cared for in their own home and this is also the general policy in many European countries. However, without changes in present health care systems, the current standards cannot be maintained.

Article 7- According to Alzheimer's disease International (2009), the global prevalence of dementia, predicted at 35 million in 2010, is expected to almost double every 20 years. While researchers search for the "magic bullet" that will slow, halt, or reverse the deterioration wrought by Alzheimer's disease (AD), millions of individuals with this disorder are languishing in nursing homes and exhausting family caregivers. Bereft of former roles and responsibilities that formed their identity and gave meaning to their lives, persons with dementia typically become socially withdrawn and isolated and dependent on paid caregivers, busy nursing home staff, or overburdened family members to structure and supervise their time and activities. It is not surprising that planning and supervising activities take a back seat to more urgent care giving tasks such as personal care, meal preparation, medical needs, and other family, work, and household responsibilities. Apathy and depression are too often the consequences of the lack of opportunity for persons with dementia to experience success at challenges and to make meaningful societal contributions.

Article 8- This study is based on the general finding that non-pharmacological factors such as interior design and architectural characteristics of environments can help reduce symptoms of Dementia of the Alzheimer Type (DAT) (Zeisel, Silverstein, Hyde, Levkoff, Lawton and Holmes, 2003). Zeisel *et al.*'s research with 427 participants of American origin identifies associations between characteristics of the architectural environment in fifteen special care units (SCU) and symptoms of agitation, aggression, depression, social withdrawal, as well as psychotic symptoms.

Article 9- The perspective on care for chronic persons with dementia, and therefore also the care for chronic *psychogeriatric* persons with dementia, such as people with Alzheimer's disease and other types of dementia, has changed profoundly over the last 40 years. Today, the emphasis is no longer only on medical-hygienic issues, but also on psychosocial aspects such as: guiding the person in accepting his disease, coping with the consequences of the disease, and ultimately on the quality of life. The setting of new goals in care has led to the development of a range of new care and treatment methods

Article 10- Because of the personal nature of this article, it is largely written in the first person. I thank the many persons who, over many years, have worked with me and discussed this approach to the treatment of dementia.

Recently, Beck, Levinson, and Irons (2009) traced the origins of J. B. Watson's famous experiment with "Little Albert," and their detective work led to the discovery of the person who probably was the infant in Watson's laboratory and shown in his films of conditioning experiments. In a similar manner, this article traces the origins of the use of Montessori educational techniques as interventions for persons with dementia. In my case, however, I have a distinct advantage over Beck, Levinson, and Irons. They had to make inferences and deductions based on records, circumstantial evidence, and the sometimes erroneous or conflicting evidence presented by the memories of persons associated with events that occurred almost 90 years ago. In my case, I only have to contend with omissions or false memories generated in my own mind over the course of the last 32 years of my life experiences. However, it is hoped that the reader will be indulgent, and that the tracing of the origins of this intervention will serve as an inspiration to younger researchers to be open to interruptions in their careers and to serendipity.

Article 11- Persistent sleep disturbances are common in persons living with Alzheimer's disease (AD), affecting up to 44 per cent of subjects in clinic [1] and community-based samples [2-4]. These fragmented sleep/wake cycles are characterized by frequent daytime napping, prolonged night-time wakefulness, and multiple nocturnal awakenings, often resulting in increased and inappropriate levels of nocturnal activity, including wandering about in either a seemingly aimless or disorientated fashion or in pursuit of an indefinable or unobtainable goal [5]. For family caregivers, being awoken at night by a relative's wandering and other aberrant motor, vocal or verbal behaviours is one of the most disturbing aspects of care [2] and are a major risk factor for earlier institutionalisation [6-9]. It has been estimated that such behaviour occurs in around 30 per cent of subjects in nursing homes and is strongly associated with the severity of dementia and diminished visuoperceptive and navigational abilities [10].

Articler 12- Psychosocial interventions for dementia have often been developed without a sound theoretical, empirical and clinical basis, and most evaluations of these interventions have had serious methodological limitations (Woods et al., 2005). In our earlier work, the Cochrane Review on Reality Orientation (RO) was used to develop an evidence based Cognitive Stimulation Therapy (CST) programme for dementia (Spector et al., 2000; 2001; 2003). The results of a randomised controlled trial (RCT) of CST compared favourably with trials of cholinesterase inhibitors for Alzheimer's disease, in terms of the size of the effects on cognition (Spector et al, 2003) and the economic analysis showed that CST was likely to be cost-effective (Knapp et al, 2006). The NICE guidelines (NICE-SCIE, 2006) recommended that people with mild/moderate dementia should be 'given the opportunity to participate in a structured group cognitive stimulation programme'. Cognitive stimulation approaches may have long-term effects (Zanetti et al., 1995; Metitieri et al., 2001) and a 16 week pilot study of maintenance CST (Orrell et al., 2005) following the initial 7 weeks of CST, found a significant improvement in cognitive function (MMSE) and identified the need for a large-scale, multi-centre RCT. Best practice is to develop interventions systematically, using the best available evidence and appropriate theory (Craig at al., 2008). This highlights the need to link intervention development with evaluation and design issues during the early stages of phase 1 or development of an intervention. This study focuses on the developmental stage of the Medical Research Council guidelines (2008) for the development and evaluation of complex interventions (Figure 1). Modelling a complex intervention prior to a full-scale evaluation can provide important information about the design of both the intervention and the evaluation (Clancy et al., 2002; Wortman, 1995; Nazaret et al., 2002). The aim was to develop a programme of Maintenance CST for dementia, as a complex long-term intervention in preparation for its evaluation in a large RCT. The three main steps for the development of the programme (MRC, 2008) were: identifying the evidence; identifying and developing theory and modelling process and outcomes.

Article 13- Dementia is characterized by acquired and persistent impairment of multiple cognitive domains that is severe enough to interfere with activities of daily living, occupation, and social interaction (Grabowski & Damasio, 2004). Affected cognitive domains include memory, attention, executive function, language and communicative function, and visuospatial abilities. Alzheimer's disease (AD) is the most common cause of dementia in older adults over the age of 65 years, accounting for approximately 50% of clinical diagnoses of dementia (Alzheimer's Association, 2010). There is substantial evidence that cognitive interventions for persons with dementia (PWD) are efficacious and can facilitate maintenance or improvement of performance on discrete cognitive tasks and on functional activities of daily living (Bayles & Kim, 2003; Bourgeois et al., 2003; Camp, 1989; Mahendra, 2001; Mahendra & Arkin, 2003; McKitrick, Camp, & Black, 1992). Given the rapidly rising incidence of dementia and the limited benefit from existing pharmacological treatments using acetylcholinesterase (ACE) inhibitors and N-methyl-D-aspartate (NMDA) antagonists, it is imperative that researchers continue to aggressively develop and study outcomes of innovative, non-pharmacological interventions. Further, it is noteworthy that there is emerging empirical evidence supporting better outcomes for PWD following a synergistic combination of pharmacological and nonpharmacalogical interventions, as compared to drug treatments alone (Chapman et al., 2004; Requena et al., 2004; Requena et al., 2006). In this paper, we report the outcomes of computer-assisted spaced retrieval training (SRT) for teaching face-name associations to persons with dementia. Spaced retrieval training is described in the next section, followed by a brief review of existing research on its application for designing interventions for persons with dementia.

Article 14- The increase in prevalence of Alzheimer's disease and related dementias (ADRD) and the lack of curative therapies is fuelling the development of non-pharmacological therapies (NPT) to improve quality of life of both people with dementia (PWD) and their caregivers (Woods 2003). Offering NPTs to PWD has two main objectives: a) convey as many positive experiences as possible while minimizing the negative ones whilst the PWD is in a session.and b) provide clinically relevant carryover effects in domains like cognition, function, behaviour or mood, amongst other.

Article 15- People are becoming increasingly aware that providing informal care to persons with chronic diseases is a heavy task [1]. This is particularly true when caring for people with dementia, because dementia deeply affects both the person concerned with the illness and his or her social environment [2]. Caring for a person with dementia frequently has negative physical, mental and social consequences for the informal carer [3-9]. These negative consequences turn out to be related with earlier institutionalization of the person with dementia [10-16].

Article 16- The groups addressed to the relatives involved with the care of persons living with dementia are generally organized by the Alzheimer's Associations [1,2,3] and can be classified in three categories: *a*) Psycho - educational groups which give information about the illness and the strategies to cope with the Behavioral and Psychiatric Signs and Symptoms of Dementia (BPSD); *b*) Support groups with a professional leader, which want to give psychological help to caregivers; *c*) Self-help groups, with or without a professional leader.

EDITORIAL

Elisabetta Farina

It was worth the trouble to wait for this third issue of "Non-pharmacological therapies in dementia".

The opening paper is an exciting methodology article by the London-Bangor group: these Authors have deeply influenced the domain of psychosocial therapies in dementia by creating a program of cognitive stimulation whose efficacy was demonstrated through a randomized study in 2003. The article contained in this issue describes the developmental stage of an evidence-based Maintenance Cognitive Stimulation Therapy program for dementia, according to Medical Research Council guidelines. The methodology used by the Authors is robust, really well constructed and detailed: therefore this paper can represent a reference for other groups who want to develop new treatments on solid bases in this field. In my opinion, a particularly relevant point in the article is the effort to marry the research for a rigorous scientific methodology with a humanistic view of care (e.g. with reference to the person-centered care of Kitwood), which means that they also try their best for taking into account the view of both people living with dementia and their carers in order to develop the therapy. I'm particularly happy about it because this evolution in the domain of non-pharmacological therapies in dementia demonstrates something which I previewed and foresaw years ago: that is that scientific medicine, cognitive psychology, neuropsychology and human values can be merged in a more holistic and comprehensive view of dementia therapy to ameliorate outcomes and quality of life of people living together this condition. Then one could also add art, culture and much more to create even a better recipe. This point of view, when shared by all the professional categories dealing with people living with dementia, would allow to join their efforts and to achieve the best results in term of efficacy of care, if we give the term "care" an all-inclusive meaning (furthermore in this view of care psychosocial therapies are not at odds with useful drug treatments). Sure, to adopt this view, different caring categories should give up that typical attitude dictated by professional jealousy. This is particularly true in our case – of medical doctors- a professional category who isn't always used to work in team. But let's imagine an ideal world where people who receive the diagnosis of Alzheimer's disease are directly guided by the physician also to turn their steps towards the non-pharmacological option (along with the pharmacological one, why not). A world where governments are convinced by now – thanks to studies carried out with good methodology-that these therapies are effective and *cost*-effective.

The views of people with dementia are also taken into account by Maria Wolff Center group, Spain, in the third article even if in a different way. In fact, this paper presents an easy-to-use instrument for measuring the affective and social experience of people with dementia while undergoing non-pharmacological interventions (NPT), the NPT experience scale (NPT-ES). This scale could indeed become a useful tool for therapists' store of knowledge, allowing them to self evaluate the quality of their interventions, to select the most appropriate non-pharmacological therapy for every person with dementia, and to save involved people an unpleasant experience and the negative effects of therapy. We must never forget that non-pharmacological therapies have to be proposed- of course in the most attractive way- but not imposed and that the subjective experience of concerned people could be very different from what we (professionals) are expecting.

On the other hand, the fourth article (written by a very active and prolific Dutch group operating for many years in the domain of psychosocial therapies for people living with dementia) takes into account the views of carers on different types of support offered in meeting centers in the Netherlands. How are satisfaction and effectiveness of the offered support related to characteristics of carers? Meiland et al. try to give a preliminary answer. In order to optimize the interventions and to make them cost-effective, it's important to try and understand which kind of support is more effective and psychologically useful for a specific category of caregivers (e.g. children versus spouses, higher educated carers versus lower educated ones).

The fifth article also focuses on caregivers by presenting an original self–help group named ABC. This group, conducted by a professional leader, is based on a new method which was developed in Italy and presented here in English for the first time: the Conversational and Enabling Approach (CEA). CEA is based on focusing the attention on the words exchanged between patient and caregiver during daily life and aims at favoring verbal expression in spite of the speech impairment and the deterioration of the communication function of speech due to dementia. To overcome the well-known sense of impotence and frustration which frequently goes with the experience of caregiving, ABC Group proposes to participants to become expert caregivers as a way out from impotence tunnel. In this way CEA aims at helping for the well-being of both: caregiver and patient. The Author also presents the results of a preliminary study finding that the method can indeed change caregivers' verbal behavior even if not their burden -measured with the Caregiver Burden Inventory-. Maybe other groups all around the world will be interested to and by this proposal and they'll be able to perform further studies to test this new method.

The last (or, in this case: the second) article is not the least! On the contrary I've particularly enjoyed the original article by Nidhi Mahendra presenting the results of a computer assisted spaced retrieval training for faces and names of people with dementia. Spaced retrieval technique has been used in several studies to teach face-name associations to persons with dementia. But, as a plus, this article contains several points of novelty and interest, first of all the use of a laptop computer: Mahendra has succeeded in "introducing" a laptop computer in the life of a group of participants whose age ranged from 75 to 93 (!) and who had no (or limited) experience on PCs (except for one). I appreciated the fact that the computer was first introduced for cognitive stimulating games selected by participants; then only when people with dementia got familiarity with the electronic tool and learned that they could even enjoy (at the point that four participants decided to buy a personal computer!), the laptop was used for face-name associations learning. Another interesting point is that it seems to exist a transfer - even if limited- of learning in participants' everyday life. A further one is the fact that the Author explored learning both for unfamiliar and familiar - but forgotten - associations: in fact the finding that no difference is evident there is puzzling and deserves further investigations. Finally the article also contains an interesting summary of literature findings about spaced retrieval which could be very useful for professionals interested in implementing this technique in their centers.

So, have a nice reading: I hope that "Non-pharmacological therapies in dementia" will become as a friend and a helpful one for your professional life!

In: Dementia: Non-Pharmacological Therapies
Editor: Elisabetta Farina, pp. 1-14

ISBN: 978-1-61470-736-3
© 2012 Nova Science Publishers, Inc.

MUSIC THERAPY IN DEMENTIA

*Alfredo Raglio**

Sospiro Foundation and INTERDEM Group
(Psycho-Social Intervention in Dementia)

ABSTRACT

The article aims at a possible definition of music therapy and underlines the principal differences between the generic and the therapeutic use of music in the field of dementia. The article begins with a brief review about the most recent studies in the international literature, followed by the presentation of the reasons of the efficacy of the music therapeutic approach in the persons living with Alzheimer's disease or with dementia. In addition, the article describes a music therapy approach based on the free sonorous-music improvisation and on the psychological intersubjective perspective. In conclusion, you can read the description of some research studies realized with rigorous methodological criteria (scientific approach), and in Appendix 1 a case report regarding music therapeutic treatment of a person with a diagnosis of mixed dementia of mild level (clinical approach).

Keywords: Music – music therapy –dementia – evidence based practice – scientific approach.

INTRODUCTION

The use of music and sonorous-music elements in the field of dementia has been, for some years, much widespread, although the application experiences are very different in relation to the purposes and contents of the proposals. The contexts in which musical activities are proposed to people with dementia are numerous. Their main goal is to create a situation of wellbeing and socialization through various music proposals (rhythmic use of instruments, singing, movement associated with music, etc.). There are also the experiences of listening to music: music is potentially evocative, stimulates memories or states of mind through moments of verbalization after listening to music; further, music is used in order to facilitate the recognition of environments or structured moments of the day; finally, listening

* Prof. Alfredo Raglio, Music therapist, researcher, Via Belfiore 2 – 26100 Cremona (Italy) raglioa@tin.it; musicoterapia@fondazionesospiro.it +390372620264; +393387291944

to music (classical music, favourite music, etc.) is used in the belief that it can effectively reduce behavioral disorders and enhance mood or socialization (Raglio, 2008a).

This assumption raises a question: are music therapy and music experience applied to a pathological condition the same thing?

It is possible to believe that music itself has beneficial effects, but I think it is time to consider how little this is related to the concept of therapy. This concept is linked to the possibility of acting on the reduction of symptoms or on the prevention/stabilization of complications resulting from them (secondary and tertiary prevention), with consequent impacts on the general quality of life of the person (Smith and Lipe, 1991; Aldridge, 1993; Kneafsey, 1997). It seems clear that the benefits of therapy should be repeated regularly, last in time and should be explicitly based upon an explicative theory (Schön et al., 2007). It is also important to understand, through further clinical applications, what subjects can find any therapeutic effect in music therapy treatment. Beside the general potential benefits of music, often defined as "music therapy" although in the absence of the above mentioned conditions, there is a definition of "music therapy" that is acknowledged and proposed by the international music therapy community[1]. This definition refers to some elements that are deemed essential in order to consider music therapy as a potential therapeutic intervention involving the use of sonorous-music elements:

– The presence of a qualified care-worker (the music therapist)
– A music therapy model based on a theoretical and methodological background
– The presence of a structured setting
– Aims (which aspire to become stable and lasting over time) linked to changes of the person or changes of parts of his/her functions
– The constant reference, in therapeutic treatment, to an intrapersonal and / or
– interpersonal plan (Raglio et al., 2009a).

Regarding to the training of music therapists, it refers to music and relational skills that characterize those who work in this area. This specific training (structured according to widely consolidated and shared criteria that are defined by the principal music therapy associations, e.g. the World Music Therapy Association, the European Music Therapy Confederation, the American Music Therapy Association, etc.) takes place through specific courses which are in many countries university-based. The choice of a music therapeutic model appears as a fundamental element characterizing each intervention based on the therapeutic relationship.

Even in music therapy, like in other therapeutic approaches, it is important to define a space-time frame and a set of rules ("therapeutic setting") to promote the therapeutic action and change. The music therapeutic treatment aims at the establishment of a relationship, and

---

[1] Music therapy is described as the use of music and/or of its components (sound, rhythm, melody and harmony) by a qualified music therapist, in individual or group relationships, in the context of a formally defined process, with the aim of facilitating and promoting communication, relationships, learning, mobilization, expression, organization and other relevant therapeutic goals intended to meet physical, emotional, mental, social and cognitive needs. The main finality of music therapy is that of developing potentialities and/or rehabilitating an individual's functions so that he/she might achieve an improved integration on the intra- and interpersonal levels and therefore an ameliorated quality of life through prevention, rehabilitation or therapy (World Federation of Music Therapy, 8th World Conference on Music Therapy, Hamburg, 1996).

the sonorous-musical element is the means that helps create this relationship, that is the very core of the discipline.

A BRIEF REVIEW

In general, literature supports the effectiveness of music therapy in the field of dementia through data and documented experiences that mixed musical and music therapeutic experiences. However, there are gaps and shortcomings in the methodological criteria of the studies. These often shows a low scientific level of evidence: randomized controlled studies almost lack and they are poorly defined in terms of content and of process and outcomes evaluation. For these reasons research in this direction is encouraged (Koger and Brotons, 2000; Vink et al., 2004). Positive effects of music and music therapy were found on psychological and behavioral disorders (Clendaniel and Fleishell, 1989; Gerdner and Swanson, 1993; Casby and Holm, 1994; Goddaer and Abraham, 1994; Brotons and Pickett-Cooper, 1996; Denney, 1997; Clark et al., 1998; Groene, 1999; Raglio et al., 2001, 2006, 2008, Snowden et al., 2003; Svansdottir et al., 2006), on cognitive abilities (Smith, 1990; Rauscher et al., 1993 , 1997, Johnson et al., 1998; Koger and,Brotons, 2000), on social and relational skills (Clair and Bernstein, 1990; Brotons et al., 1997; Koger et al., 1999; Koger and Brotons, 2000; Raglio et al., 2001, 2006, 2008), on depressive symptoms (Hanser and Thompson, 1994; Fox et al., 1998, Snowden et al., 2003, Guétin et al., 2009) and on the overall quality of life of the person (Smith and Lipe , 1991; Aldridge, 1993; 1994; Kneafsey, 1997; Pacchetti et al., 1998). Positive influence of music and music therapy was also found on the caregiver's emotional distress and defeat (Clair and Ebberts, 1997; Clair, 2002; Brotons and Marti, 2003).

Music therapy treatment, in fact, can trigger a new way to communicate with persons with dementia, creating the opportunity to retrieve a relational-emotional dimension that is otherwise impossible to achieve.

It also seems important to stress that, since in dementia you face a significant cognitive deficits, the sound-music element may constitute a more intact and still available material in the brain, both in terms of listening and of production (Aldridge, 1994; Glynn, 1992; Braben, 1992; Polk and Kerstesz, 1993; York, 1994; Lipe, 1995; Raglio et al., 2001; Sacks, 2006).

Particularly interesting are also some studies carried out at the Japanese School of Nursing of Mie Prefectual College of Nursing that demonstrate, through controlled clinical trials, how music therapy acts positively and consistently on behavioral disorders and decreases levels of stress in people living with dementia (Suzuki, 2004; 2005).

The novelty of these studies is given by combining traditional assessment tools (such as Mini Mental State Examination, Gottfries-Brane-Steen Scale , Multidimensional Observation Scale For Elderly Subjects) (Folstein et al., 1975; Gottfries et al., 1982; Helmes et al., 1987) and biological indicators such as the Chromogranin A and Immunoglobulin A for the detection of stress and of the immunological status.

Other studies have investigated the possible correlation between the effects of music therapy in general and the changes of some physiological parameters. Kumar et al. (1999) showed an increase of melatonin in blood in 20 persons with dementia undergoing music therapy sessions for 1 month. Kubota et al. (1999) have studied lymphocytes "natural killers"

(NK) on a group of persons with dementia undergoing music therapy treatments. The lymphocytes NK cells are immunological indices: quantity and numerical changes in their activities are closely linked to resistance to viral infections, to the occurrence of cancer and to the rapidity of formation of metastases. From the outcomes it is clear that the musical activities conducted in this study (to sing or to play an instrument) have contributed to an increase in NK. Long-term effects of music therapy were investigated according to psychological and physiological parameters by Takahashi et al. (2006). The authors studied a group of elderly people with dementia and measured physiological parameters such as blood pressure and, through a saliva sample, the level of cortisol, the adrenocortical hormone whose level increases with stress. The results of the study led to the conclusion that music therapy has a homeostatic effect, that is of pressure regulation, and therefore music therapy can be considered as a preventive therapy to heart and brain diseases. In relation to the levels of cortisol, there were no significant differences between pre- and post-therapy to six months, one year and two years.

Two recent reviews focus their attention on some of the most significant aspects that concern the research in the field of music therapy: the methodological questions and the contents proposed in the music therapeutic experience. Vink et al. (2004) in their recent Cochrane Review concerning the application of music therapy in dementia, analyzed 354 studies of which only 5 are included in their revision. Only these studies, in fact, follow the scientific methodological criteria for the inclusion in the review (randomized controlled trials that reported clinically relevant outcomes associated with music therapy in treatment of behavioural, social, cognitive and emotional problems of older people with dementia). Raglio et al. (2009a) focus their attention not only on the methodological aspects of research, but also on the contents of the music therapeutic interventions, reporting studies that show a suitable methodological structure but also approaches that use therapeutic models of intervention.

A POSSIBLE APPLICATIONAL MODEL: MUSIC THERAPY AND THE INTERSUBJECTIVE PERSPECTIVE

The Theory

A key point for music therapy is the biological-relational significance of sound, that is the fundamental principle in the organization and regulation of the individuals' development (Stern, 1985).

The sound elements indeed contain the archaic and innate aspects from which the communicative-relational potentiality arises.

The psychological concepts of "intersubjectivity" and "regulation of emotions" explain the idea that the individual uses innate skills that promote the interpersonal relationship and contribute to the emotional and cognitive development (Tronick, 1989; Trevarthen, 2001).

Music therapy sets up an archaic communication linked to sensory and expressive pathways of which the sound can be the vehicle.

Therefore, sound may be an element of great importance in determining the "affect attunement" described by Stern (1985), able to create "meeting moments" (Stern, 2004) in the relationship. Through sound, new intersubjective fields are developed that modify the relationship and induce the co-creation and the sharing of relational and emotional experience.

The interaction between the music therapist and the person with dementia, through musical instruments (percussions, glockenspiels, xylophones, etc.) and the modulation of sonorous parameters (intensity, dynamic, agogic, etc.), facilitates the processes of organization, co-regulation and attunement of the emotional components (Beebe, 1998; 2005; Fogel, 1993).

From a therapeutic point of view, this allows us to understand each other, to define our own position in the relationship and to share the intersubjective experience. That can help the individual feel recognized and redefine himself reflecting another one, consolidating and renewing his own identity (Stern , 2004). The outcomes of this intervention may lead to increase communication-interpersonal skills, to reduce psychological and behavioral disorders and to improve the quality of life of the person with dementia.

The Method

Also from the methodological point of view we are observing an effort to systematize the music therapy intervention aimed at persons with dementia (Raglio et al., 2001; Villani et al., 2004).

The treatment proposed here appears to be non-invasive and therefore there are no specific contraindications. The treatment is particularly indicated for people with a moderate-severe stage of dementia (from 1 to 3 level of the Clinical Dementia Rating) (Morris, 1993), also with severe behavioral disorders. For this reason the music therapy treatment can be addressed to a single person or to small groups (3-4 participants). It is important to ensure the willingness of the person with dementia to undergo the treatment, but also to verify the suitability for intervention through a specific music therapy assessment. It is possible to grasp, in the specific setting, the person's sensitivity to the sonorous-music element, and his willingness to develop a relationship with the music therapist.

The therapeutic contract explains to the person undergoing intervention the content, the purposes and how the treatment will be conducted.

The sessions (with a bi- or tri-weekly cadence, and an established duration that generally does not exceed 30 minutes) take place in a not very large room, acoustically isolated and without interfering or potentially disturbing stimuli.

The instrumental setting should be essential, easily accessible and should possibly remain unchanged over time.

The music therapist's behaviors are generally not verbal, not directive and based on the empathetic listening.

Verbal communication is used where it is necessary to direct the person in the music therapeutic setting or to soothe and calm down behaviors.

During the session, the music therapist will try, through the free use of sound and of musical instruments (improvisation) (Benenzon, 1981), to build a relationship with the person with dementia, facilitating the expression and the sharing of his emotions.

The intervention evaluation can be made with qualitative (clinical approach) or quantitative (scientific approach) methods. The evaluation concerns the "process" (what happens in the music therapy session) and the "outcomes" (which are found outside the setting).

For the process evaluation, protocols or observational schemes are used that produce comments/data on sonorous-music interactions and on the relationship between the music therapist and the person with dementia in the session; to evaluate the outcomes of the treatment, clinical tools are used to assess changes in functional, cognitive and behavioral areas.

The music therapist can decide the conclusion of the treatment observing the following conditions: the person with dementia has reached a stabilisation of the results that leads the music therapist to think that no further results can be achieved. In the other case, the natural development of the disease makes the prosecution of the treatment difficult or impossible.

Effectiveness of Music Therapeutic Approach in Dementias

In this field (as for other diseases in which, even if for different reasons, the communication functions that are more recent in ontogenetic development are compromised) we can conceive the possibility of reactivating and expanding archaic expressive and relational abilities. These abilities persist along the whole life-span as forms of interpersonal experience, alternative to the verbal communication.

It is on these bases that the sonorous-music elements can build a communicative bridge for persons with dementia. In fact, music therapy can be considered a non-verbal communication form and may prescind from symbolic and abstractive abilities and from culture-bound learning processes.

Through music therapy, therefore, it is possible to activate relational and expressive ways of natural (and archaic) origin that are most likely still present in persons with cognitive impairment. Music therapy can help the person with dementia maintain a sense of identity and to recognize the environment. In psychological terms, it determines a regression, shared and guided by the therapist: this regression facilitates a larger adaptation of the person with dementia because it allows him to create more harmonius inner frames that is to better organize and manage his emotional competences. I also think that this can be better pursued through an active approach (sonorous-music improvisation) which involves essentially non-verbal / sonorous-music aspects in the relationship between the person with dementia and music therapist. The receptive techniques (music listening), in music therapy, involve on the contrary verbal and elaborative competences that lack in the person with dementia, especially in the medium-advanced stage of the disease. In this case, listening to music can trigger emotions that the person is unable to manage and contain, leading to states of discomfort and/or disorder. Music therapy can induce a better organization of the emotional components of the personality and at the same time, since music is also a mental activity, can stimulate cognitive functions such as attention, sensory-motor co-ordination and abilities of stimulus discrimination.

In dementias, music therapy can influence mental and behavioral disorders, induce organizational processes and the (co-)regulation of emotional components and possibly promote new learning strategies, while improving relational and social aspects, and therefore the overall quality of life of the sufferer.

RESEARCH IN MUSIC THERAPY: A SCIENTIFIC APPROACH

Music therapy is moving towards a systematic process by determining an increase of scientific criteria in the field.

This implies discussions regarding theoretical and methodological aspects and a rigorous effort to make the relationship between theory and practice more coherent; such effort should also introduce research as a foundation element in the discipline.

In fact, music therapy, in a similar way to other areas of knowledge of recent application, can be better defined as a practice that is based on empirical aspects applied to different diseases through the use of sound and music.

Since music therapy focuses on the therapeutic relationship, there are still many gaps in the theoretical formulation and in the contents of the interventions.

Often, as quoted before, the presence of music together with a disease (in our case dementia) leads to use the term "music therapy", without considering the specifity of music therapy intervention, which is instead related to theoretical basis, enforcement aspects, specific contents and verifiability of the results.

I believe that this background can help find an adequate definition of music therapy and encourage suitable application.

Raglio et al. (2009a) highlight 3 key areas which define the scientific approach for music therapy intervention:

(a) defining the contents of the intervention (reference to the theoretical application model)
(b) assessment of the process (analysis, with specific evaluation instruments, of the changes in the therapeutic setting)
(c) assessment of the results (reference to the conditions of randomization and of control).

A randomized controlled study (Raglio et al. submitted), referring to these criteria, compares a treatment based on cycles of music therapeutic sessions with the analogous study (Raglio et al., 2008) based on a continuous music therapeutic regimen. Both studies assess music therapy effectiveness in reducing behavioral and psychological symptoms in persons with dementia. Sixty persons with dementia were enrolled in this study. The music therapeutic model is related to the sonorous-music improvisation and the intersubjective psychological approach (Raglio et al., 2009b). All of them underwent a multidimensional assessment including Mini Mental State Examination, Barthel Index and Neuropsychiatric Inventory (Folstein et al., 1975; Mahoney et al., 1965; Cummings et al., 1994). The experimental group underwent 3 cycles of 12 active music therapy sessions each (administered within 1 month), 3 times a week. Each session lasted 30 minutes and involved a group of 3 persons with dementia. Each cycle of treatments was followed by 1 month of wash-out. This intervention structure was led for a total duration of 6 months. Each session was videotaped with a fixed camcorder; the videotapes were analyzed by music therapists non directly involved in the process through an observational scheme. The control group received only educational and entertainment activities (occupational activities, reading a newspaper, physical activities, etc.). In this study, in the Neuropsychiatric Inventory evaluation of the experimental group, significative effects over time are shown ($F_{7, 357} = 9.06$, $P < 0.001$), and also between groups ($F_{1, 51} = 4.84$, $P < 0.05$). The comparison between this study and the previous one shows that in both cases the music therapy treatment significantly reduces behavioral and psychological symptoms of dementia. Both investigations show an analogous Effect Size (d = 1,91 vs d = 1,87), comparing the scores between the baseline and the end of the treatment in each study. This indicates the possibility of effectively conducting a music therapeutic treatment through cycles of sessions with the involvement of more people and lower intervention costs.

The data of these studies suggest the effectiveness of music therapy: however, the evaluation of the results is very complex, particularly for the lack of standardized and validated instruments, for the difficulty of selecting homogeneous samples from a clinical point of view, and the tendency to decline of people with dementia. Another problem is the difficulty of measuring general changes found in everyday life of persons with dementia. The assessment tools do not seem to be always adequate to analytically detect changes determined by music therapy treatment in behavioral and psychological aspects.

CONCLUSION

I believe that music therapy should make a greater effort in the definition of applicational models (theoretical background, techniques and procedures to verify the interventions) in order to produce an "evidence based practice" (Mace, 2001; Vink et al., 2003; Raglio, 2008b).

It is also clear that there are still gaps in the methodological research, such as the paucity and the insufficient clinical definition of the sample, the limited duration of interventions and the lack of standardized and validated instruments aiming at evaluating the therapeutic process.

Moreover, there is a lack of controlled and randomized-controlled studies.

The increase of such studies can certainly lead to a scientific validation of the intervention and thus to recognize to music therapy a therapeutic dignity.

I think, moreover, that in the evaluations of the results we should remark in a more appropriate and refined way the changes in the relationship and in the emotional-affective area; this can be done also using observational techniques out of the music therapy setting (Raglio et al., 2009a).

Studies which also use biological evaluations as indicators of efficacy (Kubota, 1999; Kumar, 1999; Suzuki, 2004; 2005; Takahashi, 2006) seems to be promising. Biological indicators of efficacy are extremely important, they can be measured with a non invasive practice, like the traditional evaluations in persons with dementia and allow greater objectivity and measurability in the evaluations of changes.

These considerations may be a stimulus for future studies in order to highlight the potentiality and specificity of music therapy intervention, whose positive effects are already evident in clinical applications.

APPENDIX 1: A CASE REPORT

Mr. G. has a diagnosis of mixed dementia (Alzheimer's disease associated with cerebrovascular disease) of mild level (CDR = 1)(Morris, 1993) according to the NINCDS-ADRDA (Mckhann et al., 1984) criteria, with a significant inclination to loneliness. Mr. G. has no deficit in motor skills and he walks independently and without any support.

He has been attending an Integrated Day Center after having memory disorders and prolonged periods of social withdrawal. The presence of depression and apathy in an early period leads Mr. G. to stay in bed all day, without attending any activity organized by the Center's educators. In addition to this, a strong state of anxiety emerges that is increased by the presence of dementia.

After a few months the patient begins to take part in the activities of the Center, although he often tends to isolation from the group, and his involvement in such activities is never spontaneous. Mr. G. is suspicious and shows a consequent resistance to any attempt of involvement done by the physicians and/or by the caregivers.

The music therapist asks Mr. G., through a preliminar interview, for willingness to attend one session of evaluation, in order to hypothesize the beginning of therapeutic treatment. Mr. G. shows resistance and doubts about the usefulness of this intervention, the transfer necessary to go to the room of music therapy and his ability in the use of musical instruments. Mr. G. accepts, however, to attend in the sessions of assessment.

These sessions are designed to verify the level of agreement to non-verbal communication and sensitivity of the person in relation to sonorous-music elements. During the music therapeutic assessment, particular attention is given to the approach of the person to musical instruments and his tolerance and acceptance of the music therapeutic setting. During the first session of assessment, 7 minutes after the beginning Mr. G. firmly expresses his will to stop the activity.

A further interview reassures Mr. G., especially in relation to his idea of being unable to use the musical instruments.

In the second session of assessment Mr. G. accepts the non-verbal setting and uses the musical instruments spontaneously. Nevertheless, Mr. G. uses verbal communication to ask confirmations and assurances about the use of some musical instruments. The session has approximately a duration of 20 minutes. The changes shown by Mr. G. during the music therapeutic evaluation induce the music therapist to begin the treatment. Mr. G. is informed of the decision in an interview which defines the purpose and the application form for his participation in the intervention.

The 30 sessions of the treatment are bi-weekly and have a duration of 30 minutes each; each session is recorded from a camcorder in order to assess, later, the relational and sonorous-music dynamics emerged in the music therapeutic setting.

The rhythmic-melodic instruments used during the sessions (percussions, glockenspiels, xylophones, ethnic instruments, etc.) are easy to play and their semicircular placement makes their use by Mr. G. easier.

The music therapeutic improvisation technique is used with the purpose to activate a relationship based on the expression and sharing of emotional states, in order to create moments of affect attunement.

During the treatment there are significant changes in the relationship between Mr. G. and the music therapist. These changes concern in particular the use of musical instruments: in the initial stage of the treatment the sonorous-music elements are used by Mr. G. with cognitive and exploratory intention; the productions of Mr. G. are characterised by many rhythmic stereotypes to the entire duration of the sessions, without any variations. Between the music therapist and Mr. G. a syntonic production arises, that is characterised however by a formal share of sonorous-music parameters, more than by a real emotional share. Mr. G. must often be reassured and calmed down verbally. The verbalizations divert the attention of Mr. G. from non verbal and sonorous-music interaction. Initially, Mr. G. frequently asks to suspend the sessions before the prescribed time, but the music therapeutic relationship gradually changes Mr. G.'s behaviors. He shows greater willingness in the relationship and this appears even in his sonorous-music production. The production, in fact, becomes more and more varied and dynamic, contextually to the reduction of sonorous-music stereotypes and verbalizations. This promotes the direct contact with Mr. G. and his greater emotional expression. Sonorous-music moments of attunement make Mr. G. more quiet and involve him emotionally, leading to empathetic moments of relationship.

The sessions analysis, made through the Music Therapy Checklist (Raglio et al., 2007), shows an increase of the attuned sonorous-music production (especially in relation to the duration of the sonorous-music interactions), often accompanied by a greater emotional involvement of Mr. G. (visual contacts, smiles, syntonic body movements according to sonorous-music production, etc.).

In addition, disattuned productions without a relational meaning decrease during the whole music therapeutic process.

The monitoring of anxiety and depression, made by the State Trait Anxiety Inventory (STAI) (Spielberger et al., 1970) and by the Geriatric Depression Scale (GDS) (Brink et al., 1982), shows some important changes after the treatment. Both scores of the two scales of assessment decrease significantly after the treatment (STAI score before the treatment = 38 and STAI score after the treatment = 23; GDS score before the treatment = 6 and GDS score after the treatment = 1)and tend to increase slightly between the first and the second follow-up (respectively to 1 month and 3 months after the end of the sessions). Moreover, there are also very positive results concerning prompt effects of the sessions on the symptom of anxiety (comparison between before and after the treatment)

From the behavioural point of view, Mr. G., generally shows a greater level of agreement towards the sessions and the occupational and rehabilitative activities. Mr. G. is more participating and motivated in relation to these activities.

The session duration gradually increases: the first session of assessment has a short duration (7 minutes), whereas the last session has a long duration (33 minutes).

This experience suggests that music therapeutic intervention based on an improvisational/ intersubjective approach has encouraged and facilitated the contact with Mr. G., allowing him to express his emotions, through sonorous-music and non-verbal communication. The empathetic moments and the emotional modulation and calibration in the relationship between the music therapist and Mr. G. have triggered an emotional (co-)regulation process. This process has led to significant changes in the relational and clinical aspects, both inside and outside the music therapeutic setting.

REFERENCES

Aldridge, D. (1993). Music and Alzheimer's disease--assessment and therapy: discussion paper. *Journal of the Royal Society of Medicine*, 86, 93-95.

Aldridge, D. (1994). Alzheimer's disease: rhythm, timing and music as therapy. *Biomedicine and Pharmacotherapy*, 48, 275-281.

Beebe, B., and Lachmann, F.M. (1998). Co-constructing inner and relational processes: self and mutual regulation in infant research and adult treatment. *Psychoanalytic Psychology*, 15, 1-37.

Beebe, B., Knoblauch, S., Rustin, J., and Sorter, D. (2005). *Forms of intersubjectivity in infant research and adult treatment.* New York: Other Press.

Benenzon, R.O. (1981). *Manual de Musicoterapia.* Barcelona: Editorial Paidos Iberica.

Braben, L. (1992). A song for Mrs Smith. *Nursing Times*, 88, 54.

Brink, T.L., Yesavage, J.A., Lum, O., Heersema, P., Adey, M.B., and Rose, T.L. (1982). Screening tests for geriatric depression. *Clinical Gerontologist*, 1, 37-44.

Brotons, M., and Pickett-Cooper, P. (1996). The effects of music therapy intervention on agitation behaviors of Alzheimer's disease patients. *Journal of Music Therapy*, 33, 2-18.

Brotons, M., Koger, S., and Pickett-Cooper, P. (1997). Music and dementias: a review of the literature. *Journal of Music Therapy*, 34, 204-245.

Brotons, M., and Marti, P. (2003). Music therapy with Alzheimer's patients and their family caregivers: a pilot project. *Journal of Music Therapy*, 40, 138-150.

Casby, J.A., and Holm, M.B. (1994). The effect of music on repetitive disruptive vocalizations of persons with dementia. *The American Journal of Occupational Therapy*, 48, 883-889.

Clair, A.A., and Bernstein, B. (1990). A preliminary study of music therapy programming for severely regressed persons with Alzheimer's type dementia. *Journal of Applied Gerontology*, 9: 299-311.

Clair, A.A., and Ebberts, A.G. (1997). The effects of music therapy on interactions between family caregivers and their care receivers with late stage dementia. *Journal of Music Therapy*, 34, 148-164.

Clair, A.A. (2002). The effects of music therapy on engagement in family caregiver and care receiver couples with dementia. *American Journal of Alzheimer's Disease and Other Dementias*, 17, 286-290.

Clark, M.E., Lipe, A.W., and Bilbrey, M. (1998). Use of music to decrease aggressive behaviors in people with dementia. *Journal of Gerontological Nursing*, 24, 10-17.

Clendaniel, B.P., and Fleishell, A. (1989). An Alzheimer day-care center for nursing home patients. *The American Journal of Nursing*, 89, 944-945.

Cummings, J.L., Mega, M., Gray, K., Rosemberg-Thompson, S., and Gornbein, J. (1994). The Neuropsychiatric Inventory: comprehensive assessment of psychopathology in dementia. *Neurology*, 44, 2308-14.

Denney, A. (1997). Quiet music. An intervention for mealtime agitation? *Journal of Gerontological Nursing* , 23, 16-23.

Fogel, A. (1993). *Developing through relationships: origins of communication, self and culture.* Chicago: University of Chicago Press.

Folstein, M.F., Folstein, S.E., and McHugh, P.R. (1975). Mini-mental state. Practical method for grading the cognitive state for the clinician. *Psychiatry Research*, 12, 189–198.

Fox, L.S., Knight, B.G., and Zelinski, E.M. (1998). Mood Induction with Older Adults: a Tool for Investigating Effects of depressed Mood. *Psychology and Aging*, 13, 519-23.

Gerdner, L.A., and Swanson, E.A. (1993). Effects of individualized music on confused and agitated elderly patients. *Archives of Psychiatric Nursing*, 7, 284-291.

Glynn, N.J. (1992). The music therapy assessment tool in Alzheimer's patients. *Journal of Gerontological Nursing,* 18, 3-9.

Goddaer, J., and Abraham, I.L. (1994). Effects of relaxing music on agitation during meals among nursing home residents with severe cognitive impairment. *Archives of Psychiatric Nursing,* 8, 150-158.

Gottfries, C.G., Brane, G., Gullberg, B., and Steen, G. (1982). A new rating scale for dementia syndromes. *Archives of Gerontology and Geriatrics*, 1, 311-30.

Groene II, R. (1999). The Effect of Therapist and Activity Characteristics on the Purposeful Responses of Probable Alzheimer's Disease Participants. *Journal of Music Therapy*, 35, 119-136.

Guétin, S., Portet, F., Picot, M.C., Pommié, C., Messaoudi, M., Djabelkir, L., Olsen, A.L., Cano, M.M., Lecourt, E., and Touchon, J. (2009). Effect of music therapy on anxiety and depression in patients with Alzheimer's type dementia: randomised, controlled study. *Dementia and Geriatric Cognitive Disorders,* 28, 36-46.

Hanser, S.B., and Thompson, L.W. (1994). Effects of a music therapy strategy on depressed older adults. *Journal of Gerontology*, 49, 265-269.

Helmes, E., Csapo, K., and Short, J. (1987). Standardization and validation of multidimensional observation scale for elderly subjects (MOSES). *Journal of Gerontology,* 42, 395–405.

Johnson, J.K., Cotman, C.W., Tasaki, C.S., and Shaw, G.L. (1998). Enhancement of spatial-temporal reasoning after a Mozart listening condition in Alzheimer's disease: a case study. *Neurological Research*, 20, 666-672.

York, E. (1994). The development of a quantitative music skills test for patients with Alzheimer's Disease. *Journal of Music Therapy*, 31, 280-296.

Kneafsey, R. (1997). The Therapeutic Use of Music in a Care of the Ederly Setting: a Literature Review. *Journal of Clinical Nursing*, 6, 341-346.

Koger, S.M., Chapin, K., and Brotons, M. (1999). Is Music Therapy an Effective Intervention for Dementia? A Meta-Analytic Review of Literature. *Journal of Music Thera*py, 36, 2-15.

Koger, S.M., and Brotons, M. (2000). Music therapy for dementia symptoms. *Cochrane Database of Systematic Reviews*, CD001121, 2-3.

Kubota, N., and Hasegawa, Y. (1999). Change in NK cell activity in the elderly through music therapy. *The Journal of Japan Biomusic Association*, 17, 183-187.

Kumar, A.M., Tims, F., Cruess, D.C., Mintzer, M.J., Ironson, G., Loewenstein, D., Cattan, R., Fernandez, J.B., Eisdorfer, C., and Kumar M. (1999). Music Therapy increases serum melatonin levels in patients with Alzeheimer's disease. *Alternative Therapeutic Health Medicine*, 5, 49-57.

Lipe, A.W. (1995). The use of music performance tasks in the assessment of cognitive functioning among older adults with dementia. *Journal of Music Therapy*, 33, 137-151.

Mace, C., Moorey, S., and Roberts, B. (2001). *Evidence in the psychological therapies: a critical guide for practitioners*. New York: Brunner-Routledge.

Mahoney, F.I., and Barthel, D. (1965). Functional evaluation: the Barthel Index. *Maryland State Medical Journal*, 14, 61-65.

Mckhann, G., Drachman, D., Folstein, M.F., Katzman, R., Price, D., and Stadlan, E. (1984). Clinical diagnosis of Alzheimer's Disease: report of NINCDS-ADRDA Work Group under the auspices of Department of Health and Human Service Task Force on Alzheimer's Disease. *Neurology*, 34, 934-44.

Morris, J.C. (1993). The clinical dementia rating (CDR): current version and scoring rules. *Neurology*, 43, 2412.2414.

Pacchetti, C., Aglieri, R., Mancini, F., Martignoni, E., Nappi, G. (1998). Active Music Therapy and Parkinson's Disease: Methtods. *Functional Neurology*, 13, 47-67.

Polk, M., and Kertesz, A. (1993). Music and language in degenerative disease of the brain. *Brain and Cognition*, 22, 98-117.

Raglio, A. Manarolo, G., and Villani, D. (2001). Musicoterapia e Malattia di Alzheimer: proposte applicative e ipotesi di ricerca. Torino: Cosmopolis.

Raglio, A., Ubezio, M.C., Puerari, F., Gianotti, M., Bellelli, G., Trabucchi, M., and Villani, D. (2006). L'efficacia del trattamento musicoterapico in pazienti con demenza di grado moderato-severo. *Giornale di Gerontologia*, 54, 164-169.

Raglio, A. (2008a). La musicoterapia nel paziente demente. *Giornale di Gerontologia*, 56, 328-330.

Raglio, A. (2008b). Musicoterapia e scientificità: dalla clinica alla ricerca. Milano: Franco Angeli.

Raglio, A., Bellelli, G., Traficante, D., Gianotti, M., Ubezio, M.C., Villani, D., and Trabucchi, M. (2008). Efficacy of music therapy in the treatment of behavioral and psychiatric symptoms of dementia. *Alzheimer Disease and Associated Disorders*, 22, 158-162.

Raglio, A., and Gianelli, M.V. (2009a). Music therapy for individuals with dementia: areas of interventions and research perspectives. *Current Alzheimer Research*, 6, 293-301.

Raglio, A., and Oasi, O. (2009b). La musicoterapia in una prospettiva intersoggettiva. Quaderni di Gestalt, Franco Angeli, in press.

Rauscher, F.H., Shaw, G.L., and Ky, K. (1993). Music and spatial task performance. *Nature*, 14, 611.

Rauscher, F.H., Shaw, G.L., Levine, L.J., Wright, E.L., Dennis, W.R., and Newcomb, R.L. (1997). Music training causes long-term enhancement of preschool children's spatial-temporal reasoning. *Neurological Research*, 19, 2-8.

Sacks, O. (2006). The power of music. *Brain,* 129, 2528-2532.

Schön, D., Akiva-Kabiri, L., and Vecchi, T. (2007). *Psicologia della Musica*. Roma: Carocci.

Smith, D.S. (1990). Therapeutic Treatment Effectiveness Documented in the Gerontology Literature: Implications for Music Therapy. *Music Therapy Perspectives*, 8, 36-40.

Smith, D.S., and Lipe, A.W. (1991). Music therapy practices in gerontology. *Journal of Music Therapy*, 28, 193-210.

Snowden, M., Sato, K., and Roy-Byrne, P. (2003). Assessment and treatment of nursing home residents with depression or behavioral symptoms associated with dementia: a review of the literature. *Journal of the American Geriatrics Soc*iety, 51, 1305-1317.

Spielberger, C. D., Gorsuch, R.L., and Lushene. R.E. (1970). *Manual for the State-Trait Anxiety Inventory*. Palo Alto, Consulting Psychologists Press.

Stern , D. (1985). *The Interpersonal World of the infant*. New York: Basic Book.

Stern, D. (2004). *The Present Moment in Psychotherapy and Everyday Life*. London: Norton and Company Ltd.

Suzuki, M., Kanamori, M., Watanabe, M., Nagasawa, S., Kojima, E., and Ooshiro, H. (2004). Behavioral and endocrinological evaluation of music therapy for elderly patients with dementia. *Nursing and Health Sciences*, 6, 11-18.

Suzuki, M., Kanamori, M., Nagasawa, S., and Saruhara, T. (2005). Behavioral, stress and immunological evaluation methods of music therapy in elderly patients with senile dementia. *Nippon Ronen Igakkai Zasshi*, 42, 74-82.

Svansdottir, H.B., and Snaedal, J. (2006). Music therapy in moderate and severe dementia of Alzheimer's type: a case-control study. *International Psychogeriatrics*, 18, 613-21.

Takahashi, T., and Matsushita, H. (2006). Long- Term Effect of Music Therapy on Elderly with Moderate/Severe Dementia. *Journal of Music Therapy*, 43, 317-333.

Trevarthen, C., and Aitken, K.J. (2001). Infant *Intersubjectivity: Research, theory, and clinical applications. Journal* of Child Psychology and Psychiatry, 1, 3-48.

Tronick, E.Z. (1989). Emotions and Emotional Communication in Infants. *American Psychologist*, 44, 112-119.

Villani, D., and Raglio, A. (2004). Musicoterapia e demenza. *Giornale di Gerontologia*. 52, 423-428.

Vink, A.C., and Bruinsma, M. (2003). Evidence Based Music Therapy. *Music Therapy Today* (online, http://musictherapyworld.net), 4, 5.

Vink, A.C., Birks, J.S., Bruinsma, M.S., and Scholten, R.J.S. (2004). Music therapy for people with dementia. *Cochrane Database of Systematic Reviews*, 4, CD003477.

In: Dementia: Non-Pharmacological Therapies
Editor: Elisabetta Farina, pp. 15-25

ISBN: 978-1-61470-736-3
© 2012 Nova Science Publishers, Inc.

French Clinical Practice Guidelines for Non Pharmacologic Interventions in Alzheimer's Disease and Related Conditions Issues and Perspectives

Jocelyne de Rotrou, Laurence Hugonot,
Olivier Hanon and Anne-Sophie Rigaud*
Broca Hospital, 54-56 rue Pascal 75013 Paris.

ABSTRACT

In this paper, the French context of non drug therapies for persons suffering from dementia is first described as well as recent guidelines recommended by the working group of the High Authority for Health (HAS[1]). Their interest and limits are also discussed.

Secondly, the authors present the advancement of two French main studies - 1/ The AIDMA study which demonstrates that a psycho-social intervention programme benefits families of patients diagnosed with a dementia, by improving Alzheimer's disease understanding and coping strategies. In addition, an increase of the depression was observed in the group which did not follow the programme, while the programme-group remained stable. - 2/ ETNA 3 study (current research) which evaluates long-term efficacy of three non drug interventions (cognitive stimulation, reminiscence therapy, made-to-measure therapy). These studies represent an important contribution to the development of non drug interventions adapted to the patient-caregivers dyads.

In addition, the authors emphasize the non drug interventions current issues, perspectives and methodological aspects. They highlight recent theoretical evolution and practices of their field of competency since 1986: cognitive stimulation. They focus on computerized ecological cognitive stimulation in the increasing domain of Gerontechnology.

Keywords: Alzheimer's disease management, guidelines, psycho-educational programmes, cognitive stimulation.

---

* Corresponding author: Jocelyne de Rotrou, CMRRIF (Centre Mémoire de Ressource et de Recherche Ile de France), Hôpital Broca, 54-56 rue Pascal. 75013 PARIS. Phone : +33 1 44 08 35 07. Fax : + 33 1 44 08 35 10. Email : jocelyne.derotrou@brc.aphp.fr
[1] HAS working group coordinated by Pasquier, F., Thomas-Antérion, C., Laurence, M.

Introduction

As the number of patients diagnosed with a dementia increases, so does the need for managing cognitive impairment, behavioural and psychological symptoms. During the past 20 years, a significant amount of knowledge, new theoretical and practical approaches have been developed. Multiple therapeutic trials have led to the marketing of symptomatic drugs, including cholinesterase inhibitors for patients with mild-to-moderate Alzheimer's Disease. At the same time, and complementary to drug therapies, various non-drug, individual or group interventions, have been designed for patients and/or caregivers (Doody et al. 2001, Brodaty et al. 2003, Seux 2008).

In France, as well as in many other countries, therapeutic nihilism in dementia management has definitely given way to a growing concern with a multidisciplinary approach to dementia care. AD management has become an ethical requirement: it is well established that medical teams can no longer disclose a dementia diagnosis without proposing pharmacologic treatment in conjunction with non pharmacologic treatment. However, there still is a paucity of evidence-based studies in the growing field of non-drug therapies, when compared with the large body of controlled studies attempting to show the efficacy of pharmacotherapy (Waldemar et al.2007).

Responding to the increasing awareness of patients' loss of autonomy and family carers' burden and needs, several French Government Alzheimer's Plans have been set up (/www.plan-alzheimer.gouv.fr). A clear consensus has been established for timely diagnosis and pharmacologic therapy leading to the development of memory centres (MC) and Memory Resource and Research Centres (MRRC). To date there are 520 MC (in 2009) and 25 MRRC (in 2008) in France (/www.plan-alzheimer.gouv.fr). Cooperation between these centres should make possible early differential diagnosis of dementia and consequently early management.

Although the average benefits of specific anti-dementia drugs appear modest, these drug therapies are strongly recommended by French specialist physicians. A recent report from the French HAS has emphasized the drug therapies' "structuring role" (www.has-sante.fr): their prescription represents a privileged opportunity for patients and carers to be offered long-term and individualized medico-psycho-social management. In addition, the HAS Department of Good Clinical Practice published guidelines validated by a working group of experienced neurologists, psychiatrists, geriatricians, general practitioners, neuropsychologists and speech therapists.

These guidelines aim to enhance and standardise practices relating to the diagnosis and treatment (including drug and non drug interventions and follow-up) of patients suffering from Alzheimer's disease or a related condition, at any stage apart from the end-of-life period.

A- French Clinical Practice Guidelines

The HAS working group considers that non-drug interventions are an important part of the patient's care irrespective of whether he or she lives independently or in a care facility. This position has been reached despite the lack of evidence for their efficacy because of methodological difficulties in performing studies. The working group specifies that non-drug interventions must always be performed by trained staff and form part of a care or rehabilitation programme.

Various forms of non-drug interventions can be considered:

1) Interventions relating to quality of life
These interventions depend on physical and mental comfort and on a suitable environment. This requires home help and an adequate staffing level in care facilities.

2) Speech and language therapy
The aim of this therapy is to maintain and adapt the patient's communication skills and to help his or her family and carers to adjust their behaviour to take into account the patient's difficulties. The main purpose is to continue communicating with the patient in order to prevent any reactive behaviour disorders.

Speech and language therapy is recommended for conditions in which language is one of the first functions to be affected (semantic dementia, progressive primary aphasia).
It also addresses problems with swallowing.

3) Cognitive interventions
a)-Cognitive stimulation is an ecological cognitive-psycho-social intervention relating to everyday situations. The activities which are provided place the patient in real or simulated situations (moving around the local area, washing/toilet use, using the telephone, etc.). It can be offered at various stages of AD and adjusted to take into account the patient's disorders. Its purpose is to delay the loss of autonomy in everyday activities. The programme includes a section for patients and a section for carers. Treatment is started by psychologists, psychomotor specialists, or trained speech and language therapists, and is continued by carers in the patient's home or in an institution.
Cognitive stimulation must be clearly distinguished from activity sessions, memory workshops or other occupational activities.
b)-Cognitive rehabilitation is a neuro-psychological re-education method aimed at offsetting a deficient cognitive process. It can be provided to patients with mild AD and moderate stages of certain focal degenerative disorders. It must be tailored to the individual patient and performed by trained staff.

4)Interventions relating to motor activity
Physical exercise (especially walking) could have a positive impact not only on the patient's physical abilities and in preventing the risk of falling, but also on certain cognitive parameters, functional skills, and some aspects of behaviour. Physiotherapists, psychomotor specialists, and occupational therapists can be called on to assist.

5) Interventions relating to behaviour
Non-cognitive symptoms can lead to major distress and dangerous behaviour. They must be analysed to identify the factors that may trigger, aggravate or improve such behaviour.

Music therapy, aromatherapy, multi-sensory stimulation, orientation rehabilitation, reminiscence therapy, animal-assisted therapy, massage, simulated presence therapy (a video of the patient's family) and light therapy could improve certain aspects of behaviour.

6) Interventions relating to practical difficulties and programmes of education and support for family and professional carers

Both family and professional carers should be given information about the disease, its treatment and the existence of families' associations.

Carers must be offered a choice of interventions, by families' associations, local information and coordination centres, day care centres, networks, etc.

Specific help must be offered to carers who are experiencing psychological distress.

B – INTEREST AND LIMITS OF FRENCH GUIDELINES

These recent guidelines have witnessed substantial changes in physicians' mentality and practices and have confirmed the interest of the French Government in non-drug intervention.

They also express the growing interest of clinical neurologists, psychiatrists, geriatricians, willing to cooperate with primary care physicians and other professionals or community care providers, specially trained in dementia management.

However, all these non-drug therapies have an important financial cost. Thus, while French HAS recommends non-drug therapies, their impact on family caregivers and/or patients remains an issue.

In other words, either non-drug interventions benefit patients and/or families and therefore could be financially more supported by the French Government; or, non-drug interventions have none or too little impact in comparison with their cost and the questions to ask would be: should they be stopped, reduced or be more adapted to patients' and families' needs, more innovatively?

In any case, an evidence-based statement of their efficacy remains to be strengthened in France. Therefore, in our opinion, the reasons why the HAS recommends the non-drug interventions is based on different considerations: -1/ their usefulness is recognized by a growing number of professionals involved in such practices, as well as persons with dementia and families. 2/ researchers are encouraged to carry out more scientific studies- and 3/ their impact on persons with dementia and/or caregivers is becoming supported by recent data (Spector et al. 2003, Olazaran et al. 2004, Acevedo and Loewenstein 2007). In North America, two studies have just published some results. The 3-country randomised controlled trial of a psychosocial intervention for caregivers combined with pharmacological treatment for persons living with Alzheimer disease demonstrated that effective counselling and support interventions can reduce symptoms of depression in caregivers when patients are taking Donepezil (Mittelman et al. 2008). The New York University caregiver intervention study indicated that institutionalization alone can reduce caregiver burden and depressive symptoms, but enhanced counselling provides additional long-term benefits (Gaugler et al. 2008).

The lack of data has led to the French HAS encouraging researchers and clinicians to carry out controlled studies and to it financially supporting some main research projects including AIDMA and ETNA-3.

C - MAIN CURRENT STUDIES IN FRANCE

By recognizing AD as a major public health issue and a social plague, the last French Government Alzheimer's Plan has focused on family carers of patients with dementia in order to reduce their burden and distress. Within this context, the Broca Hospital MRRC was able to achieve the first French multi-centre randomized controlled trial, entitled AIDMA. This study began in 2004 and has now been completed.

1. AIDMA: A psycho-educational programme designed to support and train carers of Alzheimer's disease ambulatory patients. Brief summary and first results.

Results of combined non pharmacologic interventions and antidementia drugs are lacking. Given that combined interventions are recommended, we addressed the issue of their impact on family carers and/or patients. The question was: does a programme for family carers combined with pharmacotherapy for patients improve outcomes in patients and/or families?

AIDMA included 15 French memory centres in charge of enrolling "patient-family carer" dyads fulfilling defined inclusion criteria. All patients diagnosed as having mild-to-moderate dementia were treated with antidementia drugs. Dyads were randomised in 2 parallel groups. Group I: caregivers followed an educational programme which consisted of 12 group sessions over a 3 months period. Each session (once a week) lasted 2 hours. Group II: carers did not follow the programme. The dyads were assessed 3 times by blinded psychologists, at baseline, at 3 months (end of programme) and 6 months follow-up. Significant differences were observed for the programme-group on the disease understanding and the coping strategies. In addition, an increase of the depression was observed in the group which did not follow the programme, while the programme-group remained stable (de Rotrou et al. 2009).

Beyond confirming the relevance of psycho-educational programmes for improving disease understanding and coping strategies, AIDMA results also suggest that expectations from families and a better involvement of patients in the relationship with their carer should be balanced. Health and social professionals probably expect too much from families and not enough from patients.

In contrast to the Mittelman's "3-country study", it is noteworthy to mention that in AIDMA, families and patients were not depressed at baseline (depression was an exclusion criterion), apart from normal depressive reactions related to their patient's difficulties.

Nevertheless AIDMA first results undoubtedly raise the important question of the relevance of evaluation criteria. As in studies assessing pain or anxiety, subjective self-rating scales, such as visual analogue scales (VAS) evaluating the understanding of AD, stress and coping strategies, appear more appropriate in comparison with usual scales for depression, anxiety or burden. In AD further research on VAS as well as on specific questionnaires evaluating the relationship between patients and carers would allow increased sensitivity of measures in order to identify changes. To our knowledge, assessment tools of the relationship changes between patients and caregivers are lacking.

2. ETNA 3 study: Efficacy Assessment of Three Non Pharmacological Therapies in Alzheimer's Disease.

ETNA3 study evaluates long-term efficacy of 3 non-drug therapies (cognitive stimulation, reminiscence therapy, made-to-measure therapy) on the progression rate of patients with mild and moderate dementia (Dartigues et al. 2006). These therapies are offered to the patients and a psycho-social programme is offered to the family caregivers. The interventions are compared to a control group who is offered only a psycho-social programme for the family caregivers. Two hundred patients are expected in each group. The main objective of ETNA3 is to discover if such interventions allow the onset of severe dementia to be delayed. To date (September 09) 624 patients have been included.

In the flourishing but costly area of non-drug interventions, one of the major goals of ETNA 3 is both to provide a state of the art overview of cognitive stimulation, reminiscence therapy and individualized therapy and to investigate their cost-effectiveness in comparison with important expenses supported by the French health care and social systems and also by the patients' families.

D - CURRENT ISSUES AND PERSPECTIVES

In the field of dementia management, while more controlled studies are obviously necessary to legitimate the use and development of non-drug therapies, addressing the most realistic and relevant questions appears just as necessary. Compared with issues addressed 20 years ago in the first trials on drug therapies, scientific published data as well as empirical data need to gain accuracy in defining the key issues and the expected outcomes. From a realistic point of view, up to now, non-drug interventions in AD are not thought to improve, or even stabilize in the long-term, cognitive or non-cognitive symptoms.

In summary, our research projects and clinical experience are in agreement with recent meta-analyses and highlight some of the following key issues which remain to be addressed:

- *Regarding patients*, do non-drug interventions reduce the impairment slope compared with no therapy? More specifically, which aspects of this impairment slope? Which cognitive or non cognitive functions could remain unchanged with adequate therapies and for how long? Who are the non-drug responders and non responders and for which interventions?
- *Regarding caregivers*, which type of psycho-educational programme benefits which caregiver or which profile of patient- caregivers dyads?
- Do non-drug interventions apart from educational programmes improve outcomes in persons with dementia and/or caregivers compared with no such interventions?
- Are there changes in the patient-caregiver relationship, independently from cognitive or non-cognitive symptoms impairment?

Different work groups have focused on another type of key issues for researchers and clinicians requiring guidance (Vernooij-Dassen et al. 2005):

- Does improvement of the relationship between primary care physicians, specialist physicians and community care providers benefit patients and/or caregivers?
- What economic model of care could better impact on dementia management?

To date such questions remain unanswered or partially unanswered, and perhaps unconsidered or underestimated.

Furthermore, the answers have to take into account different economic, cultural or ethical configurations specific to different countries. International focus groups are very helpful to differentiate universal questions from the specific ones depending on each country, in order to improve the design of controlled studies and the choice of expected outcomes.

E- METHODOLOGICAL ASPECTS

As a matter of fact, drug and non drug therapies evaluation share difficulties such as patient heterogeneity for instance. But molecules usually being tested belong to the same pharmacological class, as previously mentioned. The evaluation of non-drug therapies, has to deal with the heterogeneity of interventions as well as the heterogeneity in patients. Considering psychosocial programmes, for example, their content, the number of sessions, the family carers-patients dyads' profile, vary substantively. There is important variability in the objectives of studies and domain-specific outcomes. The background and clinical experience of professionals in charge of non-drug therapies can also introduce variability in the results. In such heterogeneous conditions, results cannot be concordant. When compared with drug therapies, having a clear overview of the work carried out in the field of non-drug interventions is not easy. Is it relevant to identify the efficacy of non-drug and drug interventions using the same evaluation criteria for patients? Is the methodology of drug trials suitable for non drug interventions? Non-drug interventions studies should be of sufficient size and design if specific evaluation criteria are required.

F- COGNITIVE STIMULATION: FRENCH CHARACTERISTICS

In France, since 1986 Broca Hospital (Paris) has been particularly involved in the concept of cognitive stimulation within the broad area of ageing (de Rotrou et al. 2002; 2006; 2009, Wenisch et al. 2005; 2007; Cantegreil et al. 2005; Rigaud et al.2008). Our research results as well as our clinical experience have contributed to the evolution of the concept and theoretical and practical advances concerning the understanding of patients' functional status and residual resources. Initially, cognitive stimulation was classified alongside Reality Orientation Therapies (ROT). The theoretical evolution and practices lead us to consider cognitive stimulation programmes differently from ROT. In cognitive stimulation, the theoretical background relies on the two main following concepts: the priming effect and the exposure effect based on implicit memory (Warrington 1974, Seamon et al. 1995). We have adapted these concepts to dementia. This means that exercises focused on ecological situations are performed with psychologists during the programme sessions and then reinforced in real life by trained and psychologically supported families (as previously described in HAS guidelines). Priming and exposure effects play a facilitatory role which enables patients' better involvement and compliance in real life (de Rotrou 2009).

To our knowledge, cognitive stimulation programmes are widely used in France and appear of great practical importance in other countries (Ball et al. 2002; Spector et al. 2005; Woods et al. 2006; Bier et al. 2007, Matsuda 2007, Acevedo 2007).

Today we are specifically interested in the following aspects of non-drug interventions:

- Design of more adequate evaluation tools relating to the specific non-drug intervention and according to the patients' profile and the patient-caregiver dyad.
- Emphasis on specific methodological and statistical approaches for non-drug intervention evaluation in comparison with specific drug therapy trials.
- Gerontechnology with a focus on computerized ecological cognitive stimulation programmes (Rigaud et al.2008 a, 2008 b; Faucounau et al.2009) adapted to the pattern of the patient's dementia, and in conjunction with support programmes for family carers, by means of a website for instance.

In computerized cognitive stimulation programmes, cognitive exercises for patients simulate real life situations in order to help maintain autonomy in activities of daily living. Computerized support programmes provide caregivers with theoretical information about healthy and pathological ageing in the field of cognition as well as advice on "how to help the patient" or "how to behave with the patient". Both programmes for patients and caregivers are gathered in sessions (e.g. 30 minutes) several times a week for several months (e.g. 3 months). As far as the evaluation of the benefits is concerned, computerized cognitive stimulation programmes for patients and support programmes for caregivers have shown promising results. However the evaluation has been restricted to small numbers of people and short term effects so far. Thus, benefits need to be evaluated both in patients and caregivers by means of randomized trials with a large number of participants and assessed in the long term.

CONCLUSION

Available scientific and empirical data raise the possibility that non pharmacologic interventions may be effective in treating patients' cognitive impairment and behavioural disorders and in preventing their state worsening. Data also more and more confirm that different types of psycho-educational programmes might be of therapeutic value for caregivers.

Further studies are needed to provide evidence-based results showing which non-drug therapies are of clinical benefit for which patients and/or caregivers. In dementia management, available data emphasize the urgent need to address the correct issues and specific outcomes, taking into account our current knowledge of Alzheimer's disease.

REFERENCES

Acevedo, A., and Loewenstein, D.A. (2007). Nonpharmacological Cognitive Interventions in Aging and Dementia. *Journal of Geriatric Psychiatry and Neurology; 20 (4),* 239-249.

Ball, K., Berch, D., Helmers, K., Jobe, J., Leveck, M., Marsiske, M., Morris, J., Rebok, G., Smith, D., Tennstedt, S., Unverzagt, F., Willis, S. (2002). Effects of cognitive training interventions with older adults. *JAMA; 288(18),* 2271-81.

Bier, N. Desrosiers, J., Gagnon, L. (2006). Cognitive training interventions for normal aging, mild cognitive impairment and Alzheimer's disease. *Can. J. Occup Ther; 73(1),* 26-35.

Brodaty, H., Green, A., Koshera, A. (2003). Meta-Analysis of psycho-social interventions for caregivers of people with dementia. *JAGS; 51(5),* 657-64.

Cantegreil-Kallen, I., De Rotrou, J., Gosselin, A., Wenisch, E., Rigaud, A-S. (2002). The role of cognitive stimulation in diagnosing mild cognitive impairment subjects at risk for Alzheimer type dementia. *Brain Aging; Vol. 2 (4),* 15-19.

Dartigues, J-F. (2007). Efficacy Assessment of Three Non Pharmacological Therapies in Alzheimer's disease (ETNA3). *http://clinicaltrials.gov/ct2/show/NCTOO646269*

Doody, R.S., Stevens, J.C., Beck, C., Dubinsky, R..M., Kaye, J.A., Gwyther, L., Mohs, R.C., Thal, L.J., Whitehouse, S.T., P.J., DeKosky,S.T., Cummings, J.L. (2001). Practice parameter: Management of dementia (an evidence-based review): report of the Quality Standards Subcommittee of the American Academy of Neurology. *Neurology; 56,* 1154-1166.

De Rotrou, J., Cantegreil-Kallen, I., Gosselin, A., Wenisch, E., Rigaud, A-S. (2002). Cognitive stimulation: a new approach for Alzheimer's disease management. *Brain aging; 2,* 48-53.

De Rotrou, J., Thévenet, S., Richard, A., Cantegreil-Kallen, I., Wenisch, E., Chausson, C., Moulin, F., Batouche, F., Rigaud, A-S. (2006). Impact d'un programme psycho-éducatif sur le stress des aidants de patients Alzheimer. *L'Encéphale*; 32, 650-655.

De Rotrou, J., and Wenisch, E. Stimulation cognitive et vieillissement. (2009). In Masson (Ed.), *Gérontologie préventive : Abrégés de Médecine.* 468-483.

De Rotrou, J., Cantegreil-Kallen I., Wenisch, E., Chausson, C., Jegou, D., Grabar, S., Rigaud A-S. (2009). Combined interventions in dementia. Results of AIDMA: A French controlled study. Submitted.

Faucounau, V., Wu, Y-H., de Sant'Anna, M., de Rotrou, J., Rigaud, A-S. (2009). Cognitive intervention programmes in patients affected by mild cognitive impairment: a promising intervention tool for MCI? *Journal of Nutrition, Health and Aging.* In Press.

Gaugler, J.E., Roth, D.L., Haley, W.E., Mittelman, M.S. (2008). Can counselling and support reduce burden and depressive symptoms in caregivers of people with Alzheimer's disease during the transition to institutionalization? Results from the New York University caregiver intervention study. *JAGS; 56 (3),* 421-428.

Günther, V.K., Schäfer, P., Holzner, B.J., Kemmler, G.W. (2003). Long-term improvements in cognitive performance through computer-assisted cognitive training: a pilot study in a residential home for older people. *Aging Ment Health; 7,* 200-206.

Hofman, M., Rösler, A., Schwarz, W., Müller-Spahn, F., Kraüchi, K., Hock, C., Seifritz, E. (2003). Interactive Computer-Training as a therapeutic Tool in Alzheimer's disease. *Comprehensive Psychiatry*; 44, (3), 213-219.

Matsuda, O. (2007). Cognitive stimulation therapy for Alzheimer's disease: the effect of cognitive stimulation therapy on the progression of mild Alzheimer's disease in patients treated with Donepezil. *Int. Ppsychogeriatrics;* 19(2), 241-252.

Mittelman, M.S, Brodaty, H., Wallen, A.S., Burns, A. (2008). A three-country randomized controlled trial of a psychosocial intervention for caregivers combined with pharmacological treatment for patients with Alzheimer disease: effects on caregiver depression. *Am J Geriatr Psychiatry;* 16 (11), 893-904.

Olazarán, J., Muñiz, R., Reisberg, B., Peña-Casanova, J., del Ser, T., Cruz-Jentoft, A.J, Serrano, P., Navarro, E., García de la Rocha, M.L, Franck, A., Galiano, M., Fernández-Bullido, Y., Serra, J.A., González-Salvador, M.T, Sevilla, C. (2004). Benefits of cognitive-motor intervention in MCI and mild to moderate Alzheimer disease. *Neurology ; 63,* 2348-2353.

Rigaud, A-S., de Rotrou, J., Duron, E., Faucounau, V., Seux, M-L., Hanon, O. (2008). Alzheimer's disease : a vision of future. *In Envejecimiento, Dependencia, Demencias y Nuevas Tecnologias,* José Carlos Millan Calenti, Edition Instituto Gallogo de Iniciativas Sociales y Sanitarias, Graficas Garabal ; 167-181.

Rigaud, A-S., Faucounau, V., De Rotrou, J., De Sant'Anna, M., WU, Y-H. (2008). [New technologies and cognitive stimulation]. *Soins Gerontol* ; (74), 29-32.

Seux, M-L., de Rotrou, J., Rigaud, A-S. (2008). Les traitements de la maladie d'Alzheimer. *Psychiatr Sci Hum Neurosci. ; 6,* 1-9.

Seamon, J.G., Williams, P.C., Crowley, M.J., Kim, I.J., Langer, S.A., Orne, P.J., Wishengrad, D.L. (1995). The mere exposure effect is based on implicit memory: effects of stimulus type, encoding conditions, and number of exposures on recognition and affect judgments. *Journal of experimental psychology. Learning, memory, and cognition. American Psychological Association, 21(3),* 711-721.

Spector, A., Thorgrimsen, L., Woods, B., Royan, L., Davies, S., Butterworth, M., Orell, M. (2003). Efficacy of an evidence-based cognitive stimulation therapy programme for people with dementia : randomised controlled trial. *Br. J. Psychiatry; 183,* 248-254.

Tarraga, L., Boada, M., Modinos, G., Espinoza, A., Diego, S., Morera, A., Guitart, M., Balcells, J., Lopez, O.L, Becker, J.T. (2006). A randomised pilot study to assess the efficacy of an interactive, multimedia tool of cognitive stimulation in Alzheimer's disease. *J. Neurol Neurosurg. Psychiatry; 77,* 1116-1121.

Vernooij-Dassen, M., Moniz-Cook, E.D., Woods, R.T., De Lepeleire, J., Leuschner, A., Zanetti, O., de Rotrou, J., Kenny, G., Franco, M., Peters, V., Ilife, S. and the Interdem group. (2005). Factors affecting timely recognition and diagnosis of dementia across Europe: from awareness to stigma. *International Journal of Geriatric Psychiatry*; 20, 377-386

Waldemar, G., Dubois, B., Emre, M., Georges, J., McKeith, I.G., Rossor, M., Scheltens, P., Tariska, P. and Winblad, B. (2007). Recommendations for the diagnosis and management of Alzheimer's disease and other disorders associated with dementia: EFNS guideline. *European Journal of Neurology;* 14 e1- e26.

Warrington, E.K., Weiskrantz, L. (1974). The effect of prior learning on subsequent retention in amnesic patients. *Neuropsychologia;* 12 , 419-428.

Wenisch, E., Stoker, A., Bourrellis, C., Pasquet, C., Gauthier, E., Corcos, E., Banchi, M.T., De Rotrou, J., Rigaud A-S. (2005). A global intervention programme for institutionalized demented patients. *Rev. Neurol; 161(3),* 290-298.

Wenisch, E., Cantegreil-Kallen, I., De Rotrou, J., Garrigue, P.., Moulin, F., Batouche, F., Richard, A., De Sant'Anna, M., Rigaud, A-S. (2007). Cognitive stimulation intervention for elders with MCI compared with normal aged subjects: preliminary results. *Aging Clin Exp Res*; 19, 316-322.

Woods, B., Thorgrimsen, L., Spector, A., Royan, L., Orell, M. (2006). Improved quality of life and cognitive stimulation therapy in dementia. *Aging Mental Health; 10 (3)*, 219-226.

In: Dementia: Non-Pharmacological Therapies   ISBN: 978-1-61470-736-3
Editor: Elisabetta Farina, pp. 27-42   © 2012 Nova Science Publishers, Inc.

RECREATIONAL THERAPY INTERVENTIONS: A FRESH APPROACH TO TREATING APATHY AND MIXED BEHAVIORS IN DEMENTIA

Linda L. Buettner and Suzanne Fitzsimmons*

Health and Human Performance
University of North Carolina at Greensboro
Greensboro, North Carolina.

ABSTRACT

The purpose of this study was to examine the ability to prescribe recreational therapy interventions for the treatment of neuropsychiatric behaviors in institutionalized older adults with dementia. This project took place in five long term care facilities in the southeast United States over a period of three years. Findings indicate that 10% of the participants had "pure agitation" while 30% had "apathy only," and the majority, 60%, had mixed behaviors of apathy combined with agitation. Individually tailored recreation therapy interventions were efficacious for all behavior types. Analysis determined that the improvement in both apathy and agitation, during the treatment phase was highly significant at the p<0.000. Interestingly by targeting treatment during periods of apathy for those with mixed behaviors, agitation was also reduced, providing a new approach for non-drug interventions.

Keywords: Apathy, agitation, recreation therapy, interventions, mixed behaviors.

INTRODUCTION

Apathy is defined as the loss of motivation not attributable to cognitive impairment, emotional distress, or reduced level of consciousness (Marin, 1991). Apathy occurs in approximately 71% of individuals with Alzheimer's disease (AD) within five years of diagnosis (Boyle and Malloy, 2004). Individuals living with AD with apathy require more management and support, given their reliance on others to schedule their activities and initiate tasks even when they are still physically capable of performing them. Studies examining the

---

* Contact Author: Linda L. Buettner, Ph.D, LRT, CTRS. Professor Therapeutic Recreation/Gerontology RTH/Health and Human Performance University of North Carolina at Greensboro Phone:336-334-4131 Fax: 336-334-3238 Email: llbuettn@uncg.edu

relationship of apathy to neuropsychological measures showed apathy was consistently associated with more severe functional impairments, more severe cognitive deficits, higher levels of burden and distress in caregivers, along with increased resource utilization (Landes, Sperry, Strauss, and Geldmacher, 2008; Starkstein, Ingram, Garau, and Mizrahi, 2005). Apathy is a negative symptom in AD that is often overlooked by healthcare providers, yet one that if left untreated, leads to more rapid than expected functional decline (Starkstein, Jorge, Mizrahi, and Robinson, 2006). The causes of apathy are described as complex and related to underlying pathology, atrophy of the frontal lobes, and their connections to the temporal lobes (Levy and Dubois, 2006). Damage to these areas of the brain reduces the individual's the ability to initiate, sequence, and complete tasks without assistance.

SIGNIFICANCE

Approximately 5.2 million people have Alzheimer's disease (AD) or related disorders in the United States. It is estimated that by the year 2030, the prevalence will be 7.7 million, with an anticipated 13.2 million by 2050 (Hebert, Scherr, Bienjas, Bennett, and Evans, 2003). Overall prevalence of AD appears to double for every 5-year age group beyond age 65 (National Institutes on Aging, 2005). We know, however, that people living with AD and their care providers are highly interested evidence based programs to improve troubling symptoms and manage their disease (Alzheimer's Association, 2006).

Currently there is no cure for Alzheimer's disease or other related disorders, therefore many individuals require extensive long-term services, often involving costly in-home services and out of home placements when function declines. There are approximately 1.5 million nursing home residents in the United States today, and this number is expected to double by the year 2020 with the growth in dementia (Clark, 1996; Feder, Komiar, and Niefeld, 2000). Apathy is exhibited by up to 92% of those afflicted throughout the entire course of the disease (Landes, Sperry, Strauss, and Geldmacher, 2008; Starkstein, Ingram, Garau, and Mizrahi, 2005; Clark and RF, 2000; Feder, Komiar, and Niefeld, 2000) and contributes to serious problems such as declines in functional status, social engagement, and physical activity (Starkstein, Jorge, Mizrahi, Robinson, 2006). Additionally, functional decline due to apathy contributes significantly to cost of care (Buettner, 2006; Buettner and Fitzsimmons, 2003) and is a major source of caregiver concern (Thomas, Clement, Hazif-Thomas, and Leger, 2001). Thus it is important to develop safe, efficacious, and cost effective interventions that maintain function and promote quality of life by responding to apathy in a timely way. We believe if interest and engagement levels can be maintained over time through evidence-based recreational therapy interventions, ADL (activities of daily living) function may remain longer, and the period of time for costly care may be compressed.

RECREATION THERAPY

Recreation therapy is a physician ordered, individualized and time limited intervention provided by a licensed or certified therapeutic recreation specialist (CTRS) to improve function or behavior. It is based on each individual's assessment and designed to treat a specific problem, concern or impairment. A recreational therapist utilizes a wide range of interventions and techniques to improve the physical, cognitive, emotional, and social and leisure function of their clients. Recreational therapists assist clients to develop skills, knowledge and behaviors for daily living and community involvement. The unique feature that makes recreation therapy different from other therapies is the use of highly motivating recreational modalities within the designed intervention strategies. Incorporating client's interests, and the client's family and/or community makes the therapy process meaningful, relevant, and engaging. Recreational therapy is individualized to each person, their past, present and future interests, functional abilities, needs, and desired lifestyle making it an excellent option to treat apathy.

APATHY

Apathy has profound consequences on both persons living with AD and caregivers and affects their ability to stay active. Zawacki and colleagues (2002), examined the relationship of behavioral disturbance and dementia severity to activities of daily living and dementia. A series of stepwise regression analyses was conducted to examine the extent to which dementia severity, apathy, disinhibition, and executive dysfunction predict ADLs (total, basic, and instrumental). For total ADLs, apathy accounted for 36% of the variance and dementia severity accounted for an additional 15%. For basic ADLs, apathy accounted for 27% of the variance. Dementia severity, executive dysfunction, and disinhibition were not significantly associated with basic ADLs. For instrumental ADLs, dementia severity accounted for 37% of the variance and apathy accounted for an additional 14%. These findings highlight the importance of apathy as an independent factor associated with functional independence. Individuals with limited capacity to regulate their apathy independently are likely to have significant functional impairments. These researchers suggest environmental modifications that provide structure, practice, and cueing may be beneficial for improving independent functioning in individuals with apathy. Little research has been performed on the effects of treatments directed at reducing apathy. Cholinesterase inhibitors have shown some efficacy for reducing apathy in some patients (Mizrahi and Starkstein, 2007). Unfortunately, these pharmacological interventions lack efficacy in the majority of the cases (Schuyler, 2007). Adult day programs, recreational therapy, reminiscence therapy, cognitive-based programs and discussion groups have shown a positive effect on apathy (Lerner, Strauss, and Sami, 2007). Research data supports the use of socialization, music, physical, and art programs for apathy by increasing social interactions, communication, and engagement (Verkaik, van Weert, and Francke, 2005). Apathy has also been associated with poorer treatment response in rehabilitation settings and with pharmacological interventions for cognition. In geriatric inpatients apathy correlated with lack of participation in rehabilitation with an r=0.372 (p<0.05) (Thomas, Clement, Hazif-Thomas, and Leger, 2006). In community dwelling individuals with AD apathy was more common in those who did not show a behavioral response to donepezil (Mega, Masterman, O'Connor, Barclay, and Cummings, 1999). Unfortunately, donepezil lacked efficacy in the majority of the participants with apathy (Schuyler, 2007). In community dwelling individuals with AD, caregiver distress correlated with Neuropsychiatric Inventory-rated apathy with an r=0.5 (p<0.001) (Kaufer, Cummings,

Christine, Bray, Castellon, and Masterman, et. Al, 1998). In preliminary preparation for the intervention trial we report in this paper we examined of two specific types of behaviors, apathy and agitation, that commonly occur in persons with dementia. In the analysis of baseline data, we explored the times and the types of behaviors occurring in 141 older adults living in the community, assisted living, and nursing home settings during a baseline evaluation period (Buettner and Fitzsimmons, 2006). The occurrence of apathetic and agitated behaviors was monitored throughout the day for a 5-day period. The results suggested that in all stages and settings, a combination of apathy and agitation (60%) is the most common phenomenon, and that the predominant behavior actually fluctuates during the course of the day. Study participants with "apathy only" were 30% while those with "pure agitation" alone was much less than we anticipated at 10%. These findings that argue most dementia patients have "mixed behaviors" (apathy and agitation) suggest the use of individualized non-pharmacological interventions based on carefully monitored behavior patterns may provide a more sensitive approach. Apathy presents either as a symptom or a syndrome, and is frequently reported in frontal lobe and basal ganglia pathology, as well as a host of neuropsychiatric, medical and drug-induced conditions without detectable structural brain abnormalities, including early stage dementia, delirium, depression, traumatic brain injury, and schizophrenia. The relationship between non-cognitive symptoms such as apathy and cognitive deficits in AD is not clear (Derouesné, Piquard, Thibault, Baudouin-Madec, and Lacomblez, 2001). There is growing evidence that apathy often co-occurs with depression, but also represents a distinct clinical syndrome that should be considered in the differential diagnosis and treatment process. It appears non-cognitive and cognition symptoms in AD stem from different biological and psychological mechanisms (Lerner, Strauss, and Sami, 2007).

Marin (1991) describes the diagnostic criteria for apathy as a lack of motivation related to the individuals' previous level of functioning, and the presence of at least one symptom belonging to each of the following three domains: diminished goal directed motor behavior, diminished goal directed cognition, and lack of emotional responsivity to positive or negative events. Each of the three areas is conceptualized on a continuum from "Not at all characteristic" to "A lot Characteristic" in the questions of the Apathy Evaluation Scale (AES) (Marin, Biedrzycki, and Firinciogullari, 1991). The symptoms cause clinically significant distress or impairment in social, occupational, or other important areas of functioning. The symptoms are not due to diminished level of consciousness or the direct physiologic effects of a substance (e.g., abuse of a drug or side effect of a medication). To operationalize the concept of apathy three areas are observed as signs of motivation or the lack thereof (apathy). Motor apathy is described as the tendency not to initiate a new motor activity unless externally prompted. Diminished overt behavior falls along a range of observable behavior from a small noticeable change in social or occupational functioning to profound deficits in the ability to initiate any movement at all. On the opposite end of the behavioral spectrum is motor restlessness. Ideally an intervention for motor apathy would offer interesting opportunities for successful motor performance. In each recreational therapy intervention session used in this study, sensory motor and physical performance tasks were introduced, that required visual spatial, gross motor, and fine motor activities from participants. The facilitator demonstrated the task and adapted the motor activities and cueing to achieve maximal engagement from each participant. Cognitive apathy is defined as indifference; a generalized loss of interest, decreases in goal-directed thought content, diminished motivation associated with executive functions, and at times decreased verbal fluency. In mild diminished goal-directed thought content is observed as decreased interests, plans, or goals for the future.

In severe cases there is an absence of goal-related thought content and verbal response. On the opposite end of the behavioral spectrum is verbally repetitive behavior with poor attention. In each recreational therapy intervention session participants were presented with interesting yet novel thought provoking activities to plan and to perform. Each recreational activity required interaction with the environment and solving a simple problem to complete a recreational task. Emotional apathy is defined as diminished amount of emotion, or complacency, relative to the importance of some goal-directed thought or event. Mild diminished emotional responses to goal related events are observed as mild indifference or shallow responses to important life events. In more severe emotional apathy no emotional response is observed at all in response to important life events.

On the other extreme of neuropsychiatric behaviors, patients may display excessive crying or anger responses out of proportion to the situation. In each recreational therapy session a group interaction was introduced that allowed for a positive exchange with another person, communication, and teamwork. The model for apathy and our intervention is displayed in Figure 1.

In summary apathy has been associated with a number of adverse outcomes such as premature loss of ADL function, poorer treatment response, and higher levels of caregiver distress. Apathy and agitation, or "mixed behaviors" often occur in the same day for individuals with dementia.

This recreational therapy intervention trial aimed to address apathy symptoms which overtime could improve engagement levels, improve outcomes during treatment, reduce caregiver stress, and improve quality of life for families with the ultimate goal of reducing cost of care. Specifically we hypothesized: 1). Recreational therapy interventions (RTIs) will improve apathy among long term care residents with dementia and neuropsychiatric behaviors, and 2). By providing RTIs during periods of apathy other neuropsychiatric behaviors will also improve.

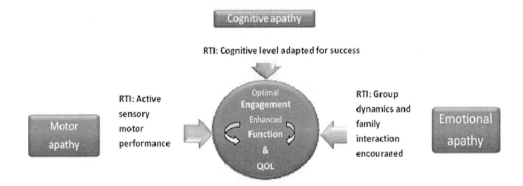

Figure 1. Concept of apathy and RTIs.

METHODS

The purpose of this study was to examine the ability to prescribe recreational therapy interventions for the treatment of neuropsychiatric behaviors in institutionalized older adults with dementia. This project took place in five long term care facilities in the southeast United States over a period of three years. This study used an experimental design with one intervention and one delayed intervention control group. Following the collection of baseline data on days 1-5, participants were randomly assigned to one of the two groups. Six participants were involved at a time, three in the treatment and three in control group. The intervention group received individually prescribed therapeutic recreation five days a week for two weeks. The delayed intervention group received usual nursing home care and a 20-minute social visit from a research team member daily for two weeks, followed by the individually prescribed therapeutic recreation program for two weeks in a later round of the study. Thus every participant in the study received the intervention and served as a wait list control. During baseline each participant was observed for activity levels, behavior patterns, and assessed for recreational preferences, cognitive and physical ability, and a recreational therapy intervention was created for each individual. Data were collected using paper-and-pencil behavior scales completed by trained nurse reviewers blinded to group assignment five days prior to initiation of the treatment-control condition and again 3 days after the treatment-control condition ended. Participants were also videotaped and later coded for engagement levels. Coders were graduate research assistants trained by the researchers. This process was repeated until 107 participants took part in the treatment group. To determine the category of behavior, apathy or agitation, of each participant, data were gathered on type of behavior the participant exhibited throughout the day for five days. This was coded for eight time periods in two-hour blocks. The time periods evaluated started at 6 AM and ended at 10 PM. Recreational interests, functioning level, and current participation levels were also gathered. This project included 107 participants recruited from five different long-term care residences in the southeast US. Inclusion criteria: 1) 65 years of age or older; 2) diagnosis of dementia in the medical record; 3) Mini-mental State Examination (MMSE) (Folstein, Folstein, and McHugh, 1975) score of 24 or less; 4) signed consent by guardian and assent by participant: 5) stable on current medications; and 6) identified by staff as having either behaviors of apathy or agitation. Table 1 details descriptive information about participants by group. It is important to realize that all participants received the intervention and that all participants served as wait-list controls. Thus the description of the participants is statistically very similar. Table 2 provides percentages of all participants in each cognitive diagnostic category.

MEASURES

Apathy: Marin and colleagues (1991) have been prime contributors to both the delineation and the assessment of the observable components of motivation vs. apathy. When examining the available measurement tools the construct validity is strongest for the Apathy Evaluation Scale (AES) (Marin, Biedrzycki, and Firinciogullari,1991). It is an 18-item scale that can be administered by a clinician as a semi-structured inventory, or reported by a caregiver as a paper and pencil scale, or self reported on a self-rated scale. The AES internal consistency has an alpha range from 0.86-0.94. We utilized the clinician delivered inventory throughout this project to measure apathy with interrater agreement rates ranged between .92 and .96.

Agitation: The Cohen-Mansfield Agitation inventory (CMAI) is a 29-item caregiver rating questionnaire for the assessment of agitation in elderly persons (Cohen-Mansfield, 1986). It includes descriptions of 29 agitated behaviors, each rated on a 7-point scale of frequency. Inter-rater agreement rates ranged between .88 and .92.

Geriatric Depression Scale: The Geriatric Depression Scale (GDS) (Yesavage, Brink, Rose, Lum, Huang, Adey, et al., 1983) is a screening tool for identifying depressive symptoms in older adults. It is especially useful in clinical settings to facilitate assessment of depression in older adults, especially when baseline measurements are compared to subsequent scores.

Time and Engagement: Treatment sessions were videotaped and evaluated by trained research assistants who coded minutes and percentages of engagement for each participant. Total minutes of engagement were recorded for each participant session. Engagement was then coded by observing interaction with recreational items, the facilitator, or others in the session video tape and graded on a 0-100% scale over the course of the intervention. Interrater agreement rates averaged .98.

Table 1. Overall Descriptives of Participants by Group

	N	Range	Min	Max	Mean	Std. Dev
Treatment Group						
Months at facility	107	122.00	2.00	124.00	25.75	20.60
Age of subject	107	34.40	67.50	101.90	86.18	6.91
total meds	107	14.00	.00	14.00	6.67	3.21
MMSE	107	26.00	.00	26.00	8.39	7.95
Global det. scale	107	5.00	2.00	7.00	5.43	1.07
GDS	99	14.00	.00	14.00	3.75	3.11
Pre-test Agitation	107	2.75	1.00	3.75	1.79	.55
Pre-test Apathy	107	4.25	37.00	54.25	49.92	9.02
Post-test Agitation	107	2.70	1.00	3.70	1.58	.47
Post test Apathy	107	4.75	39.25	55.00	41.80	9.27
Control						
Months at facility	107	122.00	2.00	124.00	25.75	20.60
Age of subject	107	34.40	67.50	101.90	86.18	6.91
total meds	107	14.00	.00	14.00	6.66	3.22
MMSE	107	26.00	.00	26.00	8.42	7.97
Global det. scale	107	5.00	2.00	7.00	5.43	1.07
GDS	99	14.00	.00	14.00	3.75	3.11
Pre-test Agitation	107	2.77	1.00	3.77	1.82	.57
Pre-test Apathy	107	4.25	37.00	54.25	49.92	9.98
Post-test Agitation	107	2.75	1.00	3.75	1.80	.56
Post test Apathy	107	4.25	39.00	54.25	51.11	9.01

Table 2. Chart diagnosis of sample

Dementia Type	
	Participants
Alzheimer's	41
	38.3%
Vascular dementia	7
	6.5%
Parkinson's dementia	5
	4.7%
Mixed dementia	11
	10.3%
Unspecified	41
	38.3%
Other	2
	1.9%
Total	107
	100.0%

INTERVENTION

Participants were assessed using the Global Deterioration Scale (Reisberg, Ferris, de Leon, and Crook., 1982) for current functioning level and the Farrington Leisure Interest Survey (Buettner and Martin, 1995) for recreational interests. We also screened for depression using the Geriatric Depression Scale (GDS). The principal investigator (PI) or co-principal investigator (Co-PI) prescribed the therapeutic recreation intervention based on the data from these assessments. Recreational activities were adapted for functional level of the participant as needed. The assessments also involved interviews with family members and nursing staff; observation of resident behavior and chart review. Each participant received 2 weeks of individualized recreation therapy services that lasted approximately 30 minutes per day, five days per week. The interventions were individualized based on function, need, and recreational interests. Some sessions consisted of several different types of interventions in order to determine what intervention was most efficacious for that participant. After the treatment period was complete the research team left a care plan for the nursing home staff so they were aware of successful approaches and could continue them. The research team used approximately 72 different recreational intervention types over the course of the project. The research team remained consistent throughout the project. This team included a doctorally prepared Gerontologist/Certified Therapeutic Recreational Specialist, an advanced practice geriatric nurse practitioner with a certificate in recreational therapy, and a gerontology/recreational therapy graduate student assistant. Data were collected each time an intervention was attempted which totaled 1825 intervention attempts. Specific data collected during these attempts included time involved in minutes, level of engagement, encouragement needed, and participation.

When possible, RTIs were scheduled to take place a few minutes before the most prevalent neuropsychiatric behavior occurred for the participant. For an example if a participant had mixed behaviors with several hours of apathy in the late morning followed by late afternoon short period of agitation the he intervention was provided just prior to the apathy period. The information collected during the baseline period allowed for time to be added in the prescription. In general, apathy peaked in late morning (10AM - 12 noon) and then again in the late afternoon (4PM-6PM). Agitated behaviors gradually increased throughout the day with a peak between 4:00 and 8:00 p.m. At times this precise scheduling did not occur due to participant involvement in dining, personal care, appointments and other facility functions (Buettner and Fitzsimmons, 2006).

ANALYSIS

A variety of statistical methods were used to examine the data in this study. The demographic data analysis used descriptive statistics. Correlations were used to explore key relationships and t-tests were used to evaluate changes in neuropsychiatric behaviors. The specific results are reported below. Relationships between baseline facility activity participation and Pretest CMAI, Pretest Apathy, MMSE, and the Geriatric Depression Scale (GDS) were explored using ANOVA. This analysis indicated a highly significant relationship between pretest apathy and level of observed activity level prior to the intervention (See Table 3).

Table 3. Relationship between Facility Activity Participation and Pretest CMAI, Pretest Passivity, MMSE, and GDS

		Sum of Squares	df	Mean Square	F	Sig.
DX	Between Groups	1.447	4	.362	1.191	.319
	Within Groups	31.001	102	.304		
	Total	32.449	106			
Pre-test	Between Groups	16.165	4	4.041	4.351	.003
apathy score	Within Groups	94.727	102	.929		
	Total	110.891	106			
Depression	Between Groups	1.449	4	.362	1.536	.197
DX	Within Groups	24.065	102	.236		
	Total	25.514	106			
MMSE	Between Groups	524.549	4	131.137	2.168	.078
	Within Groups	6168.965	102	60.480		
	Total	6693.514	106			

Post hoc tests indicate that the only significant difference is between: Frequent Appropriate and Little or None in Pretest Apathy.

Participants who scored high on apathy were more likely to have "little or no activity" involvement during the baseline evaluation period ($p < .01$). However no relationship between activity involvement was found with depression ($p = .20$) or mental status ($p = .08$). Thus we identified that apathy was negatively related to the amount of activity engagement reported prior to the study. Apathy scores were analyzed using a t-test for independent samples with a two-tailed significance at the α = .05 level. On the AES assessment tool, higher scores indicate greater apathy levels. The suggested cut off score on the AES for apathy is 42. The control phase pre-test mean of 49.9 increased slightly at the post-test to 50.1, indicating a slight but not significant increase in apathetic behaviors. The treatment phase pre-test mean of 49.9 decreased to 41.8 at the post-test denoting a marked decrease in apathy. The analysis of this variable determined that the difference in apathy means for the treatment phase was highly significant at the $p < 0.000$ level. Table 4 shows changes in apathy score for the treatment and control conditions.

Table 4. RTIs Pre-Post Differences for apathy

Group	n	Mean	Sig.(2 tailed)
Pre-Treatment	107	49.9	.000***
Post- Treatment		41.8	
Pre-Control	107	49.9	.957
Post-Control		50.1	

P>.0001.

CHANGE IN AGITATION

The CMAI scores were analyzed for change in agitated behaviors using a t-test for independent samples with a two-tailed significance at the α = .05 level. The control phase pre-test means of 1.81 decreased slightly at the post-test to 1.80, indicating a slight but not significant decrease in agitation. The treatment phase pre-test mean of 1.79 decreased to 1.58 at the post-test, showing a highly significant decrease in agitation. It is important to note for the majority of participants with mixed behaviors, or a combination of apathy and agitation, the RTIs focused on engagement just before apathy occurred. Change in agitation is reported on Table 5. The CMAI scores significantly improved for this subgroup despite the focus on apathy. Overall, the analysis of this variable determined that the difference in mean CMAI score for the treatment phase was highly significant at the $p < 0.000$ level. The mean percent of time engaged in the RTI was 84% of the time overall. When this was broken down by severity of cognitive impairment those with mild impairments (MMSE<18) were engaged 96% of the time. Those with moderate impairments (MMSE 9-17) were engaged 94% of the time. Those with severe impairments (MMSE >9) were engaged 74% of the time. Table 6 shows the percent time engaged by severely of impairment. An examination of minutes of engagement by behavior type indicates the RTIs were engaging for participants with agitation, apathy, and mixed behaviors; with those experiencing agitation as the primary problem remaining engaged for the longest period of time. Table 7 shows average minutes engaged by type of behavior. For this paper we were specifically interested in participants with apathy or mixed behaviors of apathy and agitation. When we examined the most effective recreational activities for apathy or mixed behaviors we divided the sample by level of impairment and reported both engagement percentages and time in minutes engaged in the recreational activity. These findings are detailed on Table 8.

Table 5. RTIs and Pre-Post Differences Agitation

Group	n	Mean	Sig.(2 tailed)
Pre-Treatment	107	1.79	.000***
Post- Treatment		1.58	
Pre-Control	107	1.82	.452
Post-Control		1.80	

P>.0001.

Table 6. Time engaged by behavior type

Target behavior	Mean minutes engaged	Number of RTI sessions	Std.Dev
Agitation	30.5	450	18.1
Apathy	27.5	477	15.5
Mixed	24.3	899	13.6
Mean total time	26.7	1826	15.5

Table 7. Percent engagement by level of impairment

Level of cognitive impairment	Mean % engagement	Number of RTI sessions	Std.Dev
Mild	96%	450	18.1
Moderate	94%	477	15.5
Severe	74%	899	13.6
Total	84%	1826	15.5

**Table 8. Engagement Level by Impairment
with Apathy or Mixed Behaviors**

Engagement %: Mild (MMSE >18) With Passivity or mixed behaviors				
		N	Engagement %	Time in Minutes
1	AAT	4	100%	38
2	Wheelchair bike	12	100%	36
3	Group Singing	7	100%	29
4	Discussion Group	10	100%	28
5	Photography	4	100%	28
6	Jewelry Making	5	100%	27
7	Tetherball	11	100%	26
8	Nature	6	100%	15
9	Cooking	10	96%	53
10	5 stage sensory	6	79%	21

Table 8. (Continued).

Engagement %: Moderate (MMSE 9 - 17) With Passivity or mixed behaviors				
		N	Engagement %	Time in Minutes
1	Wheelchair bike	34	100	31
2	Flower arrangement	13	100	13
3	Nature	14	100	13
4	Crafts	11	97	27
5	Cooking	30	96	44
6	Jewerly Rummage Box	13	93	35
7	Music	10	93	31
8	Discussion	19	90	24
9	Singing	34	88	28
10	Tetherball	42	87	27
Engagement % Severe (MMSE <8) With Passivity or mixed behaviors				
		N	Engagement%	Time
1	Walking program	10	100	15
2	Fashion Design	11	98	20
3	Wheelchair bike	32	94	31
4	Flower arrangement	14	93	16
5	Air mat	18	89	34
6	Group Singing	29	89	29
7	Crafts	12	87	25
8	AAT	18	87	22
9	Cooking	42	85	35
10	Discussion	43	85	24

CONCLUSION

This research clearly demonstrated the significant impact of RTIs on both types of behavioral symptoms most commonly found in dementia. It also indicates the majority of participants had mixed behaviors, showing symptoms of both apathy and agitation, making interventions difficult to prescribe. Recreational activity that promotes mental and physical engagement is a basic human need and not often utilized therapeutically with individuals with dementia. Unfortunately, long term care residents with dementia have a very low rate of meaningful activity participation because they often experience high levels of apathy and lack the ability to initiate engagement. In previous research we found only six percent of nursing home participants received three appropriate activities per week (Buettner and Fitzsimmons, 2006). Few studies have been devoted to testing the effectiveness of individualized recreational therapy activities in comparison to control conditions for reducing specific neuropsychiatric symptoms and no studies were found that reported on apathy mixed with agitation. Nevertheless, the results from a previous small body of work are promising and lay the foundation for the findings in this study. There is good evidence from the past to support individualized music interventions, animal assisted therapy, and exercise to engage nursing home residents with dementia and passive behaviors (Ancoli-Israel, Martin, and Kripke,2002; Beck, Modlin, and Heithof,1992;Churchill, Safaoui., and McCabe,1999). Additional studies have examined recreational interventions to reduce agitation. Buettner, Lundegren, Farrell, Lago, and Smith (1996) evaluated a program of individualized recreation therapy interventions vs. traditional activities on agitated behaviors of nursing home residents with dementia in a quasi-experimental cross-over design. The results showed that there was a significant improvement in strength, flexibility, and a reduction in agitation during the recreation therapy and no change in any variables during the traditional large group activity sessions. This was the first indication that individualized recreation therapy had promise for reducing behavior problems. In another more interdisciplinary intervention the researchers (Buettner and Ferrario, 1998) evaluated a randomized trial of a highly structured program of sensorimotor activities developed by a recreation therapist, which was integrated into the daily plan of care for the randomly selected experimental group. The intervention program applied and integrated nursing and recreation therapy principles on a special care unit. While significant positive outcomes were reported using standardized measures of cognition, function, mood, and agitated behavior only a narrative description of engagement levels was reported and no measure of apathy took place. For many years the most common approach for treating neuropsychiatric behaviors in dementia has been prescribing medications. Sink and colleagues (2005) found in a review of clinical trials that the evidence does not support this off label use of antipsychotics. They recommend that many other causes for behaviors should be investigated and that medical and care staff should try nonpharmacological treatment first. More recently Ballard (2009) and colleagues suggest antipsychotic medications double the risk of stroke and do not improve quality of life for people with dementia. These studies show the importance of finding nonpharmacological approaches. Finding trained personnel and efficacious interventions as an alternative to has been seen as a problem in the past. This study of recreation therapy interventions for apathy, agitation, and mixed behaviors provides support for the use of individualized recreational interventions and has demonstrated significant improvements in agitation and apathy after a 2-week trial. We were surprised that apathy and mixed behaviors were more prevalent than agitation in our sample. Moreover, the practice of providing "as needed" medications for behaviors may also need further study. We found that the majority of participants in this study had a combination of apathy and agitation and that by targeting periods of apathy the agitation also improved. This is a very different way of approaching the problem of disturbing behaviors in dementia. We recommend training all staff to offer individualized recreation as an outlet, an opportunity to move and express oneself, and as a way to improve quality of life for people with dementia and behaviors. Whether targeting apathy, agitation, or the combination of both the ultimate goal is the same. The outcome should be an engaged and meaningful life. Recreational activities are inherently rewarding, provide social contacts for isolated individuals, and an opportunity to exercise. By using a method that targets the time of day of treating neuropsychiatric behaviors with a recreational therapist prescribing and establishing the intervention other staff theoretically could provide the follow up services.

A high percentage of individuals with Alzheimer's disease and related dementias have both apathy and agitation, making pharmacological treatment difficult. There is a significant relationship between apathy and an inactive lifestyle. Both agitation and apathy respond predictably and consistently to individualized recreation therapy interventions. By targeting periods of apathy for interventions there was also a significant improvement in agitation in participants with mixed behaviors. The types of effective recreational activities varied depending on cognitive level and the recreational interventions offered were highly engaging for participants for between 15-38 minutes.

REFERENCES

Alzheimer's Association (2006). Early stage task force. Retrieved February 20, 009 from: http://www.alz.org/about_us_milestones.asp.

Ballard, C. Hanney, ML, Theodoulou ,M, Douglas, S., McShane, R, Kossakowski, K, Gill, R, Juszczak E, Yu, L, Jacoby, R.(2009). The dementia antipsychotic withdrawal trial (DART-AD): long-term follow-up of a randomized placebo-controlled trial. The *Lancet Neurology*, (8), 151 – 157.

Boyle, P.A., and Malloy, P.F. (2004). Treating apathy in Alzheimer's disease. *Dementia and Other Geriatric Cognitive Disorders,*17, 91-99.

Buettner L.(2006). Peace of mind: A pilot community based program for people with memory loss. *American Journal of Recreation Therapy*. (3), 33-41.

Buettner, L. and Martin, S.(1995). *Therapeutic Recreation in the Nursing Home.* State College, Pa: Venture Publishing, Inc.

Buettner, L., and Fitzsimmons, S.(2003). *Dementia Practice Guidelines for Recreational Therapy: Treatment of Disturbing Behaviors.* Alexandria, VA: American Therapeutic Recreation Association.

Buettner, L., and Fitzsimmons, S.(2006). Mixed behaviors in dementia: A need for a paradigm shift. *Journal of Gerontological Nursing,* 32(7), 15-22.

Clark, RF.(1996). *Home and Community-Based Care in the USA*. U.S. Department of Health and Human Services. Retrieved from: http://aspe.hhs.gov/daltcp/reports/usexampl.htm

Cohen-Mansfield, J. (1986). Agitated behaviors in the elderly II: Preliminary results in the cognitively deteriorated. *Journal of the American Geriatrics Society, 34*(10), 722-727.

Derouesné, C., Piquard, A., Thibault, S., Baudouin-Madec, V., and Lacomblez, L.(2001). Noncognitive symptoms in Alzheimer's disease: A study of 150 community-dwelling patients using a questionnaire completed by the caregiver. *Rev Neurol (Paris),* 157, 162-77.

Feder, J., Komiar, H., and Niefeld, M.(2000). Long-term care in the United States: An overview. *Health Affairs,* 19, 40-56.

Folstein, M., Folstein, S., and McHugh, P.(1975). 'Mini-Mental State': A practical method for grading the cognitive status of patients for the clinician. *Journal of Psychiatric Research,* 12, 189–198.

Hebert, L.E., Scherr, P.A., Bienjas, J.L., Bennett, D.A., and Evans. D.A. (2003). Alzheimer disease in the US population: Prevalence estimates using the 2000 census. *Archives of Neurology,*60(8), 1119-1122.

Kaufer, D.I., Cummings, J.L., Christine, D., Bray, T., Castellon, S., Masterman, D., and et al. (1998). Assessing the impact of neuropsychiatric symptoms in Alzheimer's disease: The neuropsychiatric inventory caregiver distress scale. *Journal of American Geriatric Society*, 46,210–215.

Landes, A.M., Sperry, S.D., Strauss, M.E., and Geldmacher, D.S. (2008). Apathy in Alzheimer's disease. *Journal of the American Geriatric Society*, 49, 1700-1707.

Lerner, A.J., Strauss, M., and Sami, S.A.(2007). Recognizing apathy in Alzheimer's disease. *Geriatric*, 62(11), 14-17.

Levy, R.,and Dubois, B.(2006). Apathy and the functional anatomy of the prefrontal cortex–basal ganglia circuits. *Cerebral Cortex,*16, 916-928.

Marin, R.S. (1991). Apathy: A neuropsychiatric syndrome. *Journal of Neuropsychiatry and Clinical Neuroscience*, 3, 243-254.

Marin, R.S., Biedrzycki, R.C., and Firinciogullari, S.(1991). Reliability and validity of the apathy evaluation scale. Psychiatry Research, 38(2), 143-162.

Mega, M., Lee, L., Dinov, I., Mishkin, F., Toga, A., and Cummings, J.(2000). Cerebral correlates of psychotic symptoms in Alzheimer's disease. *Journal of Neurology and Neurosurgical Psychiatry*, 69(2), 167–171.

Mega, M., Masterman, D., O'Connor, S., Barclay, T., Cummings, J.(1999). The spectrum of behavioral responses to cholinesterase inhibitor therapy in Alzheimer disease. Achieves of Neurology, 56,1388–1393.

Mizrahi, R., and Starkstein, S.E.(007). Epidemiology and management of apathy in patients with Alzheimer's disease. *Drugs and Aging*, 24(7), 547-54.

National Institutes on Aging (2005). Progress report on Alzheimer's disease 2004-2005, new discoveries, new insights. Retrieved from: http://www.nia.nih.gov/Alzheimers/ Publications/ADProgress2004_2005/

Reisberg, B., Ferris, S.H., de Leon, M.J., and Crook., T. (1982). The global deterioration scale for assessment of primary degenerative dementia. American Journal of Psychiatry, 139, 1136-1139.

Schuyler, D.(2007). Recognition of Apathy as Marker for Dementia Growing. *Applied Neurology*, 3(10), 8-13.

Sink, K., Holden, K., and Yaffe, K. (005). Pharmacological Treatment of Neuropsychiatric Symptoms of Dementia, *JAMA*, 293,596-608.

Starkstein, S.E., Ingram, L., Garau, M.L., and Mizrahi, R. (2005). On the overlap between apathy and depression in dementia. *Journal of Neurology, Neurosurgery, and Psychiatry*, 76, 1070-1074.

Starkstein, S.E., Jorge, R., Mizrahi, R., and Robinson, R.G. (006). A prospective longitudinal study of apathy in Alzheimer's disease. *Journal of Neurology, Neurosurgery, and Psychiatry,*77, 8-11.

Thomas, P., Clement, J.P., Hazif-Thomas, C., and Leger, J.M. (2001). Family, Alzheimer's disease and negative symptoms. *International Journal of Geriatric Psychiatry,*16, 192-202.

Verkaik, R., van Weert, J.C., Francke, A.L.(2005) The effects of psychosocial methods on depressed, aggressive and apathetic behaviors of people with dementia: A systematic review. *International Journal of Geriatric Psychiatry*, 20, 301-314.

Yesavage, J.A., Brink, T.L., Rose, T.L., Lum, O., Huang, V., Adey, M.B., and Leirer, V.O., (1983). Development and validation of a geriatric depression screening scale: A preliminary report. *Journal of Psychiatric Research,* 17, 37-49, 1983.

Zawacki, T.M., Grace, J., Paul, R., Moser, D.J., Ott, B.R., Gordon, N., and Cohen, R.A.(2002). Behavioral problems as predictors of functional abilities of vascular. *Journal of Neuropsychiatry Clinical Neuroscience,* 14, 296-302.

In: Dementia: Non-Pharmacological Therapies
Editor: Elisabetta Farina, pp. 43-59

ISBN: 978-1-61470-736-3
© 2012 Nova Science Publishers, Inc.

LIFE REVIEW WITH PEOPLE WITH DEMENTIA IN CARE HOMES: A PRELIMINARY RANDOMIZED CONTROLLED TRIAL

Sarah Morgan[1] and Robert T. Woods[*2]
[1] Bro Morgannwg NHS Trust, Wales, UK.
[2] Clinical Psychology of Older People, Bangor University, Wales, UK.

ABSTRACT

There is little empirical evidence on the impact of reminiscence work in general, and life review therapy in particular, with people with dementia. People with mild to moderate cognitive impairment living in care homes were randomly allocated to a life review intervention (n=8) or a treatment as usual comparison condition (n=9). The intervention was carried out with people individually and culminated in the creation of a life story book detailing information from the reviewer's life. Measures of depression and autobiographical memory were taken for all participants at the pre, post and 6 week follow up assessment stages. The life review participants improved significantly more on the Geriatric Depression Scale short-form (group x time interaction F $(2,15)$=13.97; p=0.009), with a mean 3.25 point reduction in depression scores at the 6 week follow-up assessment; in contrast, depression scores of control participants showed no change. In comparison to the control group, the life review participants were also significantly more able to recall personal facts from their lives at follow up (group x time interaction F $(2, 15) = 5.92$; p=0.007). Case vignettes of the life review process and its impact are presented, and clinical issues discussed. Life review was often not an easy process for the participant, and is demanding of therapeutic skills in relation to the powerful emotions and feelings of loss it may elicit. The life story book was typically viewed positively, with the life review process and the therapeutic relationship valued at its completion. This study is the first to associate an improvement in autobiographical memory in dementia with a reminiscence intervention, and is indicative of a possible psychological therapy for depressed mood in dementia, which is believed to be highly prevalent in care homes.

Keywords: Reminiscence; dementia; autobiographical memory; depression; life review; care homes.

---

[*] Correspondence to: Professor Bob Woods, DSDC Wales, Bangor University, Ardudwy, Holyhead Road, Bangor LL57 2 PX, Wales, UK. b.woods@bangor.ac.uk

INTRODUCTION

In recent years there has been a growing interest in reminiscence work with older adults. There appears to be a general assumption that reminiscence work has a positive impact on those who participate, including people with dementia (e.g. Woods and McKiernan, 1995; Gibson, 2004). However, the evidence to date with older adults with dementia has been very limited and offers little insight into these approaches. Only five studies could be included in the revised Cochrane review of reminiscence work in dementia (Woods et al., 2005), each evaluating a different modality of reminiscence work, and the results from these did not allow firm conclusions to be drawn. In light of the widespread application of these techniques, the effects of clearly specified reminiscence approaches need to be carefully evaluated.

The current study evaluates a specific type of reminiscence work, namely life review. This therapeutic approach involves an in-depth, structured, evaluation of the life span, and is usually conducted on a one to one basis. Butler (1963) argued that life-review forms the final developmental task in life, with its focus on 'integrity versus despair', in Erikson's (1950) model of life-span development. Haight (1992a) developed a life review protocol or Life Review Experiencing Form (LREF) to facilitate life review by assisting the person in progressing through and resolving issues at each life stage. She evaluated this approach empirically with people without cognitive impairment in a series of studies (Haight, 1988; 1992b; Haight and Dias, 1992). Improvements in life satisfaction and well being and decreases in depression were found. Life review should be distinguished from more general reminiscence work, which may have as its aim enhanced communication, enjoyment and social interaction (Burnside and Haight, 1992). Life review is seen as a psychological therapy that is highly personal, evaluative and concerns the person's identity, as manifested in autobiographical memory. Woods (1996) describes life review as 'a more appropriate approach for older people without cognitive impairment', in view of the potential cognitive and emotional demands of this form of psychological therapy. However, the use of life review has been reported in a few case-studies of people with dementia (e.g. Jarvis, 1998; Pietrukowicz and Johnson, 1991; Bailey, Kavanagh, and Sumby, 1998) and Hirsch and Mouratoglou (1999) reported positive effects on the person's mood. Lai, Chi and Kayser-Jones (2004) report a large randomized controlled trial of individualized reminiscence work with people with dementia who were residents of a nursing home. Residents in a comparison group took part in 'friendly discussions' with staff for the same amount of time as those in the reminiscence condition, whilst a further control group received no intervention. The authors conclude that residents participating in the reminiscence condition, described as a life-story book approach, showed improved well-being following the intervention. Although having some overlap with life review work, the absence of an emphasis on *evaluation* of past memories may be an important difference.

Haight, Gibson and Michel (2006) evaluated an intervention also involving the production of a life storybook, but clearly based on an individual structured life review. The intervention was delivered by care staff, who received training and weekly supervision. Randomisation and evaluations were undertaken by researchers – it is not clear that those carrying out assessments were blind to group allocation. Thirty one people with dementia participated, 16 of these being randomised to receive treatment as usual. Improvements favoured the reminiscence group in terms of depression, communication, positive mood and cognition, as measured by the Mini-Mental State Exam (MMSE).

It has been claimed that life story work can ease a move into a new environment; for example, it has been used with people with learning disabilities to facilitate moves from long-stay hospitals to the community (Hussein, 1997). Haight (1999) argues that life review offers the person with dementia in such a position an opportunity to resolve 'unfinished business' whilst they still have the opportunity to do so. The approach could enable the person with dementia to maintain internal and external continuity following a move into a care home, despite the progressive effects of the dementia on the person's sense of self (Parker, 1995). A life-story book may act as an aide memoir of their life review.

Depression is very common in residents of care homes (Ames, 1991) and depression is, in any case, found frequently among people living with Alzheimer's disease and other dementias (Ballard, Bannister and Oyebode, 1996). The individual with cognitive impairment who has moved into a care home may thus be particularly likely also to show depressive signs and symptoms, inevitably leaving behind many of the possessions and cues that have contributed to their sense of identity previously. Their autobiographical memory becomes the main route by which identity might be maintained (Woods, 1998).

There is relatively little research on autobiographical memory in dementia (Fromholt and Larsen, 1991). Morris and Kopelman (1986) noted that people with dementia have difficulty with almost every aspect of memory but that remote memory appears to be more intact than recent memory. However, Fromholt and Larsen (1991) cast doubt on the idea that remote memories are relatively preserved, even in the earliest of dementia stages. The implications for this in terms of ability to retrieve memories for life review warrants further investigation. Autobiographical memories are a particular form of remote memory, regarding the person's own life. Morris (1994) suggests that the usual pattern of autobiographical memories across the life-span, with elevated recall early and late and a relative 'dip' regarding the middle-years may result in many people with dementia having virtually no recall from the middle phase of life. This might result in a virtual disconnection of early memories from more recent experiences, posing particular strain on maintaining a sense of identity. There are no investigations into the effect of life review or other reminiscence work specifically on autobiographical memory, despite this being the primary cognitive process involved.

This study therefore aimed to evaluate the effects of a life-review therapy intervention on mood and autobiographical memory in a group of people with dementia at high risk of depressed mood, having been recently admitted to a residential care home. It was predicted that the intervention would be associated with improved mood and autobiographical memory.

METHODS

Design

The study was a small-scale preliminary randomized control trial that included individuals with mild-moderate dementia living in care homes. Ethical approval was given by the North West Wales NHS Ethics Committee. Assessments were carried out pre- and post-therapy and at six week follow-up. 17 clients were randomly allocated to the intervention group or to a 'treatment as usual' control group. The intervention group took part in a structured life review as well as the pre and post assessments and the no treatment control group participants only took part in the assessments. Initial participants were randomly assigned alternately to the groups. Subsequent participants were allocated using the randomization by minimization method (Altman and Bland, 2005), which allocates the next participant in the trial according to the characteristics of those already participating, so that each allocation reduces any imbalance in the stratifying variables – in this case age and relationship to family care-giver. This method ensures balanced groups even when, as here, sample size is small.

Participants

Participants who had received a diagnosis of dementia were selected according to the following eligibility criteria, having been approached via care homes and a community dementia service:

- They consented to participate.
- They had a carer or relative who agreed to support the intervention.
- They showed a mild to moderate degree of dementia according to the Clinical Dementia Rating Scale (CDR, Hughes et al 1982), scoring 1 or 2 on this scale.
- Participants had to have sufficient verbal abilities to be able to participate and not be demonstrating signs of florid psychosis.
- The care home manager agreed to their participation.

Depressed mood was *not* an inclusion or exclusion criterion. Of 40 potential participants approached, 17 were eligible and agreed to take part, 11 were eligible, but either refused themselves or their relative refused, and 12 people did not meet the eligibility criteria or were too physically unwell to participate.

Assessment Procedure

At the pre and post assessment stages, participants completed measures described below. The researcher also met with the individual's carer beforehand to gain some information about the person's life, and to corroborate information obtained from the AMI. All the pre-intervention assessments were carried out, prior to randomization, by the researcher, who also guided participants through the life review. Almost half of the post-test and follow-up assessments were carried out by an assistant psychologist blind to the allocation of participants to the groups. Half of the individuals assessed by the blind assessor were from the life review group and half from the control group. The remaining assessments were carried out by the primary researcher. There were no significant differences in scores of those assessed by the researcher and the blind assessor.

The Life Review Intervention

The therapist (SM) was a clinical psychologist in her final year of a doctoral training programme, under the supervision of an experienced clinical psychologist (RTW). The life review was closely based on Haight's Life Review model and in particular the Life Review Experiencing Form (LREF, Haight, 1992a). The form was utilized to try to ensure consistency of approach between participants (Haight, 1988). The LREF allows the therapist to guide the reviewer chronologically through their life stages and allows time to focus on different life stages, including early childhood, teenage years, adulthood, and a summary section which aims to pull together the person's overall evaluation of their life. This summary section is deemed to be the most important aspect of the whole process. Haight's life review model consists of six one-hour sessions. In this study approximately 12 or more weekly sessions per individual reviewer were necessary. Sessions were shorter (30 – 60 minutes) and progress through the form was slower than anticipated. The area to be talked about was clearly defined but it was up to the reviewer to lead the focus onto the material to be discussed. Various prompts from the LREF and the person's carers were used to help the person engage in the process. Some individuals found photographs and other materials helpful in retrieving information. Follow-up sessions were framed according to the previous session's content and a life story-book was developed by the therapist between sessions and used as the intervention proceeded. This information was taken to sessions for the reviewer to edit – the reviewer retaining editorial control over the content of the book.

Measures

Two primary outcome measures were utilized:

Geriatric Depression Scale- Short Form (GDS-SF; Sheikh and Yesavage, 1986). The fifteen item Geriatric Depression Scale has been widely used with people with dementia, and is recommended by Moniz-Cook et al. (2008) as a self-report scale to assess changes in mood in early dementia. A cut-off score of 5 and above is usually taken to indicate depressed mood. This was the only indicator of depressed mood used in the study.

Autobiographical Memory Interview (AMI; Kopelman, Wilson and Baddeley, 1990). The AMI was developed by Kopelman et al. (1990) to provide an assessment of recent and remote memory of personal events and facts. The AMI consists of two subscales, the Personal Semantic Schedule, (PSS) and the Autobiographical Incident Schedule (AIS). The PSS requires participants to recall facts from their life span, relating to childhood, early and later adult life. The AIS assesses the same three time periods, but participants are required to recall three specific incidents from each life stage. Kopelman et al. (1990) reported inter-rater reliability correlations of 0.83-0.86. Unfortunately there appears to be no data available yet regarding test-retest reliability or other psychometric factors.

In order to ascertain that the groups were matched in relation to dementia severity, the following scale was used:

Clinical Dementia Rating Scale (CDR - Hughes, Berg, Danziger, Coben, and Martin, 1982). The CDR is a global rating tool developed to distinguish between older adults with a wide range of cognitive functioning, from healthy to severely impaired. Hughes et al (1982) reported good inter-rater reliability (r = 0.89), and also demonstrated high concurrent validity with other tests, and good test-retest reliability. It was completed following interviews with the resident, staff and family and consulting clinical records.

RESULTS

Quantitative Measures

Table 1 summarises the demographic features of the sample. The average participant was female, aged 82, a widow, who had been resident in a care home for 8 months. There were no demographic differences between the intervention and control groups (tested using independent samples t-tests for continuous variables and Fisher's exact test for categorical variables). There were no pre-test differences between groups on severity of dementia, depression or on the PSS component of the AMI. However, on the AIS subscale of the AMI. the control group were able to recall significantly fewer incidents than the intervention group (t= 2.27, p=0.038). There were no between group differences on the CDR throughout the study duration, with the groups remaining well matched on severity of dementia.

Inspection of the data did not indicate any major deviations from normality, and so a two-way analysis of variance with repeated measures on one factor (time) was carried out with each of the outcome measures to evaluate the effects of the intervention, with the group x time interaction being the critical statistic. Where main effects or interactions were significant (p<0.01), post-hoc analyses were conducted using independent and paired t-tests.

Table 1. Summary of demographic details of the sample

Variables.		Life review Group (n = 8)	Control Group (n = 9)
Mean Age		80.5 years (s.d.= 5.75)	84.44 years (s.d.=7.81)
Gender (% in	Male	25.0 (n=2)	22.2 (n=2)
Group)	Female	75.0 (n=6)	77.8 (n=7)
Marital Status	Single	25 (n=2)	22.2 (n=2)
(% in group)	Widowed	75 (n=6)	77.8 (n=7)
Mean Time Resident at Care Home		7 months (s.d.=6.48)	8.66 months (s.d.=5.22)
Severity of dementia (pre-test CDR)		Mild (CDR 1) 62.5% Moderate (CDR 2) 37.5%	Mild (CDR 1) 55.6% Moderate (CDR 2) 44.4%

Table 2 indicates the means, standard deviations, and gains in scores made over the study period at the three assessment points for the GDS-SF. Higher scores indicate increased levels of depression, with a score of five and above said to indicate depression of clinical significance. The life review group showed an overall improvement in GDS-SF scores from 7.75 to 4.5. In comparison, the control group mean increased from 6.22 to 6.55, during the course of the study.

**Table 2. Means, standard deviations and change scores
on the GDS-SF at the three assessment points**

	Life Review (n=8)				Control (n=9)			
	M	SD	Mean Change from Pre-test	SD of Change from Pre-test	M	SD	Mean Change from Pre-test	SD of Change from Pre-test
Pre-Test	7.75	3.06			6.22	2.48		
Post Test	6.25	3.20	-1.5	3.02	6.00	2.74	-0.22	1.30
Follow up	4.50	2.33	-3.25	2.05	6.67	3.77	+0.44	2.24

Figure 1 indicates that the intervention group continue to improve during the follow-up period, where the mean score moves outside the range associated with depression. There were no significant main effects of group or time, but the group x time interaction was significant ($F_{(2,15)}=13.97$; $p=0.009$). Post-hoc analyses indicated that there was a significant change in the life review group scores during the follow-up period ($t = 2.35$, $p = 0.05$) with a highly significant improvement in this group's GDS-SF scores overall, ($t = 4.48$, $p < 0.001$). At pre-test, 87.5% of the life review group scored 5 or above on the GDS (i.e. were in the range for depression), compared with 78% of the control group. At follow-up, there had been no change in depression status in the control group, but the proportion of the life review group scoring as depressed had fallen to 50%.

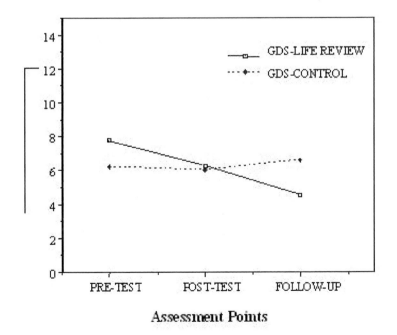

Figure 1. Mean scores on GDS-SF by group over time.

Table 3 indicates the means and standard deviations at the three assessment points for the two AMI sub-scales. Higher scores indicate the positive recall of facts or incidents. On the PSS, as Figure 2 indicates, the life review group improve markedly during the treatment phase, levelling off during the follow-up period, whilst the control group tend to show gradual decline. Again, main effects of group and time are not significant, whilst the group x time interaction effect is significant (F (2, 15) = 5.92; p=0.007). At follow-up, there was a significant difference between groups (t=2.72, p=0.016), with the life review group able to recall more personal facts. There was a trend suggesting an increase in positive recall of facts from pre- to post- testing for the life review group (t = -2.23, p=0.06) and a significant decrease overall in the amount of factual information recalled by the control group over the course of the study, (t = 7.19, p<0.001). On the AIS sub-scale, neither the main effects of group or time, nor the group x time interaction approached significance (F (2,15) = 1.27; p=0.297).

**Table 3. Means (and standard deviations) of PSS and AIS sub-scales of
AMI for life review and control groups at each assessment point**

	PSS Life REVIEW	PSS CONTROL	AIS LIFE REVIEW	AIS Control
Pre-test	25.00 (12.44)	24.83 (11.40)	11.38 (5.04)	6.22 (4.32)
Post-test	36.69 (13.10)	23.44 (15.24)	8.75 (5.99)	8.77 (5.43)
Follow-up	34.50 (12.75)	18.88 (10.88)	9.69 (7.96)	6.33 (5.10)

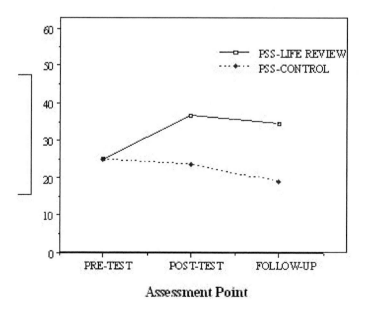

Figure 2. Mean scores on PSS subscale by group over time.

Case Vignettes

In order to provide a flavour of the process of the life review work undertaken, and its relationship to outcomes, descriptions of two cases from the life review group are presented. All names used are pseudonyms.

Case No. 1: Sian

Sian was a 79 year old woman referred to the project by the dementia team social worker. Her son was also contacted and he agreed to facilitate the process by supplying life history information. Sian had significant cognitive impairment according to a previous psychological assessment. She had recently moved to live in a residential home, prior to this she had been living alone after having lost her husband several years before. She had been admitted to the home as her son was concerned about her confused behaviour and difficulties with everyday living tasks.

At the first assessment meeting Sian was a little reluctant to take part but agreed to "have a go" at the life review. She was concerned about "telling lies" as she explained that she could not remember things as well as she used to. The doctor had, apparently, told her that this was because she had "something that begins with a 'D', and that is why I am here now because I can't manage on my own anymore". She also said that "I have nothing really special to talk about, my life has been quite ordinary, I don't know what I can tell you". Nevertheless, Sian agreed to continue with the process. Sian obtained pre-test scores of 9 on the GDS-SF and 1 on the CDR, indicative of moderate depression and mild dementia. On the AMI she had scores of 9 on the PSS and 16 on the AIS.

During the life review sessions Sian talked a great deal about the losses she had experienced including her regrets regarding the loss of her father, who had died at sea when she was a teenager. She explained that she missed her parents a great deal as well as her husband. At the sessions subsequent to those where the bereavements were discussed she said that she had been feeling particularly low in mood. During later sessions she was able to talk more of the fun and enjoyment she had experienced in her life, including memories of her husband, son and grandchildren, and how good they had been to her. She was very proud of her son and his values and was subsequently able to reflect on the good values that she and her husband had instilled in him. She was also more able to recount positive childhood experiences that she had experienced.

At the post-test assessment she explained that she hadn't particularly enjoyed the life review and had found it difficult to remember the loved ones she had lost. However, she was more able to be positive about the present and joked that she might live for another 20 years as she had friends in their 100's. At this point, Sian's GDS-SF score had fallen from 9 to 7, which was still in the range associated with depression. Her CDR had now increased to 2. Her PSS scores had increased dramatically from 16 initially to 36 at follow up, whereas her AIS scores decreased by 2.

At follow up Sian explained that everyone who had seen her life-story book had loved it. People had been coming in to her room to see it and her son had been so pleased that he wanted to keep it after she had died. He also said that he was very proud of her and of the things that she had done with her life. She said that she had to keep a careful eye on the book in case somebody took it. Her depression score had continued to decrease to be within "normal" limits at 3 points. Her PSS score dropped 5 points from the immediate follow up, but this score was still an improvement of 15 points from pre-test. Interestingly, her AIS score increased again from 7, the score obtained at immediate follow up, to 13 points.

Case No. 2: John

John was an 83 year old man who was also referred to the project by the dementia team social worker. He had recently moved to live in a residential home, prior to which he had been living alone after losing his wife. He had two sons, one of whom lived locally. He had previously lived very independently and did not have regular visits from family. He had worked for 25 years in the forces. He agreed to participate and the researcher was able to speak with his son for assistance and background information. John had been assessed as an in-patient on the dementia assessment unit and obtained a score of 16 on the MMSE (Folstein et al., 1975) having presented as uncooperative, sometimes aggressive and very disoriented and confused.

John agreed to participate but found the AMI questions difficult and became irritated. It appeared to confront him with the realisation that he could not remember some personal information and this was particularly difficult for him to accept. He rationalised this, saying that the questions related to events a long time ago: "When I was there I never took much notice of these things, I just got on with it". He also reasoned, following the recent admission to hospital and the move to the home, that "They keep on moving me around so I don't know where I am, they rush me from one place to the next; I was fine where I was". Despite his defences and his attempts to protect his self-concept, his score of 11 on the GDS-SF was clearly in the depressed range; he obtained a rating of 2 (moderate dementia) on the CDR. On the autobiographical memory interview he had scores of 11 on the PSS and 4 on the AIS.

At the start of every session, John would begin by saying that he was not happy "being in a place like this, this isn't my home, I don't know who's it is". He explained, "I know I have a home somewhere that belongs to me but I don't know where it is, I know that this isn't my home, this isn't my bed". The initial few sessions were difficult as John could remember very little from his past and his son seemed to withdraw from the process. This came to a head at the fifth session when John shouted "You come here and ask me these stupid questions and stare at me with your stupid blank face, leave me alone, don't come back, leave me in peace". Prior to this confrontation, the process had felt very uncomfortable and it did seem inappropriate to continue with the LREF questions. Following this session, in respect of his wishes, the researcher did not return to visit for several weeks. However, this presented a difficult ethical situation in terms of leaving him in a state of anger and partial insight into his memory difficulties and not offering the opportunity and support to work though these issues. It is possible that John was projecting his sense of anger with himself onto the researcher. Accordingly it was decided to re-visit him, and in fact he was happy to see the researcher again. On reflection, it seemed that the researcher had previously failed to "hold" John's anger at his predicament and it is possible that a failure to go back to reappraise the situation would have been a further threat to his sense of personhood (Kitwood, 1996).

Subsequent sessions were more comfortable for both parties, with a focus on the generation of the life story book. John was well travelled and sessions were geared towards discussing places where he had travelled and the issues that were relevant for him then, including marriage and the Second World War. Consequently, rather than being a neat progression through the LREF, the sessions focused on specific aspects of John's life that were most easily accessed and on which he wanted to focus.

When the final life story book had been completed, John was very pleased with the end product. He said that he was very much looking forward to reading through the book in his own time. His depression score improved by three points but was still in the depressed range at 8 points, with the AIS having improved by 2 points and his PSS by just 1 point.

At the follow up assessment John remembered a great deal more information not previously elicited on the AMI. On remarking on this, he said "Yes, I have remembered a lot more today, but that's because the book sets things off in my head, it helps me remember all sorts of things and reminds me of things I had forgotten". His depression score had continued to improve and had dropped a further 2 points to 6. John's AIS improved by another 1.5 points and his PSS score by 3.5 points. John was also able to gain some enjoyment from the book and related it to the 'This is your life' programme on TV, saying "That says it all, I couldn't have put it better myself. That's what my parents were like". The book provided him with an important connection with his past and identity, and seemed to help him to carve out a new identity for himself in the care home, with aspects of his life-story that he might not have been able to otherwise communicate to the staff. It provided him with a talking point from which to share and develop relationships which may have enabled him to counter the negative experiences of his current situation and instead to capitalize on his achievements:

> "Now I am divorced. I feel divorced from my past, from my belongings, which I have collected over the years and from my family and friends. I am isolated. I have been thrown into a place, which isn't my home…I live with people I know nothing about. People I don't know come to me and do things to me. I am confined, I would love to go out and enjoy this weather, I don't get to see it anymore...going out in a bus with strangers and driving around isn't my idea of going out. I would love to go out just for a little stroll but I would want company, I wouldn't want to go on my own. I have travelled well in my time, I have been to 21 different countries with the forces".

CONCLUSION

Summary of Quantitative Results

The life review group demonstrated an initial trend to recall more personal facts, although this trend did not continue during the follow up period. In contrast, the control group PSS scores decreased significantly over the course of the study and there were significant differences between the two groups' PSS scores at follow up. This study is believed to be the first to indicate that an improvement in autobiographical memory in dementia may be associated with any form of reminiscence work. The life story book may have acted as a tangible reminder of the person's life story, which in combination with the sessions and discussion with visitors or staff who happened to see the book, may have contributed to the relatively better performance of the life review group. This is illustrated by John's comments about the book being a good reminder of things he had forgotten. However, a similar pattern was not observed with AIS scores. This may relate to most of the information recorded in the life story-books being factual as opposed to being records of specific incidents. It is also conceivable that a greater degree of cognitive effort is required to recall or re-learn AIS as opposed to PSS information. The finding that reviewers were not enabled to retrieve specific autobiographical incidents from their past, is not consistent with the assumption often made in the literature that life review enables the individual to draw on specific memories and instances to enable them to cope more effectively with current difficulties (Pincus, 1970).

The life review group depression scores improved significantly overall, as in the study reported by Haight et al. (2006). The intervention may have offered the opportunity for some individuals to discuss and resolve old issues which may have been re-awakened as a result of the disease process and their weakened ability to defend themselves. Furthermore, the review may have allowed the person to focus on their strengths and achievements with the life story book itself ultimately serving to attract more positive social interaction, leading other people to express praise and respect for the person's achievements and life (e.g. Sian). There may, of course, have been different reasons for different participants and it might be argued that the scores decreased simply as a result of therapist contact and the impact of this social interaction as opposed to the intervention per se. However, this would not explain the continued reduction in depression scores in the life review group during the follow-up period, when there was no additional contact. It is important to note that the intervention did not lead to an *increase* in depression scores, which has been suggested in the literature (Lewis and Butler, 1974), although the process was difficult for several participants.

Clinical Observations

A number of issues emerged during the study which may be helpful to consider prior to engaging in life review with people with dementia.

Engaging Participants in the Life Review Process
It proved difficult to recruit participants, despite Butler's (1974) assertion that life review is universal. In light of this, it is important to consider factors which might hinder or facilitate engagement. Weiss (1994) suggested that for some individuals the residential home move involves the loss of physical boundaries, which may in turn encourage rigid psychosocial boundaries. This might lead to a reluctance to share experiences, as there is a danger of becoming too vulnerable, particularly pertinent to those experiencing unresolved loss. Individuals may prefer not to develop relationships as a protective mechanism. There may also be some anxiety associated with the threat of exposure of the individual to their memory problems (e.g. John). Some individuals may be in denial of their memory problems and circumstances. Consequently, it is important to consider whether it is better to be in denial of the past and of a deteriorating memory rather than risk life review, which challenges this defence mechanism. Should the person wish to engage in the process, there is a need to enable them to access alternative defences or coping strategies to ensure their safety and well-being.

Reflection on the Life Review Process as a Therapeutic and Research Exercise
The LREF initially seemed to represent a useful framework on which to base the intervention, however, there was also a need to develop an individualized approach according to the person's cognitive abilities, emotional needs, preferences and coping strategies. This was particularly pertinent with individuals who wished to discuss one life stage for longer

than anticipated. Some individuals were ruminating on and struggling with issues of loss and grief, which were then discussed and processed in the sessions (e.g. Sian). One participant in particular spent several of the sessions talking about the loss of her parents; following extensive discussion, she was able to move beyond this and began to talk about other experiences at other life stages.

Discussing negative life events in session and allowing the client to experience negative affect raised the risk of "losing the participant". There was the possibility that the negative affect could become intolerable and that the individual would be unable to utilise effective coping strategies to process it. For example, one participant talked of her unhappy marriage, but was unable to utilize the therapeutic time to help her with this and subsequently refused any more input. The danger is then that the individual is left with an overwhelming feeling of confusion and sadness and may not have the cognitive capacity to be able to appreciate from where the feeling arose, let alone how to resolve it.

Alternatively, some individuals may find it difficult to cope with the comparison between their previous self and circumstances with the reality of their current situation. Furthermore, it is important to consider that the recall of memories involved in life review may be traumatic for the individual who had a difficult childhood or life experiences. It is important to consider for whom this intervention is appropriate and currently the research provides little guidance on who might benefit. The importance of establishing the social support and coping strategies available to the person prior to engagement is reinforced. The life review process may possibly only be appropriate if the individual requests it or if they are spontaneously reminiscing; the intervention must be client led with individuals adequately prepared and informed of the possible implications. Individual attitudes to reminiscence, as identified by Coleman (1986), must be taken into account.

The Impact of the Life Story Books

The life story-book was useful for gaining a sense of continuity between sessions. Furthermore, some participants explained that they felt "listened to" and seemed to enjoy the opportunity of seeing their life story in print. However, one individual became concerned regarding how much information the researcher knew about him; he could not understand how they had acquired it, as he could not remember talking about it. Another person was confused by the details presented in the book and expressed frustration at herself for not being able to remember how things actually were. Greater involvement of relatives in the process would have been helpful in taking some pressure off the person's own memory.

Ending Life Review

Haight, Coleman, and Lord (1995) indicate the importance of the intervention in providing the person with a confidante for a short period of time. However, this could be considered harmful in the long run, especially if a state of deprivation of social contact had existed prior to the intervention. The therapist enters the individual's life, develops a relationship with them and then withdraws. The individual is left with the loss of the therapeutic relationship to contend with in addition to bereavements they might have experienced, and the implications of their deteriorating cognitive capacity and its associated losses.

Ending sessions may therefore prove difficult, for example one participant explained:

> "The only good thing in my life is you coming to talk to me, I have nothing else. I am incontinent, I live in this room day in and out. People bring me meals which I don't like and nobody takes the time to sit and talk to me. I can't walk like I used to. My family doesn't come to see me because they live away."

Several of the participants attempted to delay the signalled ending of the therapy, saying that the researcher could come back anytime, explaining that there was no hurry, that they would not be going anywhere. For example, another participant explained:

> "I don't go out into the common room anymore. There was this woman there when I used to go to sit there who was really noisy, a trouble-maker and she used to pick on me, so I started to stay in my room from then on, but its difficult because I don't really have anyone to sit down and talk to. I get lonely. You are the only person who comes to talk to me, apart from my son who visits at weekends."

There is also the possibility that the person may blame themselves that the relationship had ended; the natural end point, in terms of chronological order, for the review may not be self-evident. It is essential for the therapist to make clear and explicit cues regarding the length of involvement. The therapist may aim to facilitate the development of new relationships within the home, which can be maintained following the intervention, or engage a family member more actively in the process.

Positive Factors

Of the eight life review participants, most enjoyed the life story books, even if, like both Sian and John they found the process of creating the book and the review itself difficult. People who were formerly modest about their achievements were encouraged to show the book to members of the family and were surprised by the positive responses that they received. Interest in life story books from family members was largely positive. Furthermore, there were positive anecdotal reports from staff who explained that they were surprised at how much the individual could remember and how much the person had done in his or her life.

This study has provided evidence regarding the feasibility of the life review approach with people with mild to moderate dementia. Improvements in mood and in the personal facts element of autobiographical memory were associated with the intervention. The major methodological limitation of the study related to a number of assessments not being conducted 'blind' to treatment allocation, as they were undertaken by the therapist. In a larger-scale trial, it would be important to ensure that all assessments were blinded. Although those in the intervention group received additional therapist contact, the continued improvement in mood following the end of therapy may suggest that the social contact was not the only therapeutic factor. Further research should also aim to control for the impact of receiving a life story book, which was clearly a positive feature of the approach for several participants, and would be expected to have most impact in the post-therapy phase. It is conceivable that a life story book prepared only with input from family members, and not involving a life review process for the individual might also have beneficial effects;

comparing a group receiving such a book made without their active involvement would begin to indicate the specific role of the life review process. However, the trend to improvement in autobiographical memory during the treatment phase suggests that the life story book also is not the sole therapeutic element.

It is possible that the life review process is beneficial in helping to reduce depression in these individuals who are able to complete the whole review and work through unresolved issues and emotions. There is the risk of "losing" the reviewer before the intervention process is complete, with effects that are as yet uncertain. This work should not be entered into lightly, and it may more appropriately be carried out by staff experienced in conducting therapy with this vulnerable group of individuals or by those under close supervision.

ACKNOWLEDGMENTS

This project was undertaken in partial fulfilment of the first author's Doctorate in Clinical Psychology at Bangor University. We are grateful to Katie Harrop for assistance with assessments and Kat Algar for help with referencing. We wish to thank all the participating residents, relatives and care homes for their willingness to be involved.

REFERENCES

Altman, D. G., and Bland, J. M. (2005). Treatment allocation by minimisation. *British Medical Journal,* 330, 843.

Ames, D. (1991) Epidemiological studies of depression among the elderly in residential and nursing homes. *International Journal of Geriatric Psychiatry,* 6, 347 - 354.

Bailey, D., Kavanagh, A. and Sumby, D. (1998) Valuing The Person: Getting To Know Their Life. *Journal of Dementia Care,* Sept./Oct., 26-27.

Ballard, C. G., Bannister, C., and Oyebode, F. (1996) Depression in dementia sufferers. *International Journal of Geriatric Psychiatry,* 11(6), 507-515.

Burnside, I. and Haight, B.K. (1992) Reminiscence and Life Review: Analysing Each Concept. *Journal of Advanced Nursing,* 17, 855-862.

Butler, R.N. (1963) The life review: An interpretation of reminiscence in the aged. *Psychiatry,* 256, 65-76.

Butler, R. N., (1974) Successful aging and the role of the life review. *Journal of the American Geriatrics Society,* 22, 529-535.

Erikson, E. (1950) *Childhood and Society.* New York: W.W. Norton.

Folstein, M.F., Folstein, S.E. And McHugh, P.R. (1975) Mini-Mental State: A Practical Method for Grading The Cognitive State Of The Patient For The Physician. *Journal of Psychiatric Research,* 12,189-198.

Fromholt, P and Larsen, S.F. (1991) Autobiographical Memory in Normal Aging And Primary Degenerative Dementia (Dementia of Alzheimer Type). *Journal of Gerontology,* 46, 85-91.

Gibson, F. (2004) *The past in the present: using reminiscence in health and social care.* Baltimore: Health Professions Press.

Haight, B.K. (1988) The Therapeutic Role Of A Structured Life Review Process In Homebound Elderly Subjects. *Journal of Gerontology,* 43, 40-44.

Haight, B.K. (1992a) The structured life-review process: a community approach to the ageing client. In G. M. M. Jones and B. M. L. Miesen (Eds.), *Care-giving in dementia* (pp. 272 - 292). London: Routledge.

Haight, B.K. (1992b) Long Term Effects of a Structured Life Review Process. *Journal of Gerontology,* 47, 312-315.

Haight, B.K. (1999) An American In Vienna. *Reminiscence,* 18, 12-13.

Haight, B.K., Coleman, P. and Lord, K. (1995) The Linchpins of a Successful Life Review: Structure, Evaluation and Individuality. In B.K. Haight And J.D. Webster, (Eds.) *The Art And Science Of Reminiscing: Theory, Research, Methods, and Applications.* Washington: Taylor and Francis.

Haight, B. K., and Dias, J. K. (1992) Examining key variables in selected reminiscing modalities. *International Psychogeriatrics,* 4 *(Suppl. 2),* 279 - 290.

Haight, B. K., Gibson, F., and Michel, Y. (2006) The Northern Ireland life review/life storybook project for people with dementia. *Alzheimer's and Dementia,* 2(1), 56 - 58.

Hirsch, C.R. and Mouratoglou, V.M. (1999) Life Review of An Older Adult with Memory Difficulties. *International Journal of Geriatric Psychiatry,* 14, 261-265.

Hughes, C.P., Berg, L., Danziger, W.L., Coben, L.A. and Martin, R.L. (1982) A new clinical scale for the staging of dementia. *British Journal of Psychiatry,* 140, 566-572.

Hussein, F. (1997) Life Story Work For People With Learning Disabilities. *British Journal of Learning Disabilities,* 25, 73-77.

Jarvis, K. (1998) Recovering a Lost Sense of Identity. *Journal of Dementia Care,* May/June, 7-8.

Kitwood, T. (1996) A Dialectical Framework for Dementia. In R.T. Woods (Ed.) *Handbook of The Clinical Psychology of Ageing.* Chichester: Wiley.

Kopelman, D., Wilson, B.A. and Baddeley, A.D. (1990) *The Autobiographical Memory Interview.* Bury St. Edmunds: Thames Valley Test Company.

Lai, C. K. Y., Chi, I., and Kayser-Jones, J. (2004) A randomized controlled trial of a specific reminiscence approach to promote the well-being of nursing home residents with dementia. *International Psychogeriatrics,* 16, 33-49.

Lewis, M.I. and Butler, R.N. (1974) Life-review therapy: putting memories to work in individual and group psychotherapy. *Geriatrics,* 29, 165-173.

Moniz-Cook, E., Vernooij-Dassen, M., Woods, R., Verhey, F., Chattat, R., De Vugt, M., Mountain, G., O'Connell, M., Harrison, J., Vasse, E., Dröes, R. M., and Orrell, M. (2008) A European consensus on outcome measures for psychosocial intervention research in dementia care. *Aging and Mental Health,* 12(1), 14 - 29.

Morris, R.G. and Kopelman, M.D. (1986) The Memory Deficits In Alzheimer Type Dementia: A Review. *Quarterly Journal of Experimental Psychology,* 38, 575-602.

Morris, R. G. (1994) Recent developments in the neuropsychology of dementia. *International Review of Psychiatry,* 6, 85 - 107.

Parker, R.G. (1995) Reminiscence: A Continuity Theory Framework. *Gerontologist,* 35, 515-525.

Pietrukowicz, M.E. and Johnson, M.M.S. (1991) Using Life Histories to Individualize Nursing Home Staff Attitudes Toward Residents. *Gerontologist,* 31, 102-107.

Pincus, A. (1970) Reminiscence in aging and its implications for social work practice. *Social Work,* 15, 47-53.

Sheikh, J. I., and Yesavage, J. A. (1986) Geriatric Depression Scale (GDS): recent evidence and development of a shorter version. In T. L. Brink (Ed.), *Clinical gerontology: a guide to assessment and intervention* (pp. 165-173). New York: Haworth Press.

Weiss, J.C. (1994) Group Therapy with Older Adults in Long-Term Care Settings: Research and Clinical Cautions and Recommendations. *The Journal for Specialists in Group Work,* 19, 22-29.

Woods, R. T. (1996) Psychological 'therapies' in dementia. In R. T. Woods (Ed.), *Handbook of the clinical psychology of ageing* (pp. 575 - 600). Chichester: Wiley.

Woods, R. T. (1998) Reminiscence as communication. In P. Schweitzer (Ed.), *Reminiscence in dementia care* (pp. 143 - 148). London: Age Exchange.

Woods, R. T., and McKiernan, F. (1995) Evaluating the impact of reminiscence on older people with dementia. In B. K. Haight and J. Webster (Eds.), *The art and science of reminiscing: theory, research, methods and applications* (pp. 233 - 242). Washington DC: Taylor and Francis.

Woods, B., Spector, A., Jones, C., Orrell, M., and Davies, S. (2005) Reminiscence therapy for people with dementia (review), *The Cochrane Database of Systematic Reviews.* Chichester: Wiley.

In: Dementia: Non-Pharmacological Therapies   ISBN: 978-1-61470-736-3
Editor: Elisabetta Farina, pp. 61-70   © 2012 Nova Science Publishers, Inc.

TRANSLATING RESEARCH INTO PRACTICE: A PILOT STUDY EXAMINING THE USE OF COGNITIVE STIMULATION THERAPY (CST) AFTER A ONE-DAY TRAINING COURSE

Aimee Spector[*1], *Martin Orrell*[2] *and Elisa Aguirre*[2]

[1] Research Department of Clinical, Educational and Health Psychology,
University College London, 1-19 Torrington Place, London WC1E 6BT.
[2] Department of Mental Health Sciences, University College London,
Charles Bell House, Riding House Street, London.

ABSTRACT

Past studies evaluating training in dementia care have shown variable and limited findings, with most showing that staff training does not lead to any lasting change. This pilot study looks at the outcome of a one-day training course in Cognitive Stimulation Therapy (CST), an evidence-based therapy for people with dementia. Following the Medical Research Council's guidelines for complex interventions, this study represents 'phase IV' – the implementation of CST in practice following an earlier clinical trial. 152 people who had attended a one-day CST training course were contacted, of whom 76 responded. Respondents completed a questionnaire which established whether or not they had taken up CST groups and the obstacles that they had faced. It also included measures of attitude towards dementia (ADQ), job satisfaction (JS) and learning transfer (LTSI). The sample of 76 was divided into two groups: those who took up CST (27) and those who did not (49). Independent samples t-tests were used to compare group scores on the measures. The group taking up CST scored significantly better on work environment and ability /enabling. There were no differences between groups on the other measures and no relationship between having started a CST group and job title, place of work, gender, age or ethnicity.

There has been little research on the long-term implementation of complex interventions in practice and almost nothing in dementia care, hence this is a novel study. It showed that individuals with better learning characteristics may be more likely to take up CST following training, and simple factors such as a lack of staff time and resources may prevent people from doing CST. Future research could focus on comparing the effectiveness of different training methods in the form of a randomised controlled trial.

---

[*] All correspondence to Dr Aimee Spector, e-mail a.spector@ucl.ac.uk, tel: 0044-207-679-1844, fax: 0044-207-916-1989.

Keywords: staff, trial, phase-IV, learning theory, training.

INTRODUCTION

Improving the quality of care for people with dementia is a key priority of the National Dementia Strategy (DoH, 2008), and staff training is essential to the development of good standards of care (Innes, 2001). However, a review of training in dementia (McCabe et al, 2007) showed mixed results, with half of the studies finding no effect of staff training on the resident they provided care for, even when increases in the knowledge and skills of staff were demonstrated. The authors suggested that training can bring secondary benefits including increasing job satisfaction; reducing staff stress levels and turnover rates, possibly through an increased sense of competence, morale, and self- worth. Moniz-Cook et al. (1998) found that following a training programme, staff often went back to prior ways of working. As the title of one report suggests, 'Training is not enough to change care practice' (Lintern, Woods, and Phair, 2000).

Cognitive Stimulation Therapy (CST) is a brief, evidence-based group intervention for people with dementia. A recent clinical trial showed that it led to significant benefits in cognition and quality of life, was cost effective and that cognitive benefits are comparable to some of the dementia drugs used (Spector et al, 2003, Knapp et al, 2006). As a consequence, group CST has been recommended in the NICE guidelines (NICE, 2006) for all people with mild / moderate dementia, regardless of medication used. There has been a subsequent surge in the provision of CST, with the National Audit Office (2007) reporting the use of CST in 29% of the community mental health teams in the UK. A CST manual has now been published and (Spector et al, 2006) and a one-day training course has been established.

It is still unclear how to get training consistently into practice. Within the dementia literature, there is an appreciation of organisational factors, for example Lintern et al (2000) argued that the effectiveness of staff training programs within dementia care is dependent upon the commitment of management to the training program and whether it supports the aims and objectives of the service. The 'Transfer System' (Holton et al, 2000) has been defined as "all the factors in the person, training and organisation that influence transfer of learning to job performance". This theory assumes that the effectiveness of training and whether it leads to any subsequent changes in practice will be linked to the design and quality of the training, the personal characteristics (such as motivation) of the recipients of training and organisational factors, for example support for doing new things. However, after extensive searching, the authors could find nothing which described how the training itself and the personal characteristics of trainees may be associated with the use of the training in practice.

We have followed the Medical Research Council guidelines for the development and evaluation of complex interventions (MRC, 2000) including a systematic review of the literature to develop CST, a pilot study, a randomised controlled trial, and a longer-term study. There has been little research on the long-term implementation and evaluation of complex interventions in practice (Phase IV trials; MRC, 2000) and almost nothing in dementia care. This study evaluated the effectiveness of disseminating CST in practice, looking at the use of CST groups by staff who had attended the one day CST training course.

The aim was to investigate any association between whether or not people went on to run CST groups and other factors including the three dimensions of transfer system theory (the training, characteristics of trainees and organizational factors). The primary hypothesis was that after attending a one-day CST training course, trainees were more likely to run CST if they had a better work environment and organizational support, were more motivated, had more positive/person-centred attitudes to dementia and had higher levels of job satisfaction.

METHODS

The Training Intervention

The training involved a theoretical and research background to dementia, psychosocial interventions and CST; with the primary focus being the practical application of CST in clinical settings. Methods included a PowerPoint presentation, small group exercises, role-play and video observation. Attendants were asked to evaluate the course using a feedback form. Eight courses were run by AS, the lead researcher on the CST trial. She developed the training course and is a Clinical Psychologist and Lecturer in Clinical Psychology. Two courses were run by HD, a Consultant Clinical Psychologist who was trained by AS. There was no contact with trainees following the training.

Sample and Data Collection

The sample were 168 staff working with people with dementia, trained across ten courses in the UK from January 2007 to June 2008. All trainees were contacted by e-mail and/or post (depending on contact information available) and asked to complete a questionnaire. Sixteen had moved jobs or were no longer contactable, therefore 152 people were approached of whom 76 responded. Data were collected over a three-month period, which meant that data from the first trainees was collected approximately 18 months after the training, with a minimum period of three months for the final trainees.

Measures and Other Information

Information was gathered from feedback forms immediately following training and people were asked to rate different aspects of the training, such as the methods used and trainer's knowledge, on a Likert scale where 1 = poor and 5 = excellent. Because feedback forms were anonymous, it was not possible to match them with the participants in this study. However, across all the trainings run, scores of 4 (good) and 5 (excellent) were given for most items by most trainees. The only item which was predominantly scored as average (3) concerned the audiovisual equipment used.

The post-training questionnaire included the outcome measures described below. The factors investigated and sources of information are summarized in Table 1. The questionnaire included general information such as job title, place of work, (e.g. specialist dementia setting), gender, ethnic group, age, years working in dementia care. Information relating to CST included whether or not person had run CST groups, problems/barriers setting up groups, and any further support which would have been helpful.

Table 1. Transfer System Theory and sources of information

Domains assessed	Source of information / outcome measures
Design and Quality of Training	Feedback forms Items on questionnaire, e.g. about whether training provided necessary skills
Personal factors	Hope (ADQ) Person-centredness (ADQ) Job satisfaction (JS) Motivation (brief LTSI) Learner characteristics (brief LTSI)
Organisational factors	Environment (brief LTSI) Ability / enabling (brief LTSI) Obstacles, as reported in questionnaire

The Learning Transfer System Inventory (LTSI: Holton et al, 2000). This comprises sixty-eight items grouped into sixteen constructs which were categorized into four major groups: trainee characteristics, motivation, work environment, and ability / enabling (Noe and Schmitt, 1986). It was selected because it considers both personal and environmental factors which might impact on the administration of CST. Reliability and validity (including cross-cultural validity) is high (e.g. Holton et al, 2000; Khasawneh et al, 2006). The LTSI can be used as a diagnostic tool (to assess training needs) as well as an evaluation tool of training policies. For this survey we used a brief version of the LTSI (table 2) comprising of the sixteen items one for each construct (Holton et al, 2000). All of the items use five-point Likert-type scales from 1 (strongly disagree) to 5 (strongly agree).

Approaches to Dementia Questionnaire (ADQ: Lintern and Woods, 2001). This is a 20-item Likert scale in which staff rate their extent of agreement with different statements about dementia (e.g. "people with dementia are very much like children") from (5) 'strongly agree' to (1) 'strongly disagree'. A total score and two sub-scores, 'hope' and 'person-centredness', can be calculated. It was selected because these seem to be important characteristics in care staff, for example staff hope has been associated with quality of life in people with dementia (Spector and Orrell, 2006). Test-retest reliability is good (total = 0.76, hope = 0.70, person-centredness = 0.69) and predictive validity is good for the hope subscale.

Job Satisfaction Index *(Aspects of work inventory (AWI): Barkham et al, 1989) This is an 18-item Likert scale in which respondents rate their satisfaction with different aspects of their job on a scale from extremely dissatisfied (1) to extremely satisfied (7). Inter-rater reliability and validity are good.*

Analyses

Data were entered into SPSS version 10. Independent samples t-tests were used to compare the two groups (those who had / had not run CST groups) on the outcome measures used.

Table 2. Learning Transfer System Inventory (LTSI): Factors Items and questions

Learner characteristics	Question used
Learner Readiness	Before the training I had a good understanding of how it would fit my job-related development.
Performance Self-Efficacy	I am confident in my ability to use newly learned skills on the job.
Motivation	Question used
Motivation to Transfer	I get excited when I think about trying to use my new learning on my job.
Transfer Effort–Performance Expectations	My job performance improves when I use new things that I have learned.
Performance-Outcomes Expectations	When I do things to improve my performance, good things happen to me.
Work environment	Question used
Positive Personal Outcomes	Employees in this organization receive various 'perks' when they utilize newly learned skills on the job.
Negative Personal Outcomes	If I do not utilize my training I will be cautioned about it.
Motivation to Transfer	I get excited when I think about trying to use my new learning on my job.
Transfer Effort Performance Expectations	My job performance improves when I use new things that I have learned.
Performance-Outcomes Expectations	When I do things to improve my performance, good things happen to me.
Resistance/ Openness to Change	People in my group are open to changing the way they do things.
Performance Coaching	After training, I get feedback from people about how well I am applying what I learned.
Ability / enabling	Question used
Personal Capacity for Transfer	My workload allows me time to try the new things I have learned.
Perceived Content Validity	What is taught in training closely matches my job requirements.
Transfer Design	The activities and exercises the trainers used helped me know how to apply my learning on the job.
Opportunity to Use	The resources I need to use what I learned will be available to me after training.

RESULTS

Demographics

The questionnaire was sent to 152 people of whom 76 responded (50%). People were contacted by post and e-mail including up to three reminders, but the biggest problem was where all contact/correspondence with a group who had been trained needed to go via a single person. Of the respondents, the mean age was 43.6 years (s.d. = 10.9, range 20 – 72 years). Sixty (79%) were female and 16 (21%) were male. Forty-three (56%) worked in a specialist dementia setting. The majority of the trainees (60 / 79%) were professional staff including 26 (34%) occupational therapists, 24 (32%) nurses, 8 (11%) psychologists, and 2 (2%) physiotherapists. Of the remainder there were 5 (7%) care staff, 3 (4%) who worked for a charity, and 8 (1%) others. 33 (43%) worked in Community Mental Health Teams (CMHTs) for older people, 10 (13%) in day hospitals, 7 (9%) in care homes, 3 (4%) in day centres and 3 (4%) in the voluntary sector. 20 (27%) fell into the 'other' category which included a civic centre, ward for elderly, acute inpatient unit, university, EMI unit and in a self-employed capacity. Most respondents (91%) were white. Of the 76 respondents, 27 (35%) had run CST groups following training and 49 (65%) had not. There was no relationship between having started a CST group and job title, place of work, gender, age or ethnicity.

Quality of Training

The post-training questionnaire asked whether people felt that the training equipped them with the necessary skills for the delivery of CST. Of the 75 respondents, 65 (86%) responded 'yes' and 10 (14%) responded 'no'. People were asked to comment on what further support might be necessary to run CST effectively and 100 responses were received (some people marked more than one option). 24 (24%) wanted more support from staff, 23 (23%) regular supervision from a specialist, 17 (17%) an online forum, 16 (16%) training in other areas, 15 (15%), regular supervision, and 7 (7%) made other comments. Including the other comments, six key themes were identified to improve the set up and running of groups: support from colleagues, learning from colleagues, group facilitators training, facilitators experience running activities/groups, understanding of the groups, and work flexibility.

Characteristics of Staff Running CST Groups
Versus Those Not Running Groups

For the purpose of this analysis, the sample was divided into two groups: people who had run CST groups after training and people who had not (see table 3). Staff who had run CST groups did significantly better in terms of total Brief LTSI score and three of the subscales: learner characteristics, work environment and ability/enabling. There were no differences between the groups on scores on the ADQ and Job Satisfaction measures.

Barriers to Running CST Groups

The 27 people running CST groups said they had encountered some difficulties. 11 (37%) highlighted a lack of staff time, 6 (22%) a lack of resources, 4 (15%) not enough suitable participants, 2 (7%) no suitable room, 2 (7%) transport problems, and 2 (7%) lack of support from management. Everybody stated that they felt skilled enough to run CST.

The 49 people who did not do CST were asked to give one or more reasons as to why groups did not run. Of the 62 responses 27 (55%) mentioned lack of staff time, 9 (18%) lack of resources, 7 (14%) no suitable room, 7 (14%) not enough suitable participants, 6 (14%) transport problems, 4 (8%) not feeling skilled enough, and 2 (4%) lack of support from management.

Table 3. Group differences using independent samples t-tests

Measure	'Did CST' group	'Did not do CST' group	Independent samples t-test: Difference
Brief LTSI total	2.5 (0.4)	2.8 (0.3)	P = 0.002*
Brief LTSI motivation	2.3 (0.7)	2.4 (0.6)	P = 0.27
Brief LTSI learner characteristics	2.0 (0.6)	2.3 (0.6)	P = 0.05*
Brief LTSI work environment	2.8 (0.5)	3.0 (0.4)	P = 0.04*
Brief LTSI ability / enabling	2.4 (0.6)	2.9 (0.7)	P = 0.01*
ADQ total	4.2 (0.3)	4.2 (0.4)	P = 0.85
ADQ hope	3.9 (0.6)	3.9 (0.6)	P = 0.87
ADQ person-centredness	4.6 (0.3)	4.5 (0.5)	P = 0.54
Job satisfaction	5.1 (1.0)	5.1 (0.7)	P = 0.88

*= significant (p<0.05).

CONCLUSION

This is one of the few studies in the dementia literature that looks at the outcome of training in normal practice, with most having evaluated training as part of an experimental design. As such, it offers a useful insight into how effective this training was in achieving a clearly defined goal i.e. running CST groups following the training course. This study may also be the first that has used transfer of learning theory measures in dementia care. The key finding was that people running CST groups scored significantly better on the brief LTSI than those who did not, suggesting that they had effective learner characteristics, work environment and ability/enabling. The study to some degree addressed the three areas which Holton and Baldwin (2000) suggested may affect success in putting training into practice: training factors, personal factors and environmental factors. The results suggest that the training itself was adequate enough to equip people with the skills necessary for running CST groups, with 86% of the sample stating that this was the case. However, whereas support from staff and regular supervision were highlighted as the main areas in which further support would have been useful, the key barrier to running groups appears to have simply been staff time although lack of resources was also important. This fits in with informal feedback given during training, addressing concerns about having sufficient staff to prioritise CST above essentials such as personal care.

In terms of personal factors, no link was found between the groups in job satisfaction or attitudes to dementia (hope and person-centredness). Trainee characteristics on the brief LTSI which include learner readiness and performance self-efficacy, however, were greater in the group which took up CST. One must interpret these results with caution, as these patterns do not necessarily imply causation. In other words, people who are more likely to run CST groups may by nature have enhanced readiness and self-efficacy, as opposed to these characteristics enabling them to 'learn' something which they then applied in practice. Research has examined the influence of work environment factors such as interpersonal support (Bates et al 2000), opportunity to transfer (Ford et al, 1992) and culture (Tracey et al, 1995) and in this study environmental factors also appeared to play some part, with the group offering CST scoring better in 'work environment' and 'ability/enabling'. The work environment scale includes performance coaching, supervisor support, supervisor sanctions, peer support, resistance-openness to change, positive personal outcomes, and negative personal outcomes.

This study begins to address some areas of investigation in a training trial, but none are examined in depth due to the pilot nature of the project. As such, the sample size limited the meaningfulness of statistical comparison. The design and quality of the training was not addressed in any detail, although participants indicated that they viewed it as high quality and adequate to prepare them for running CST groups. The personal characteristics that we hypothesised might link to uptake of CST were not found to predict CST use. The elements were selected due to parallel drawn from other research, for example hope in care staff has shown to be associated with quality of life for the person with dementia (Spector and Orrell, 2006). However, it is possible that other factors (such as sense of competence) may be more relevant when evaluating staff training. Learning was not specifically evaluated since to do this, an individual's competence in and adherence to CST would need to be assessed (in addition to CST uptake).

The population recruited was only 50% of the sample contacted, and may not be representative of all the trainees. This could have been increased if full contact details for each trainee had been recorded on the day of training rather than relying on a single contact person. The responders may have been a more motivated group, possibly with a higher percentage of qualified staff and CST use than the full sample. Time between training and assessment of participants was variable and it may be that some of the trainees who were followed up after shorter periods would have taken up CST groups if the follow-up had been longer. The degree to which these results may generalise to trainings in other psychosocial interventions is unknown and future research may help to determine this.

This implementation study has been useful in considering the practicalities of putting CST into practice, following a one-day training course. Individuals with better learning characteristics may also be more likely to take up CST following training, and simple factors such as a lack of staff time and resources may prevent people from doing CST. Changing practice in dementia care will optimize the existing resources to improve the quality of life of people living with dementia. Future research could focus on comparing the effectiveness of different training methods, for example the current course versus training with ongoing support and supervision versus the training manual only.

In addition, studies need to examine whether the training method might influence how effectively CST is carried out by measuring competence, adherence and using simple cognitive and quality of life outcome measures such as the MMSE (Folstein et al, 1975) and the QoL-AD (Logsdon et al, 1999). It would also be interesting to examine the relationship between personal characteristics and skills in group facilitation.

CONFLICT OF INTEREST

AS runs the CST training course on a commercial basis.

DESCRIPTION OF AUTHORS' ROLES

*Aimee Spect*or developed and administered the training intervention, oversaw the design and implementation of the study, and was the main author of the paper.

Martin Orrell contributed to the design and implementation of the study and commented on drafts of the paper.

Elisa Aguirre collected the data and contributed to the write-up of the paper, making a significant contribution to the background and theory.

ACKNOWLEDGMENTS

We would like to thank Sandeep Sandhu for her hard work in collecting the data. We also thank everyone who took their time to complete the measures.

REFERENCES

Barkham, M; Firth-Cozens, JA; Hardy, GE; Reynolds, SA; Shapiro, DA; and Warr, PB. (1989). Measures of work experience for stress reduction research. SAPU Memo 1049, Department of Psychology, University of Sheffield.

Bates, RA et al. (2000).The role of interpersonal factors in the application of computer-based training in an industrial setting. *Human resource development international*, 3 (1) 19-42.

DoH (2008). Department of Health (2008) National Dementia Strategy. London; Department of Health.

Folstein, MF; Folstein, SE and McHugh, PR. (1975). Mini-mental state: A practical method for grading the cognitive state of patients for the clinician. *Journal of Psychiatric Research*, 12, 189-198.

Ford, JK; Quinones, MA; Sego, DJ; and Sorra J. (1992). Factors affecting the opportunity to perform trained tasks on the job. *Personnel Psychology, 45,* 511–527.

Holton, EF and Baldwin, T. (2000). Making transfer happen: An action perspective on learning transfer systems. *Advances in Developing Human Resources, 8,* 1–6.

Holton, EF; Bates, RA; and Ruona ,WEA. (2000). Development of a generalized learning transfer system inventory. *Human Resource Development Quarterly, 11*(4), 333–360.

Innes, A; Surr, C. (2001). Measuring the well-being of people with dementia living in formal care settings: the use of Dementia Care Mapping . *Aging and Mental Health*, 5,(3) 258-268.

Khasawneh, S; Bates, R; and Holton, E. (2006). Construct validation of an Arabic version of the Learning Transfer System Inventory for use in Jordan. *International Journal of Training and Development, 10*(3), 180–194.

Knapp, M; Thorgrimsen, L; Patel, A; et al. Cognitive Stimulation Therapy for people with dementia: Cost Effectiveness Analysis. *British Journal of Psychiatry*, 188: 574-580 (2006).

Lintern, T; Woods, B; and Phair, L. (2000). Training is not enough to change care practice. *Journal of Dementia Care*, March/April, 15-17.

Lintern, T; and Woods, B. (2001). *Approaches to dementia questionnaire*. University of Wales, Bangor.

Logsdon, R ; Gibbons, LE ; McCurry, SM ; and Teri, L. (1999). Quality of life in Alzheimer's disease: Patient and caregiver reports. *Journal of Mental Health and Aging*, 5, 21-32.

McCabe, M; Davison, T; George, K. (2007). Effectiveness of staff training programs for behavioral problems among older people with dementia. *Aging and Mental Health*, 11 (5) 505-519.

Medical Research Council (2000) A framework for the development and evaluation of RCTs for complex interventions to improve health. MRC.

Moniz-Cook, E; Agar, S; Silver, M; Woods, R; Wang, M; Elston, C; and Win, T. (1998) Can staff training reduce behavioural problems in residential care for the elderly mentally ill?. *International Journal of Geriatric Psychiatry*, 13(3), 149-158.

National Audit Office (2008). Improving services and support for people with dementia: report by the Comptroller and Auditor General. London: The Stationery Office.

NICE-SCIE (2006) Dementia: supporting people with dementia and their carers. Guideline - draft for consultation. NICE-SCIE.

Noe, RA; and Schmitt, N. (1986). The influence of trainee attitudes on training effectiveness: Test of a model. *Personnel Psychology, 39*, 497–523.

Orrell, M; Spector, A, Thorgrimsen, L; Woods, B. (2005) A pilot study examining the effectiveness of maintenance Cognitive Stimulation Therapy (MCST) for people with dementia. International Journal of Geriatric Psychiatry, 20, 446-451.

Spector, A; Thorgrimsen, L, Woods, B, Royan, L; Davies, S; Butterworth, M; and Orrell, M. (2003). Efficacy of an evidence-based cognitive stimulation therapy programme for people with dementia: Randomised Controlled Trial. Br J Psychiatry, 183: 248-254.

Spector, A; and Orrell, M. (2005) Quality of life in dementia: a comparison of the perceptions of people with dementia and care staff in residential homes. Alzheimer's Disease and Associated Disorders, 20 (3): 160-165.

Spector, A; Thorgrimsen, L; Woods, B; and Orrell, M. (2006). Making a difference: An evidence-based group programme to offer cognitive stimulation therapy (CST) to people with dementia: Manual for group leaders. Hawker Publications: UK.

Tracey, JB; Tannenbaum, SI; and Kavanaugh, MJ. (1995). Applying trained skills on the job: The importance of the work environment. *Journal of Applied Psychology, 80*, 239–252.

In: Dementia: Non-Pharmacological Therapies
Editor: Elisabetta Farina, pp. 71-91

ISBN: 978-1-61470-736-3
© 2012 Nova Science Publishers, Inc.

User-Participatory Development of Assistive Technology for People with Dementia – From Needs to Functional Requirements. First Results of the COGKNOW Project

Franka Meiland[*,1], *Annika Reinersmann*[2], *Stefan Sävenstedt*[3],
Birgitta Bergvall-Kåreborn[3], *Marike Hettinga*[4], *David Craig*[5],
Anna-Lena Andersson[6] *and Rose-Marie Dröes*[1]

[1] Dept. of Psychiatry, Alzheimer Centre,
EMGO Institute for Health and Care research,
VU University medical center, Valeriusplein 9,
1075 BG Amsterdam, The Netherlands.
[2] Heidelberger Akademie der Wissenschaften,
Karlstraße 4, 69117, Heidelberg, Germany.
[3] Centre for Distance-Spanning Healthcare,
Luleå University of Technology, SE-971 87 Luleå, Sweden.
[4] Novay, Brouwerijstraat 1, 7523 XC Enschede, The Netherlands.
[5] Belfast City Hospital/Queen's University of Belfast,
51 Lisburn Road, Belfast BT9- 7AB, Northern Ireland.
[6] Luleå Municipality/ CDH, ÄldreCentrum
The Lighthouse Lulsundsgatan 42 97242 Luleå.
Funding: European Commission's Information
Society Technologies (IST) programme under grant 034025.

Abstract

The increasing number of persons with dementia means growing demands on care and support at home, and so additional solutions are needed. In the European COGKNOW project dementia experts and technological system designers cooperate closely to develop a cognitive prosthetic device that supports persons with mild dementia in their daily functioning and improves their quality of life. The project focuses on the areas of memory, social contact, daily activities, and feelings of safety.

* Address of correspondence: Dr. F.J.M. Meiland, Department of Psychiatry, EMGO Institute, VU University medical center, Valeriusplein 9, 1075 BG Amsterdam. The Netherlands. T: +31-20-7885623. F: +31-20-6737458. E: fj.meiland@vumc.nl

The design process is user-participatory and consists of three iterative cycles. In each cycle 12 to 18 persons with dementia of the Alzheimer type and their carers at three test sites across Europe are invited to actively participate in the development process. Each cycle starts with user needs inquiry workshops and interviews, followed by (further) technological development of the device, and ends with user field tests to test the user-friendliness, usefulness and impact of the developed prototype in daily life.

This article reports on the first project phase in which a top four list of Information and Communication Technological (ICT) solutions was selected that formed the basis to develop a first prototype. The list was based on the priorities of needs mentioned by the first participants group of people with dementia (n=17) and their carers (n=17), the solutions they preferred, their disabilities, personal and situational characteristics, and the technological designers' opinions on the feasibility of developing the proposed solutions within the time frame of the project. Based on the information gathered in the user workshops and interviews, the dementia expert researchers further explained the selected ICT solutions in written scenarios. Next, a functional requirements list was composed and a first prototype was developed that offered support in four areas: *reminding* - day and time orientation support, find mobile service and reminding service; *social contact* – telephone support by picture dialling; *activities* - media control support through a music play back and radio function; and, *feelings of safety* - a warning service to indicate when the front door is open and an emergency contact service.

The results of this first project phase show that, in general, the people with mild dementia as well as their carers were able to express and prioritize their (unmet) needs, and the kind of technological assistance they preferred in the selected areas. This made it possible to compose an overall priority list for the development of a multifunctional ICT device. In next phases it will be tested if the user-participatory development and multidisciplinary approach applied result in a user-friendly and useful device that positively impacts the autonomy and quality of life of people with dementia and their carers.

Keywords: dementia, carers, needs, user-participatory development, assistive technology.

INTRODUCTION

One of the great challenges of the 21st century will be the provision of adequate care to the growing number of elderly people, and in particular, those with dementia. With an estimated 24 million people world-wide suffering from dementia at present [1], a number expected to double every twenty years, and the parallel decrease in the number of persons of the working population who are potentially available to offer formal and informal care [2], health care systems require significant adaptation to meet the future demands of persons with dementia. Because of the expected disproportional grow of institutionalized care, relatively more people with dementia will need to be cared for in their own home and this is also the general policy in many European countries. However, without changes in present health care systems, the current standards cannot be maintained.

Finding alternative strategies to provide high quality yet cost-effective care services that enable people with dementia to remain at home, in a safe and acceptable manner, is therefore of vital importance. One possible solution is the greater use of assistive technology, an umbrella term for different technological systems and devices that can assist people who have functional limitations due to age-related disabilities, such as dementia [3]. Assistive technology can offer a cost-effective means to enhance independence and quality of life in people with dementia as well as enable them to remain in their own environment, which is what they themselves generally prefer [2]. Also, support by means of Information and Communication Technology (ICT) offers the opportunity to expand the delivery of the currently advocated person-centered and tailored care by making use of intelligent equipment that 'knows' the person, their situations and needs [4]. The potential role of these new technologies in health care is recognized [5], and various ICT solutions have been developed, for instance informative websites, electronic memory aids, videophones, picture gramophones and sensor-based monitoring systems inside or outside the house [6]. Though in some studies the ICT solutions were tested with persons with dementia in real life situations [7-10], many did not (yet) test the applications in this target group. A reason for the limited testing and application of assistive technology for people with dementia is the complexity of testing devices in a group with heterogeneous disabilities and needs [11]. Problems and disabilities that may influence the potential use of technology in this target group include, for instance, memory and orientation problems, difficulties with comprehension, and with performing executive functions. ICT-solutions for persons with dementia therefore require device use to be as intuitive as possible, otherwise persons with dementia who have little insight into their difficulties will refuse to use it or deny that additional support technology is needed in the first place. Dementia affects every individual differently and each person has his own specific set of circumstances, disabilities and needs. The individual's requirements when it comes to providing a supporting technology are similarly wide-ranging. Development processes are therefore probably best pursued where technological experts and those experienced in the needs of persons with dementia act in tandem with a user-participatory developmental design process, engaging groups of persons with dementia and their carers from the start. That way, difficulties related to lack of insight and technological naivety in this group of mostly older persons are approached in a combined fashion, and the heterogeneous functional requirements for this special group are ascertained in the most suitable way.

Knowledge about abilities and disabilities of the persons with dementia and context information on living arrangements provide essential information in this regard [3,12,13]. However, of even greater importance is clear information on user-needs and preferences, as these determine whether the persons with dementia will perceive the device as useful and thus influence the extent of future engagement [3,13,14]. A thorough needs-assessment to learn more about the actual needs and wishes of people with dementia regarding ICT solutions is therefore indispensable [15-19].

The need to involve the persons with dementia in the development process motivated the present study, the COGKNOW project. COGKNOW is a 3 year, 2.7 million Euro European Framework Programme project in which integrated, user-participatory ICT-solutions are developed to help people with mild dementia navigate through their day. In this project, a team of dementia experts and technological system designers from eleven institutes in eight European countries co-operate [1].

---

[1] Participating organizations are: Telefónica (Spain), University of Ulster (Northern Ireland), Luleå University of Technology (Sweden), Novay (The Netherlands), VU University medical center (The Netherlands), AcrossLimits Ltd (Malta), Groupe des Ecoles des Télécommunications – Institut National des Télécommunications (France), University Hospital of North Norway/Norwegian Centre for Telemedicine (Norway), Belfast City Hospital/Queen's University of Belfast (Northern Ireland), Mobi Solutions OÜ (Estonia), Norbottens Läns Landsting (Sweden). See www.cogknow.eu

The COGKNOW project started from the results of a large survey on needs assessment conducted by one of the consortium partners (VU University medical center) among 230 community dwelling persons with dementia and 320 carers [20], and literature reviews on subjective needs of persons with dementia conducted by the same research group [21,22]. The COGKNOW project focuses on need areas in which this earlier research identified most unmet needs, namely memory, social contact, daily activities and feelings of safety. COGKNOW aims to study in a smaller group of persons with dementia, and their carers, what needs they specifically experience in these areas of daily life and what preferences they have regarding the development of an ICT device to support them in these areas.

To involve end-users in the design of new technologies, different methods can be used throughout the development process: interviews, surveys, focus groups or diaries; observation of end-users' behaviour in their natural context via applied ethnography; organization of design workshops to collaborate with end-users, and study (e.g. by observation and interviewing of) end-users when they use a product or service during a field study or in the lab [23].

In this article, we report on the needs and ICT solutions inventory that was carried out among people with mild dementia and their carers in the first phase of the COGKNOW project [24]. The needs and preferred ICT solutions inventory focussed on the following research questions:

- What actual (unmet) needs do people with mild dementia and their carers express in the areas of memory, social contact, daily activities and feelings of safety?
- Do people with mild dementia and their carers express preferences for specific ICT solutions to address their needs?
- Taking into account the needs, abilities, context variables and preferences of people with mild dementia and their carers, which ICT device(s) could possibly provide adequate solutions for their wishes?

METHODS

Design

The user-participatory design process consists of three iterative cycles in a three year time period (2006-2009). In each cycle 12 to 18 community dwelling persons with mild dementia and their carers, spread out over three test sites (Amsterdam, Belfast and Luleå), are invited to participate in the study. Thus, in total about 45 persons with mild dementia and their carers will participate in the study. It was decided to include a relatively small sample per site in each project cycle, because of the primarily qualitative nature of the study and the specifically planned detailed data collection. There were more practical reasons as well, such as: small needs inquiry focus groups were expected to help participants to feel candid and relaxed in describing their needs, time restrictions and limited budget for equipment costs in user field tests.

Each cycle starts with an inventory among the participants of user needs and preferred ICT solutions in the selected support areas of the COGKNOW project by means of workshops and (standardized) interviews. In principle, separate workshops are organized for people with dementia and carers, to give them the opportunity to express their own opinion. In addition to the workshops, domiciliary individual interviews are conducted using standardized questionnaires to collect information that could be relevant in developing an ICT solution, such as personal background and context characteristics, cognitive functioning (disabilities), (unmet) needs, and experienced autonomy. The results of the workshops and interviews are used as input for the (further) technological development of the device. Each cycle ends with user field tests in which the developed prototype is tested with people with dementia, and a thorough, so-called Human factors impact analysis is carried out on the user-friendliness, usefulness and (in the last iteration also on) the impact of the prototype on the daily life of people with dementia and their carers. In this way participants contribute to the design process as well as to the implementation and evaluation process.

The study was approved by the relevant medical ethical authority of each research site.

Sample and Setting

In this first project phase 17 people with mild dementia of the Alzheimer type and their carers were recruited from memory clinics and/or the Meeting Centres Support Programme for people with dementia and their carers in Amsterdam (The Netherlands), Belfast (Northern Ireland) and Luleå (Sweden)(see Table 1). Inclusion criteria were:

- People with a diagnosis of Dementia of the Alzheimer type (possible/probable) as described in the DSM-IV-TR
- Severity of dementia: Global Deterioration Stage 3,4,5: mild cognitive decline (early confusional; GDS 3) moderate cognitive decline (late confusional; GDS 4) and moderately severe cognitive decline (early dementia; GDS 5) (assessed by using the standardized Brief Cognitive Rating Scale [25]
- People are willing and able to participate actively (through individual interviews, participation in a small focus group and field test sessions) in a research project in which an ICT device is being developed that aims to support them in their memory, daily activities, social contact with family and friends and feelings of safety
- The informal carer has regular contact with /cares for the persons with dementia.

Measuring Instruments

The following standardized questionnaires were used. To inventory the needs of persons with dementia, the Camberwell Assessment of Need for the Elderly (CANE) was used (interrater reliability: $r = 0.99$; test-retest reliability: $r = 0.96$) [26,27]. Needs in 24 areas of daily living are assessed with the CANE. Background characteristics and context variables were collected with a standardized questionnaire constructed specifically for this study that was administered to the carer. Cognitive functioning was assessed with the CAMCOG ($\alpha=.97$), the cognitive scale of the Cambridge Examination for mental disorders in the elderly (CAMDEX) [28]. Experienced Autonomy of persons with dementia was assessed with the

Experienced Autonomy list [29], which was constructed specifically for the purpose of this study using seven items from the Mastery Scale [30] and five items that were adapted from the WHOQOL100 [31]. And finally the Quality of life in Alzheimer's Disease Scale was administered to the person with dementia (QoL-AD, α=.88-.89) [32].

Table 1. Characteristics of participants in the study

	Amsterdam (n=6)	Belfast (n=6)	Luleå (n=5)
Persons with dementia			
Age (mean, range)	64.0 (56-78)	72.7 (65- 86)	67.8 (60-77)
Sex			
female	3	5	3
male	3	1	2
Civil status			
married	5	3	5
divorced/widowed/single	1	3	-
Living alone	1	2	-
Cognitive disabilities			
GDS (mean, range)	3 (2-5)	3 (1-4)	3 (3-4)
Time orientation *	3	3	3
Place orientation *	0	0	1
Comprehension *	3	2	0
Reading comprehension *	0	0	0
Expression name *	4	0	2
Expression repeat *	4	5	2
Praxis *	2	5	0
Perception *	4	na	0
Difficulty performing everyday activities #	3	2	1
Difficulty with mobility #	3	5	4
Carers			
Age (mean,range)	58.5 (49-78)	53.0 (40-72)	61.4 (23 – 78)
Sex			
female	4	3	2
male	2	3	3
Relation to patient			
spouse	5	3	4
child	1	2	1
other (cousin)	-	1	-

GDS= Global Deterioration Scale.

* results on the CAMCOG indicate problems with this cognitive function, in Luleå the CAMCOG was administered to only 4 persons.

item of the Experienced Autonomy list.

The general practitioner, medical specialist or programme coordinator of the meeting centre was contacted for information on the diagnosis of dementia and a clinical judgment about the severity of dementia with the Global Deterioration Scale (GDS) (validity: $r = 0.53 - 0.83$) [25].

Procedure

Workshops guidelines, containing a checklist with the general workshop structure and the questions to be addressed, were set up in advance and applied at all test sites. To structure the workshops and to stimulate the discussion, two PowerPoint presentations were used. One showed pictures of daily life situations and activities during the day (e.g. waking up and getting dressed in the morning, having breakfast, having lunch, taking a walk outdoors, having dinner and going to bed at night). For each part of the day, it was discussed what activities persons with dementia performed, what they considered important for their quality of life, how this could be improved, and whether they experienced any problems or needs during specific parts of the day and/or with regard to specific activities in the four COGKNOW need areas (memory, social contact, daily activity and feelings of safety). All problems and needs mentioned in the four areas were listed on a flip chart and the participants were asked to prioritize them. The second PowerPoint presentation showed some examples of ICT solutions that have been developed for people with cognitive disabilities, or with dementia, in the four COGKNOW need areas (e.g. electronic calendars, pictophone and find object device). These examples where used to stimulate the participants' own ideas and the discussion on preferences of ICT solutions for the inventoried needs in the selected needs areas.

Both the workshop guidelines and the PowerPoint presentations were based on previous field and literature research on needs of people with dementia [21,22], and assistive technology successfully applied among people with cognitive disabilities or dementia [6].

In cases where participants could not, or did not want to join the group workshops, individual interviews were conducted based on the same structure and content as the workshops.

In the recruitment phase participants initially received detailed oral and written information from the personnel (neurologist, care coordinator) of the memory clinic or meeting centres, explaining the purpose and aim of the project. If they were willing to join, they were further involved in an informed consent procedure in which they were invited to participate in one project cycle of about 9 months. At the beginning of the workshops, or individual interviews, all participants again confirmed their informed consent to participate in the first project cycle.

In Amsterdam, workshops were held at the memory clinic of the VU University medical centre and led by a senior researcher (psychologist), while a junior researcher (also a psychologist), took minutes. The workshops were audiotaped and a detailed report on the workshops was written up afterwards. The two workshops (one with the persons with dementia and one with the carers) both lasted approximately three hours. Every participant received a summary of the workshop minutes afterwards. Because one couple had been on vacation during the time of the workshops, they were interviewed individually at home about their needs and preferred ICT solutions. In Belfast, the interviews were conducted by two trained dementia research nurses, who interviewed all patient-carer dyads individually at their homes and made written records. In Sweden, an assistant professor in social informatics carried out two group interviews, and three individual interviews at the participants' homes (at this site data were also recorded in the form of written notes).

After the inventory of needs and preferred ICT solutions, individual interviews were carried out at the homes of the participants, where data were collected by means of the standardized scales.

At the beginning of the project researchers and other project members directly involved with participants were specifically trained in communication skills, ethics, data storage and privacy. All collected data were anonymized, individually coded, and stored in computerized databases at the three research test sites. The key of the codes was kept in locked safety cabinets. Only anonymized data were exchanged between research sites.

Analysis

All research sites performed a descriptive analysis on background characteristics, cognitive (dis)abilities, context information, needs, experienced autonomy and quality of life of people with dementia, collected with the standardized questionnaires.

Detailed written reports were made of the audio recordings of the workshops and the workshop-interviews. A content analysis was done at each site to assess the most important needs and the most preferred ICT solutions in each of the four COGKNOW areas. Persons with dementia and carers were asked to state these priorities during the workshops. If there was no agreement on specific needs during the workshops, the most frequently (and strongly) mentioned needs were selected as having priority. The same method was used with regard to preferred ICT solutions. Two researchers at each site performed this analysis independently, and any discrepancies in the priority list were discussed until agreement was reached. Subsequently a top four list was made for the most appropriate solutions for the prioritized needs of the participants in the following way: a) the ICT solution had to (at least partly) solve the prioritized need, b) the ICT solutions that were preferred by the users were given preference, and c) existing ICT-solutions that were previously tested on persons with dementia and had been proven helpful for them were given preference. Regarding this latter consideration, a literature review on ICT solutions was studied by all researchers [6].

After that, possible scenarios were created (likely situations that the final COGKNOW ICT solution ultimately hopes to realize). The scenarios were based on the collected workshop and interview data and the top four lists from each research site. All three top four lists were then discussed with the technological partners in the project consortium to check aspects of developmental feasibility. This resulted in a joint agreement on one overall top four list of devices or functionalities to be developed and tested in a first field test, in which the emphasis would be on user-friendliness and usefulness of the ICT solution to be developed.

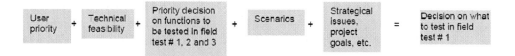

Figure 1. Types of inputs used to decide on the functionalities to be tested in field test # 1 of the COGKNOW project.

Finally, the information collected on background characteristics, cognitive (dis)abilities, context information, needs, experienced autonomy and wishes of people with dementia was used to specify the functional requirements for the agreed ICT solutions [24].

Figure 1 depicts the process of deciding which functionalities to develop for the first field test.

RESULTS

Sample Characteristics

A total of seventeen patient-carer dyads participated in the three test-sites. Table 1 shows an overview of the participants' characteristics per site.

The persons with dementia varied in age from 56 to 86 years and, except for one person in Amsterdam and two people in Belfast, all lived together with their main carer. Twelve out of seventeen people with dementia were limited in their mobility, either due to a physical complaint or due to spatial disorientation in unfamiliar surroundings. Several people with dementia at the three test sites suffered from medical complaints such as arthritis (4 people), diabetes (2 people) or hypertension (3 people). Despite mobility constraints and medical complaints, none of the participants had installed safety measures in their homes yet.

(Un)Met Needs and Wishes of Persons with Dementia

Descriptive analysis of all data on needs and wishes resulted in a detailed overview per site of met and unmet needs and wishes of people with dementia. Results of the needs inventory workshops and individual interviews were described for the four COGKNOW areas at each site.

Table 2 gives an overview of the needs of people with dementia per COGKNOW needs area.

Support for Memory

At all research sites, the predominant need in the area of memory mentioned by people with dementia as well as their carers was the need to support their forgetfulness. One person referred to her forgetting recently acquired information as her "blankety blank moments". People reported various problems with remembering, such as to take their medicine, to take along their keys or phones when leaving the house, to know where they had put items, to remember their pin codes, appointments and the day or date. "It happens almost daily that I am searching for things", one person said. They expressed a great desire to compensate for this memory loss. People with dementia also described forgetfulness when it came to switching off electric appliances, how to cook or how to carry out household activities. Some people with dementia also had a need to be supported in remembering what was being said or what had happened recently. The carers confirmed these memory problems ("he is stressing around searching for keys"). Even when they wrote down appointments in a diary to help them remember, a person with dementia could ask "five times a day: what day is today?". Carers added that the need to be reminded to close doors or switch off electric appliances was of great priority. Across all research sites carers were concerned about the potential danger of this problem for their partners and themselves.

**Table 2. Inventoried needs in the four COGKNOW areas
during workshops and individual interviews**

COGKNOW Area	Inventoried Needs
Memory	Need for being reminded of activities, appointments, location of items, pin codes, closing and/or switching off devices/doors, personal hygiene, past events and experiences (short and long term)
Social contacts	Need for support with conversations, using phone, maintaining social contact
Daily activities	Need for support with – finances, – groceries, – activities, – hobbies
Feelings of safety	Need for security and safety – cookers – turning on/off devices – closing/locking doors – finances – being alone

Support for Social Contacts

The most important need people with dementia in Amsterdam and Luleå voiced was the need to be supported in holding a conversation. Their word-finding and comprehension problems impeded initiating or maintaining conversations, either via the telephone or face to face, and made maintenance of social contacts difficult. Persons with dementia complained about "people not having time to listen" or "not being given sufficient time to express themselves". Another difficulty, exacerbating social interaction, was the growing inability to use the phone, and consequently many had given up calling family or friends. In Belfast, people with dementia did report word-finding or comprehension difficulties as a hindrance to social exchanges less frequently, but more frequently reported their forgetfulness of appointments, birthdays and names, and expressed a need to be reminded in these areas.

Carers at all research sites agreed with these needs, but in Amsterdam and Luleå they explicitly reported another social problem that was not due to the inherent disabilities caused by Alzheimer's disease: The stigma associated with dementia had led former acquaintances or friends to withdraw. While carers could understand this in a way, at the same time they wished for more (public) openness regarding the diagnosis and course of the illness so that others would feel less intimidated by it.

Support for Daily Activities

At all test sites, people with dementia reported a great need for support in carrying out daily activities more independently. In line with the degree of progression of dementia, people differed in their perceived and reported difficulty to perform daily living activities. One person with dementia explained he did "not even want to play chess anymore because it confronted me with my impairment every time I played". Other participants worried about being a burden to other people. They had not given up activities yet, but realized they might have to do so in the near future. To help participants perform activities, automatic reminders could be useful. However, the majority of the participants commented they not only needed support to initiate an activity but also to carry on with it. With that expressing the need of stepwise assistance during the performance of activities. Activities they wanted support for ranged from household chores such as doing laundry, groceries and cooking or handling financial issues to pleasurable activities such as watching the TV or listening to the radio and to hobbies such as handcrafting, drawing, dancing, reading or parlour games. Across the three research sites different priority was given to the activities people with dementia wanted support for. While people in Amsterdam and Luleå attached importance to support with carrying out pleasurable activities, people in Belfast set particular value on being supported in household chores and in being reminded of taking their medication on time.

While carers agreed with the need for support in understanding written or oral instruction mentioned by their partners, they also reported a lack of initiative that they felt was even more to blame for the difficulties with daily activities. Disorientation in time and space caused further need for support in carrying out activities.

Beyond the abovementioned needs, people with dementia voiced a need that was closely related to feelings of autonomy, namely the need to be able and allowed to drive their car. People with dementia at all sites talked about the tremendous loss of independence they associated with having had to give up driving their cars. While they understood the inevitability of giving up driving, they still mourned for the resulting restriction to their mobility.

Feelings of Safety

The need to feel safe emerged forcefully in the participants' accounts of perceived insecurity in daily life. Forgetfulness, uncertainty about appropriate behaviour in demanding situations and difficulties carrying out daily activities caused insecurity and made people with dementia feel unsafe in their lives and in their homes. This was especially true of the dangers of forgetting to switch of electric appliances, or the gas cooker, having left the front door open or being unable to handle finances, and it concerned people with dementia at all research sites. People considered it "especially disturbing" when they had to do two things at the same time, for instance the phone rings while they are cooking. Many participants had experience with burning food in the pan, which made them feel "insecure" or "unsafe". Strikingly, people with dementia also felt they faced an enhanced risk of deception due to their weakness in remembering names or recognizing faces of people they met, either in public places or alone at home. Carers' accounts of needs in this area correspond with those of people with dementia. A meaningful way to indicate an emergency situation as well as being able to offer immediate help in case of emergency was a need that carers ascribed particular priority to.

Disabilities, Personal and Context Information
Relevant for Developing ICT Solutions

Results from the interviews with persons with dementia and carers showed some dementia-related disabilities that were considered relevant for the development of an assistive technological device. These disabilities were: memory and orientation problems; poor understanding of verbal instruction; difficulties with instrumental daily activities; and recognizing or understanding the meaning of pictures. Relevant personal and environmental features were: persons with dementia living alone or with a carer; using aids like a cane; possessing technological appliances that were no longer easy to use; living in a house with multiple rooms and levels; and feeling insecure when being alone.

Final Top four list

The decision on which ICT solutions would be developed in COGKNOW was based on the workshop and interview data outlined above, inventoried priorities at each sites and overall priorities of sites: to this end a table with priorities for ICT solutions was prepared per site (see table 3), and this was discussed with the technical partners and the research site leaders, who also took into account the feasibility of developing the solutions within the project. This resulted in a final top 4 list of ICT solutions for the four COGKNOW areas.

It was decided to develop a stationary component, such as a tablet PC with touch screen, and a mobile component featuring the same functions as the stationary component but allowing the persons with dementia to make and receive phone calls outdoors as well. Only simple written instructions were to be used on the devices (the cohort's language deficits recorded on the CAMCOG showed that almost one-third of the participants had problems with verbal instructions).

For the area 'support for memory' it was decided to realize a reminding service to provide prompts to help people remember to eat meals, make phone calls, and carry out personal hygiene such as brush their teeth. Also, the day and date would be featured on the devices to support people with orientation in time. Additionally, the ICT device would contain a function that locates the mobile phone component in case the person with dementia has misplaced it.

Excerpts of one of the two scenarios, which were developed during the analyses, show a reminder service to be developed and tested in Field Test 1. It is used by a woman with dementia, who lives together with her husband.

> "When Anne was diagnosed with Alzheimer's disease, her husband Jim had the COGKNOW Day Navigator system installed, to help them both through the day. The COGKNOW Day Navigator is a tablet PC that also includes a separate mobile device, which can be used in and outside the house. The COGKNOW Day Navigator can be configured according to the particular needs of each person. Jim and Anne decided together on which reminders they considered as supporting for Anne, and Jim could easily program the chosen reminders, such as reminding Anne to eat her meals or brush her teeth as she often forgets these activities." [24]

Table 3. Top 4 list of preferred ICT-solutions by people with dementia and their carers on the three test-sites

COGKNOW area of support Focus	TOP4 Amsterdam	TOP4 Belfast	TOP4 Luleå	CONCLUSION on TOP4 for first field test after feasibility check with system designers
Support for memory Reminding and remembering	Reminder activities/ appointments/taking medicine. The solution should preferably be stationary with touch screen as well as mobile: e.g. Neuropage [9,33]	Item locator, misplacement of items is a key early, and almost universal, symptom of a dementing illness – reflected in the Belfast workshops and literature review (see SMART home, BIME (Bath Institute of Medical Engineering)	Activity reminder/ electronic calendar, stationary device with touch screen	Reminding functionality + locator mobile COGKNOW device Examples in literature: Neuropage, electronic calendar (ENABLE project: see also http://www.ihagen.no/english.htm http://www.enableproject.org/html/products.html)
Support for social contacts Enable communication with family and friends	Picture dialling function on touch screen integrated within the screen of the stationary device of the reminding system (i.e. not as a separate pictophone)	Electronic calendar with emphasis on appointments and social activities pending. Usefulness emphasized in workshops and within research community; see Forget-me-not http://www.ihagen.no/engl ish.htm	Picture dialling function on touch screen integrated within the screen of the stationary device of the reminding system (i.e. not as a separate pictophone)	Picture dialling functionality Examples in literature: - Photodialler (http://www.ellisenviro.com/news.html) - Photophone (http://www.unisar.com/shoponline.asp?point=m oreinfo&catid=&id=127)(http://www.enableproje ct.org/html/products.html) - Photo contacts (mobile): (http://www.pocketx.net/smartphone/photocontac ts.html)

Table 3. (Continued)

COGKNOW area of support Focus	TOP4 Amsterdam	TOP4 Belfast	TOP4 Luleå	CONCLUSION on TOP4 for first field test after feasibility check with system designers
Support with daily activities Help execute activities that provide pleasure, recreational activities, useful activities	Support for activities for pleasure: e.g. picture gramophone ENABLE-project [34] integrated within touch screen of activity reminder or picture of TV on touch screen that starts the TV when touched	Pill dispenser – medication management issue identified as an important "daily activity" particularly within workshops and concerning elderly persons generally [35]	Support for activities for pleasure: e.g. picture of TV on touch screen of the stationary device of the activity reminder that starts the TV when touched	Support functionality for activities for pleasure on stationary device with touch screen to turn on e.g. radio/TV media playback Examples in literature: picture gramophone (ENABLE project: http://www.enableproject.org/html/products.html
Enhance feelings of safety Prevent people with dementia from experiencing anxious or dangerous situations	Support during cooking e.g. Cooker usage monitor ENABLE project [26]. Signal on stationary and mobile activity reminder device or Warning to close door/ take things outside such as keys or simple mobile phone with or without GPS: e.g. Mobile Coach [36]	Picture telephone identified in workshop discussions and see Mobile Telecoach [36]	Reminder to turn devices off on stationary device, for example the cooker (not as a separate artefact, but as a function within the activity reminder system) or Direct or easy contact possibilities to a service or emergency line (not as a separate artefact, but as a function within the reminder system)	Warning to close and/or lock front door Reminder to take mobile phone outside Easy emergency contact

For the area 'support for social contact', a picture dialling function was agreed upon to facilitate making or receiving phone calls. The picture dialling service aims to support the persons with dementia in calling a person by simply pressing on his/her picture, either on the stationary device or on the mobile device, without having to remember or dial any phone number. In the following excerpt of a scenario, the use of the picture dialling function is illustrated:

> "Jim had inserted photographs of their children in the COGKNOW Day Navigator so that Anne could phone them easily by touching the screen when she felt alone or insecure in the absence of her husband. She is then quickly connected and if her daughter cannot answer the phone, Anne can easily contact another person using the picture dialling contact list." [24]

To support people with dementia with 'daily activities' it was decided to develop an entertainment service in the form of a radio control and music player. It enables people with dementia to engage in pleasurable activities, such as listening to music or to the radio, which they cannot carry out on their own anymore, because they have difficulty operating devices. Again, an excerpt of the developed scenarios in this case a 74 year old widower living alone:

> "The COGKNOW Day Navigator asks Martin whether he wants to listen to the music or the radio. Martin decides to listen to the radio and presses the radio picture on the touch screen of the tablet PC. For music, he simply has to touch the music notes symbol and previously programmed pieces are replayed. In case he is not content with the music piece that the system plays, all Martin has to do is double click on the music notes picture and the next song is played." [24]

For the final area, 'enhance feelings of safety', a warning service to detect open or closed doors was agreed upon. Additionally, it was decided to install an emergency call function in the system so that the persons with dementia would be able to call for help easily. The warning service should offer audio and visual warnings, available on both the stationary and the mobile device.

In the following scenario excerpt about Martin, the male widower living alone, it is explained how the warning service and emergency function could be of help.

> "Due to his forgetfulness, Martin frequently forgets to close his front door, which is then left open all day long and sometimes during the night as well. Since Martin has been using the COGKNOW Day Navigator he is reminded to close the door in case he has forgotten to do so. The COGKNOW warning service alerts Martin with a beep to close the door." [24]

> "In case Martin falls or some other emergency situation occurs, Martin can easily call for help. By simply pressing the emergency button on the stationary or mobile device, the system automatically connects him with his son, the agreed primary contact in case of emergency. If his son is not available, the system automatically connects Martin with another contact."

CONCLUSION

This article describes the development process of an ICT solution aimed to help persons with dementia experience more autonomy and an enhanced quality of life. Right from the start of the COGKNOW project, persons with dementia and their carers were involved in the development process that consists of three iterations in which user-needs are assessed and consequently discussed among clinical dementia experts and technological system designers to ensure a good translation of needs into functional requirements and design specifications. This paper focused on the first iteration of the study.

In the area of memory, persons with dementia preferred support with remembering daily activities, the location of items, and switching off devices in the home. In the area of social contact, people wished to be supported in maintaining contact with their social network. In the area of daily activities, people wanted to be supported in performing these activities more independently. The need to feel safe became apparent from persons with dementia reporting feelings of insecurity and uncertainty. Dangers resulting from forgetting to switch off appliances or close the door were particularly relevant to both people with dementia and their carers.

People with dementia and carers preferred the following ICT solutions: reminders for activities, the time and an item locator; a simple solution for contacting family members such as a picture dialling phone; assistance with turning on music or television; and an automatic switch-off for devices. Across and within the sites there were differences and similarities regarding the expressed needs and preferences, which reflect the variety of disabilities and preferences for support within the target group. Differences seemed to be related to several aspects, such as living alone or together with an informal carer, cultural differences (e.g. used to handle mobile phones), age and gender. Because of the small group size it was not possible to study this in more detail. Future research is recommended.

Finally, taking into account the (cognitive) disabilities of persons with dementia and the technical feasibility of developing solutions within the time frame of the project, it was decided that for the first prototype of the cognitive prosthetic ICT device the following functions would be developed: In the area of remembering, a day and time indication, a find mobile service and reminding service; in the area of social contact a picture dialling function; in the area of daily activities a media playback and radio function; and in the area of safety a warning device for an open front door and an emergency contact service.

The preferred ICT solutions inventoried in the study correspond partly with other studies among persons with dementia [6], e.g. aids for reminding appointments of activities like NeuroPage [33], Electronic Memory Aids (EMA) [9,37], an Electronic agenda [38] or calendar [39], and aids to find items [7]. To enhance communication, simple photo phones [40], videophones [41] or mobile phones were proposed and tested [7,8]. Technological support for leisure activities were recommended by Sixsmith et al. [40] and Wherton et al. [42], and amongst others an activity guidance system with music and sung messages [43] and a picture gramophone were tested [7]. To enhance feelings of safety, several Global Positioning Systems to locate elderly persons with cognitive impairments were developed, such as GPS Columba [44], and Keruve [45]. Also, monitoring systems inside and outside the house were tested in which alarm messages are forwarded in case of potentially dangerous behaviour of the person with dementia [46, 47]. When persons with dementia accept such solutions, these may enhance their experienced autonomy, help them to keep in contact with family and friends, help them in engaging in useful activities and enhance their feelings of safety. All these domains are considered important determinants of quality of life by people with dementia [48].

The COGKNOW system is specifically intended for persons with mild dementia, but it will be a challenge to develop a system that also helps people in the more severe stages of dementia to stay at home with the maintenance of their autonomy and quality of life. This is the aim of the European Ambient Assisted Living project ROSETTA, in which the COGKNOW system will be integrated in an activity guidance and awareness service that intends to help people with progressive chronic disabilities, such as Alzheimer's Disease and Parkinson's Disease, to live independently as long as possible [49].

Although the study was set up carefully, there were some limitations. First of all, the needs assessment was conducted among groups of people with dementia and informal carers in three Northern European countries. People from other parts of Europe were not represented in the study sample. Therefore the study results are not necessarily valid for people with dementia living in other parts of Europe. We tried to compose a varied group by randomly recruiting persons with dementia and carers who differed in characteristics that might be related to needs, e.g.: age, gender, living alone or together with the carer, type of relationship between persons with dementia and carer, and rural or non-rural living area. Nevertheless, the majority of the recruited persons with dementia were married and lived together with the carer. This may have caused an underrepresentation of needs and wishes experienced by people with dementia who live alone. Some persons in the very early stages of dementia felt they did not need support yet. On the other hand, these persons were able to articulate clearly what they found important in their daily life and imagine what might be useful to them in the future. Another limitation of the study was that not all workshops and interviews were conducted separately for people with dementia and their carers. Especially in Northern Ireland participants preferred combined home interviews. This might have led to a domination of the carers' opinion on (unmet) needs.

Our experiences in this study reflect the view that it is important to assess and understand in-depth the needs and wishes of persons with dementia and their preferences for ICT solutions. It helps to understand how to translate these needs into functional requirements when developing assistive technology for this target group. Besides that, to increase the chance of developing an ICT device that would be useful for people with mild dementia in general, the COGKNOW project focused on four need areas that in a large-scale survey of one of the COGKNOW consortium partners were identified as frequently unmet in people with dementia [20]. Subsequently, the final plans for developing assistive technology in the COGKNOW need areas were based both on the results of the user workshops and interviews in our study, and on research findings regarding the use of assistive technology in dementia as described in the literature [6, 34-36]. Finally, the project provides two more iterative cycles in which new participants will be included/recruited and user needs inquiry workshops will be conducted again.

As the development of an ICT product is a long and complex process, it is advisable to involve potential users in different phases of this process, to attune the ICT product as much as possible to the needs and wishes of the future users and to make it more user friendly and useful. Within COGKNOW, the needs and wishes of the persons with mild dementia and the carers are assessed at the start of the prototype development as well as in later stages. The developmental method applied in COGKNOW is best typified as a user-participatory approach [50], firstly because the four target areas chosen for development of the ICT device were based on findings from research on needs reported by persons with dementia themselves, secondly because the needs and potential ICT solutions were elaborated by interviewing potential end-users, and thirdly because the prototype is also evaluated by end-users by means of field tests. The data collected among the users will be used as input for the further development of the device.

We aim to develop our ICT solution for people with mild dementia living in the community. However, it is anticipated that because of the variability even in people with mild dementia, (e.g. in cognitive disabilities, mobility and living circumstances), ICT solutions need to be adaptable to needs and preferences of individual persons with dementia and their carers. These personalization aspects will be further explored in the project. In the final stage of the study the ICT solution will be evaluated on user-friendliness, usefulness and impact on autonomy and quality of life of the persons with dementia.

Besides the involvement of potential end-users, we also recommend a multidisciplinary team approach: only clinical researchers and technological system designers working together will be able to translate the needs of persons with dementia into functional requirements of assistive technology.

Another issue is the potential acceptance and implementation of the developed ICT solution in daily practice. This issue will also be addressed in the project, by studying viable business models for the COGKNOW device during workshops and interviews [51]. For instance, pricing and division of roles will be discussed among local stakeholders, insurers, patient organisations and governmental parties.

To conclude, both a user-participatory design and a multidisciplinary approach may help to develop more user friendly and useful products for persons with dementia and their carers, that will gain easier acceptance by the target group. Acceptance is an important precondition for effectively integrating technological applications as an additional means of supporting people with dementia at home.

ACKNOWLEDGMENTS

We thank all persons with dementia and their carers who participated in the workshops and interviews in Amsterdam, Belfast and Luleå. We also thank our colleagues from the University of Ulster who provided us with visual aids (images/cartoons) for the workshops. The COGKNOW project is mainly funded by the European Commission's Information Society Technologies (IST) programme under grant 034025.

REFERENCES

[1]   Ferri, C.P., Prince, M., Brayne, C., Brodaty, H., Fratiglioni, L., Ganguli, M., et al. (2005). Global prevalence of dementia: a Delphi consensus study. *Lancet, 366*, 2112-17.

[2]   Health Council Netherlands (2002). *Dementia.* The Hague: Health Council of the Netherlands.

[3]   ASTRID (2000). *ASTRID: A guide to using technology within dementia care.* London: Hawker publications.

[4]   Schuurman, J.G., Moelaert El-Hadidy, F., Krom, A., Walhout, B. (2007). *Ambient Intelligence* [in Dutch]. Den Haag: Rathenau Instituut.

[5]   Sixsmith, A.J., Gibson, G., Orpwood, R.D., Torrington, J.M. (2007). Developing a technology 'wish-list' to enhance the quality of life of people with dementia. *Gerontechnology, 26,* 2-19.

[6]   Lauriks, S., Reinersmann, A., Van der Roest, H.G., Meiland, F.J.M., Davies, R.J., Moelaert, F., et al. (2007). Review of ICT-based services for identified unmet needs in people with dementia. *Ageing Research Reviews, 6,* 223-246.

[7]   Gilliard, J., Hagen, I. (2004). *Enabling technologies for people with dementia.* Cross-national analysis report. D4.4.1. QLK-CT-2000-00653,1-69.

[8]   Ager, A., Aalykke, S., (2001). TASC: A microcomputer support system for persons with cognitive disabilities. *British Journal of Education Technology,32,* 373–377.

[9]   Wilson, B.A., Emslie, H.C., Quirk, K., Evans, J.J. (2001). Reducing everyday memory and planning problems by means of a paging system: a randomised control crossover study. *Journal of Neurology, Neurosurgery and Psychiatry, 70*(4), 477-82.

[10] Woolham, J., 2005. *Safe at Home.* In: The effectiveness of assistive technology in supporting the independence of people with dementia: the Safe at Home project, Hawker Publications, London.

[11] Orpwood, R., Gibbs, C., Adlam, T., Faulkner, R., Meegahawatte, D. (2005). The design of smart homes for people with dementia – user interface aspects. *Universal Access in the Information Society, 4,*156-64.

[12] Hagen, I., Holthe, T., Duff, P., Cahill, S. Gilliard, J. Orpwood, R., et al. (2002). A systematic assessment of assistive technology. *Journal of dementia care,10,* 26-8.

[13] Nygard, L., Starkhammar, S. (2007). The use of everyday technology by people with dementia living alone: Mapping out the difficulties. *Aging and Mental Health, 11,* 144-55.

[14] Nugent, C.D. (2007). ICT in the elderly and dementia. Editorial. *Aging and Mental Health, 11* (5), 473-6.

[15] Astell, A.J. (2006). Technology and personhood in dementia care. *Quality in Ageing, 7,* 15-25.

[16] Cash, M. (2003). Assistive technology and people with dementia. *Reviews in clinical gerontology, 13,* 313-19.

[17] Mountain, G. (2006). Self-management for people with early dementia: an exploration of concepts and supporting evidence. *Dementia, 5,* 429.

[18] Nygård, L. (2008).The meaning of everyday technology as experienced by people with dementia who live alone. *Dementia, 7,* 481-502.

[19] Sixsmith, A., Sixsmith, J. (2000). Smart technologies: meeting whose needs? *Journal of Telemedicine and Telecare, 6* (Suppl. 1), 190-92.

[20] Van der Roest, H.G., Meiland, F.J.M., Comijs, H., Derksen, E., Jansen, A.P.D., Van Hout, H.P.J., et al. (2009). What do community dwelling people with dementia need? A survey of those who are known to care and welfare services. *International Psychogeriatrics, 21*(5), 949-65.

[21] Dröes, R.M., Meiland, F.J.M., Van der Roest, H.G., Maroccini, R., Slagter, R., Baida, Z., et al. (2005). *Opportunities for we-centric service bundling in dementia care.* Amsterdam: Freeband Frux Projectpartners.

[22] Van der Roest, H.G., Meiland, F.J.M., Maroccini, R., Comijs, H.C., Jonker, C., Dröes, R.M. (2007). Subjective needs of people with dementia: a review of the literature. *International Psychogeriatrics, 19,* 559-592.

[23] Steen, M., Faber, E., Bouwman, H. (2008). Methods for human centered service design. In E. Faber, H. de Vos (Eds). *Creating successful ICT services, practical guidelines based on the STOF method.* Enschede: Telematica Instituut.

[24] Hettinga, M., Andersson, A.L., Dröes, R.M., Meiland, F.J.M., Armstrong, E., Bergvall-Kåreborn, B., et al. (2007). *COGKNOW Project, Deliverable 1.4.1. Functional Requirements Specification.* COGKNOW consortium.

[25] Reisberg, B., Ferris, S., De Leon, M.J., Crook, T. (1982). The Global Deterioration Scale for Assessment of Primary Degenerative Dementia. *American Journal of Psychiatry, 139,*1136-1139.

[26] Reynolds, T., Thornicroft, G., Abas, M., Woods, B., Hoe, J., Leese, M., et al. (2000). Camberwell Assessment of Need for the Elderly (CANE): Development, validity and reliability. *British Journal of Psychiatry, 176,* 444-452.

[27] Dröes, R. M., Van Hout, H. P.J., Van der Ploeg, E.S. (2004). *Camberwell Assessment of Need for the Elderly (CANE).* Revised Version (IV). Amsterdam: VU University medical center, Department of Psychiatry, EMGO institute.

[28] Lindeboom, J., Ter Horst, R., Hooyer, C., Dinkgreve, M., Jonker, C. (1993). Some psychometric properties of the CAMCOG. *Psychological Medicine, 23,* 213-9.

[29] Meiland, F.J.M., Dröes, R.M. (2006). *Experienced Autonomy.* VU University medical center, Department of Psychiatry, EMGO institute, Amsterdam.

[30] Pearlin, L.I., Schooler, C. (1978). The structure of coping. *Journal of Health and Social Behavior, 19,* 2-21.

[31] WHO SRPB Quality of Life group (2002). *WHOQOL-SRPB Field test instrument.* Department of Mental Health and Substance dependence, WHO, Geneva, Switzerland.

[32] Thorgrimsen, L., Selwood, A., Spector, A., Royan, L., De Madariaga Lopez, M., Woods, R.T., et al. (2003). Who's Quality of life is it anyway? The validity and reliability of the Quality of Life-Alzheimer's Disease (QoL-AD) scale. *Alzheimer Disease and Associated Disorders, 17,* 201-8.

[33] Hersh, N.A., Treadgold, L.G., (1994). NeuroPage: the rehabilitation of memory dysfunction by prosthetic memory and cueing. *Neurorehabilitation 4,* 187–197.

[34] Adlam, T., Faulkner, R., Orpwood, R., Jones, K., Macijauskiene, J., Budraitiene, A., et al. (2004). The installation and support of internationally distributed equipment for people with dementia. *IEEE Transactions on Information Technology in Biomedicine, 8,* 253-57.

[35] Nugent, C., Finlay, D., Davies, R., Pagetti, C., Tamburini, E., Black, N. (2005). *Can technology improve compliance to medication?* In S. Giroux, H. Pigot (Eds). *From Smart homes to smart Care,* IOS press, pp 65-72.

[36] Kort, S. (2005). *Mobile Coaching. A pilot study into the user-friendliness and effects of Mobile Coaching on the wellbeing of people with dementia and their informal caregivers.* MSc thesis, Amsterdam: Faculty of Psychology, Vrije Universiteit.

[37] Inglis, E.A., Szymkowiak, A., Gregor, P., Newell, A.F., Hine, N., Shah, P., Wilson, B.A., Evans, J., (2003). Issues surrounding the user-centred development of a new interactive memory aid. *Universal Access Information Society 2*, 226–234.

[38] Zanetti, O., Zanieri, G., Vreese, L.P.d., Frisoni, G.B., Binetti, G., Trabucchi, M., (2000). *Utilizing an electronic memory aid with Alzheimer's disease patients. A study of feasibility.* In: Paper presented at the Sixth International Stockholm/Springfield Symposium on Advances in Alzheimer Therapy.

[39] Holte, T., Hagen, I., Björneby, S., (1998). *Evaluation of an electronic calendar as helping aid for persons suffering from memory problems or cognitive impairment.* Report of the TED-group.

[40] Sixsmith, A., Orpwood, R., Torrington, J. (2007). Quality of life technologies for people with dementia. Topics in geriatric rehabilitation. *Smart technology, 23*, 85-93.

[41] Sävenstedt, S., Brulin, C., Sandman, P.O., 2003. Family members' narrated experiences of communicating via video-phone with patients with dementia staying at a nursing home. *Journal of Telemedicine and Telecare 9*, 216–220.

[42] Wherton, J.P., Monk, A.F. (2008). Technological opportunities for supporting people with dementia who are living at home. *International Journal of Human-Computer studies*, 571-86.

[43] Yasuda, K., Beckman, B., Yoneda, M., Yoneda, H., Iwamoto, A., Nakamura, T., (2006). Successful guidance by automatic output of music and verbal messages for daily behavioural disturbances of three individuals with dementia. *Neuropsychological Rehabilitation, 16*, 66–82.

[44] http://en.eu.medicalmobile.com/iiix/home/

[45] http://www.keruve.com/

[46] Masuda, Y., Yoshimura, T., Nakajima, K., Nambu, M., Hayakawa, T., Tamura, T., (2002). *Unconstrained monitoring of prevention of wandering the elderly.* In: Engineering in Medicine and Biology, 24th Annual Conference and the Annual Fall Meeting of the Biomedical Engineering Society (EMBS/BMES Conference). Proceedings of the Second Joint 2. pp. 1906–1907.

[47] Lin, C.C., Chiu, M.J., Hsiao, C.C., Lee, R.G., Tsai, Y.S., (2006). Wireless health care service system for elderly with dementia. *IEEE Transactions on Information Technology in Biomedicine, 10*, 696–704.

[48] Dröes, R.M., Boelens-van der Knoop, E.C.C., Bos, J., Meihuizen, L. , Ettema, T.P., Gerritsen, D.L., et al. (2006). Quality of life in dementia in perspective. An explorative study of variations in opinions among people with dementia and their professional caregivers and in literature. *Dementia, The International Journal of Social Research and Practice, 5*, 533-58.

[49] ROSETTA. (2008). *ROSETTA (Guidance and Awareness Services for Independent Living).* Research proposal Ambient Assisted Living (AAL) Joint Programme.

[50] Helander, M. (2006). *A guide to human factors and ergnomics.* (2nd ed.) UK: Taylor and Francis group.

[51] Faber, E., de Vos, H. (Eds). (2008). *Creating successful ICT services, practical guidelines based on the STOF method.* Enschede: Telematica Instituut.

In: Dementia: Non-Pharmacological Therapies
Editor: Elisabetta Farina, pp. 93-117

ISBN: 978-1-61470-736-3
© 2012 Nova Science Publishers, Inc.

PHYSICAL AND MENTAL EXERCISE PLUS WORK THERAPY FOR ALZHEIMER'S PATIENTS: A CASE-INSPIRED TREATMENT THAT SLOWED COGNITIVE DECLINE

Sharon Arkin*

University of Arizona, Dept. of Speech and Hearing Sciences
Tucson, Arizona

ABSTRACT

This article advocates for the provision of ongoing multi-component, exercise-based treatments for persons with dementia, and the use of students as interveners. The author will present a first person account of the empirical and serendipitous experiences as Alzheimer caregiver and doctoral student that led to the federally-funded Alzheimer (AD) Rehab by Students (also referred to as Elder Rehab) program she directed at the University of Arizona from 1996 through 2001[1]. Previously published information about this program and its outcomes will be reviewed. Key studies and reports in support of AD Rehab's component interventions: physical exercise, language and memory stimulation activities, and supervised volunteer work, especially those published since 2001, will be cited. Recommendations for replication and expansion of the AD Rehab program model will be offered.

Keywords: Exercise, Language, Work Therapy for Alzheimer's.

INTRODUCTION

According to Alzheimer's disease International (2009), the global prevalence of dementia, predicted at 35 million in 2010, is expected to almost double every 20 years. While researchers search for the "magic bullet" that will slow, halt, or reverse the deterioration wrought by Alzheimer's disease (AD), millions of individuals with this disorder are languishing in nursing homes and exhausting family caregivers. Bereft of former roles and responsibilities that formed their identity and gave meaning to their lives, persons with

---

* Contact Information: Retired from University of Arizona, Private practice psychologist. PsyD, 10402 E. Glenn St. Tucson, Arizona 85749. Phone: 520-760-5595; FAX: 520-298-7811; Email: arkinaz@earthlink.net

dementia typically become socially withdrawn and isolated and dependent on paid caregivers, busy nursing home staff, or overburdened family members to structure and supervise their time and activities. It is not surprising that planning and supervising activities take a back seat to more urgent care giving tasks such as personal care, meal preparation, medical needs, and other family, work, and household responsibilities. Apathy and depression are too often the consequences of the lack of opportunity for persons with dementia to experience success at challenges and to make meaningful societal contributions.

While the cognitive losses associated with AD cannot be reversed, physical fitness, communicative abilities, quality of life and mood of the person with dementia can be enhanced at the same time respite is provided to the caregiver [20]. Evidence from the AD Rehab experience suggests also that the rate of cognitive decline can be slowed [3]. All this can be accomplished at minimal cost through resources available in virtually every community: gyms and fitness centers, community agencies that need volunteers, and potential volunteers among students who (a) in some schools, must do community service as a requirement for high school graduation or as a condition of their financial aid in college or (b) who can earn independent study, service learning, or practicum credit at their college or university by working with a person with dementia, or (c) belong to religious or youth organizations that encourage community service.

The observations and interventions that led to the AD Rehab program model were largely experienced during trial and error experiments with my mother, Bee, diagnosed with probable AD during my 2nd year of doctoral studies in Chicago, and with Dick, a person with dementia I worked with in Orange County, California, during a practicum and internship, and later validated through exhaustive literature searches. Because of the personal nature of this article, it is written largely in the first person.

Guinea Pig Par Excellence: Bee Schultz 1913-1997

> Tall, striking Jewish widow, 75, semi-retired singer (Chicago Symphony Chorus) seeking outgoing, affectionate man for companionship, romance, and mutual pampering. Enjoys symphony, Scrabble, theater, schmoozing, family.

That is how I described my mom (Bee) in a personals ad I composed on her behalf a year after her husband's death and before we realized the extent of her memory impairment.

BACKGROUND

Bee was diagnosed with "very mild cognitive dysfunction consistent with early Alzheimer's Disease" (at Chicago's Rush Alzheimer Center) in June, 1988, at age 75. Bee's tested *memory* functioning was actually at the *moderate* level from the outset. Three months after her diagnosis, she introduced herself to a doorman at my brother's apartment building as Mrs. Fadim (her maiden name). At the time, I wrote in my journal, "I felt like I'd been kicked in the stomach. Her name had been Schultz for 49 years. It seemed like such an ominous sign – pointing to a deterioration/decline that I've been denying …For the first time, she expressed sadness at her inability to remember some of the good times she'd enjoyed with her family..." When I probed, I was shocked to learn that she was unable to name a single magazine she'd ever read, movie or play she'd ever seen, TV personality or show she'd ever watched, song she'd ever sung, or singer she'd ever admired. This was particularly startling given the fact I had lived in the same small apartment with her, helping her care for my dad during five months of his terminal illness. I'd attributed the sameness of the meals she prepared and lack of any but superficial routine conversation to her pre-occupation with caring for my dad.

I immediately made a date to show her videotaped family history interviews I'd conducted with her and my dad and with her and her sister, Shirley, five years previously.

From that day forward, a video camera became part and parcel of all my intervention efforts.

My siblings and I first noticed something was wrong when Bee proved unable to compose a simple thank you note to persons who'd attended our father's funeral. (She used to send us 5-6 page detailed typed letters.) Her poor memory was initially attributed to depression. However, other than a brief period of appropriate sadness over her husband's death, she showed no other signs of a mood disorder.

Bee's Strengths

While not a serious reader, Bee had an exceptional vocabulary and love of words. She always had been proficient at crossword puzzles and Scrabble and quick with puns and double entendres. As a young mother, she had coached all three of her children to become competitive spellers. Well into her dementia, during an eye examination, she recalled (correctly) upon hearing the word *retina*, that I had missed that word in a spelling bee nearly 50 years previously! In her sixties, she had worked as a proofreader. Though much of her post-Alzheimer's conversation was empty and full of platitudes, she retained an ability to make witty remarks even at the moderate-to-severe stage. At the end of a session in which she and some other men and women with dementia in her assisted living residence had been cutting up fruit and arranging platters for their dining room's dinner buffet table, a volunteer said, "Look at the fruits of your labors." Bee, who hadn't said a word the whole afternoon, piped up, "You mean the fruits of your neighbors!" Another time, in response to my sister who had been bragging about the "healthy" chicken dinner she'd just served, Bee said, "That chicken is not healthy. It is very dead!" She also had an exceptional spatial ability. Once, while she was being videotaped, I asked her to trace the number of her new apartment in the air as an aid to remembering it. She traced it *backwards,* pointed to the camera and said, "So you can see it!"

Bee's most outstanding and durable talent was music. She'd been a semi-professional choral and solo singer most of her life, most proudly as member of the Chicago Symphony chorus. Three years after her diagnosis, she resumed playing the piano after a lapse of several years, inspired by a visit to the home of Boston Philharmonic Symphony conductor Ben Zander whom she helped rehearse for a piano concert by turning the pages of his sheet music. Through determined practice, she perfected the performance of four classical pieces which, eventually, became so preservative, that the management of her residence had to remove the piano from its lobby!

Intervention

Bee became my motivation to specialize in the treatment of AD. She was a willing subject for practice in test administration and an enthusiastic "guinea pig" for various mini-experiments. For two years, I intervened personally, challenging her with word games and fluency exercises, getting her involved in swimming, social and volunteer activities, taking her on trips, and creating multi-media memory aids. One such aid was a "This is Your Life" photo-illustrated memory book with captions in the first person that she could read aloud in a conversational manner. She'd often recount associated memories as she was reading the book aloud. A short film about making such a book was produced by Michelle Bourgeois [4].

I think Bee regarded the various exercises as games, such as the ones we used to play during rides in the car when I was a child. I also think she reveled in the attention from me, the daughter who had lived far away for all of her adult life.

When my studies required me to move from Chicago, I hired a local college student to carry out rehab activities which I assigned and monitored by mail. Examples of verbal fluency and memory exercises used with Bee, plus others later incorporated into the AD Rehab treatment protocol, may be seen on the AD (Elder) Rehab website: www.u.arizona.edu/~sarkin/elderrehab.html

Sufficient exemplars of each activity for 10 treatment sessions may be found in a resource manual that is part of a continuing education correspondence course "Language-Enriched Exercise for Clients with Alzheimer's Disease"   which is available from Desert Southwest Fitness in Tucson, Arizona [5].

Bee's Research Participation

Memory Training

Bee was a subject in two published research studies. The first was on explicit learning and relearning of personally significant information via tape recorded narratives and strategically placed questions. The method was an outgrowth of work I'd done with another client, Dick, in California. One day, while videotaping Dick taking a quiz on an outing he'd recently experienced, it was apparent that he remembered almost nothing of the experience. I decided to restart the quiz, this time providing the correct answer to each question he couldn't answer. I then gave the videotape to Dick's wife and instructed her to play it for him a few times until my next visit. After having gotten only 8 items out of 19 correct initially, he got all 19 correct after four viewings of the tape.

That became the basis for a series of audiotapes I prepared for my mother to orient her to my leaving Chicago and to her imminent move to a retirement building. Because she quickly learned and retained 10 out of 10 new facts on one tape and 14 out of 15 on another after 8-10 practices, I decided to test the method, under single subject experimental conditions, as my doctoral dissertation research. Both Bee and another subject learned or relearned and retained 2 sets of 6-10 personally significant facts after six practice sessions for each set [6]. Similar results were achieved in 22 replications, seven of them by students working with AD Rehab participants [7, 8, and 9]. Portions of a sample script may be seen in Appendix A.

Bee was proud of her achievements in memory training and participated with me in demonstrations at a national psychology conference and at an Alzheimer support group meeting.

Implicite Learning

Bee's second experimental involvement was in an implicit learning experiment in which repeated exposure to a category of items on a picture naming and quiz study task resulted in subsequent production on a verbal fluency test of items from that category that had been on the study task, but never previously produced on 18 pre-exposure fluency tests. Significant explicit learning also occurred on the study task [10]. This experiment was subsequently replicated successfully with seven Elder Rehab participants using a different category of objects [11]. The study task which, in the two research projects, consisted of pictures of and questions about clothing and jewelry and animals, respectively, was used during the Elder Rehab project using the categories *modes of transportation* and *occupations*.

Progression

Three and a half years after Bee's initial diagnosis, David Bennett, her neurologist at Chicago's Rush Alzheimer Center wrote: "Basically, there was no change over the previous testing, and her (test) scores actually remain relatively unchanged over the last few years since she's been coming here...." Six months previously, he'd noted, "Conversational language remains fluent and generally coherent, and performance on various linguistic tasks remains within the average to superior range."

A report by Rodman Shankle, neurologist with the University of California/ Irvine's Alzheimer's Disease Diagnostic and Treatment Center, who assessed her in December, 1989, and again in October, 1991, noted in 1991 that her annual decline on the Mini-Mental State exam [12] was one point, whereas "usually we expect to see a 3 to 4 point drop...for every passing year." Bee hovered at the mild to moderate stage for about 7 years. By 1995, 7 years after her initial diagnosis, her MMSE score had dropped to 14 from 24. After that, her decline became more rapid. Mood was positive, but insight very poor during those first years. She'd respond to questions about her current activities with answers that were true of her pre-dementia life, but no longer true. Curiously and chillingly, she demonstrated insight when she was at the severe stage and almost mute. I overheard her mutter: "I'm not here anymore; I'm dead already."

Bee died two weeks shy of her 84th birthday, nine years after she was tentatively diagnosed with AD. Brain autopsy confirmed the diagnosis. Her brother, three years her senior, who died three months before her, was also found to have the plaques and tangles associated with AD, though he'd also had bipolar disorder and had a history of excessive drinking. Her younger sister, who died in August, 2009, at age 86, had just begun to exhibit signs of dementia. Her brain autopsy indicated the presence of Alzheimer's type pathology. The brains of all three siblings are part of the multi-site Alzheimer's Disease Genetics Research Study and I and my two siblings and first cousin have all agreed to participate in that study through the Rush Alzheimer Center.

Volunteers in Partnership: Precursor to AD Rehab by Students

The AD Rehab program grew out of a small pilot project that took place in 1994 during my post-doctoral fellowship at the department of Speech and Hearing Sciences at the University of Arizona. With the guidance of my department head, Audrey Holland, a renowned physiologist, I developed a language-focused intervention that drew upon her academic and my practical experience. Named "Volunteers in Partnership" or "VIP", the program ran for two semesters, each with six early stage persons with dementia who were matched one-to-one with undergraduate students from the speech and hearing sciences and psychology departments [13]. Each semester, the program provided participants with ten weekly sessions of 30-40 minutes of language-strengthening exercises administered by their student partner. Settings for the interventions were several non-profit community agencies where each 2-person team contributed an hour of volunteer service each week. During the first semester, all the volunteer work was done at a child daycare center near campus. Participants read stories to small groups of children. During the second semester, volunteer sites also included a nursing home, a community food bank, and an animal shelter.

Outcome measures were language-oriented: performance on a discourse battery, analyzed by a system developed for this project and used later in the AD Rehab program [14, 15], a proverb interpretation task, and a picture description task. The picture descriptions were scored according to guidelines in the manual of the Aphasia Diagnostic Battery (ADP) [16]; proverb interpretations were scored according to guidelines published by Ulatowska and colleagues [17]. Small to massive gains in number of substantive on-topic statements were achieved by seven out of 11 participants who completed the program.

Eight improved on picture description and eight on proverb interpretation [13]. Stimulus questions contained in the discourse battery and the proverbs and picture description task used may be seen in Appendix B.

AD Rehab by Students

The AD Rehab program had three main components: physical fitness training, cognitive-linguistic exercises, and supervised volunteer work. A sub-group of 7 of the first 11 participants also participated in the author's previously-described audio-assisted biographical memory training [8, 9]. Occasionally, a cultural or recreational activity was substituted for a session of volunteer work.

The major change in the AD Rehab program from its predecessor was the addition of the physical exercise component. This addition, which turned out to be the component most valued by the caregivers and the greatest source of pride for participants, was unplanned. It came about after I noticed that a new state-of-the-art fitness center was being installed at the University Medical Center at the University of Arizona. It occurred to me that regular physical exercise would be beneficial whether or not the other interventions worked. I asked the Center's director if my study participants could work out there twice a week with one-to-one supervision by their student partner or family members. He readily agreed. Furthermore, he helped me design a suitable regimen of aerobics, flexibility, balance, and weight training, consistent with guidelines of the American College of Sports Medicine for the elderly [18] and assigned staff to help me train each semester's new cohort of students.

Rational for a Multi-Component Intervention

When The AD Rehab program was conceived back in 1995, the terms multi-component and non-pharmacological had not yet entered the common parlance of Alzheimer researchers or clinicians. Research focus back then was on drug studies. As I was a non-physician, drugs were not in my toolkit and, in any case, were not yet in general use for managing AD. As a caregiver and doctoral student, intern, and post-doc, I had experimented with interventions and found some that persons with dementia enjoyed and caregivers appreciated.

All of them had involved one-to-one attention from a student, structured conversational interaction, and involvement in activities outside the home and/or being helpful to others. Several important practical considerations influenced the design of the AD Rehab protocol. Using community volunteer sites for interventions permitted the tailoring of treatment to the respective interests of participants, educated the community to the preserved skills of people with dementia, and gave respite to caregivers. The structured language exercises eliminated the need for students to struggle to "make conversation" with individuals whose ability to initiate and sustain non-repetitive substantive discourse was impaired. When the exercise component was added, the language exercises served to prevent boredom and provide distraction from fatigue during lengthy sessions on the treadmill and exercise bike.

The positive experiences with the VIP program elements were enough for me to want to test them formally. The VIP program took place while I was in an already-funded post-doc position and did not require any justification other than the approval of my department head, who had participated actively in designing the project.

However, the obtaining of a grant to fund AD Rehab and the demands of academic writing required a search of the literature to provide a theoretical rationale for the AD Rehab multi-component program model.

Rational for Language Stimulation Activities

Epidemiological research has found that involvement in cognitively stimulating activities is associated with a reduced risk of developing dementia. Verghese et al., who studied 469 adults in the Bronx, NY between 1980 and 1983, found specific associations between reading, playing board games, and playing a musical instrument and the lowered risk [19]. Wilson et al., who studied members of Catholic religious orders for seven years, found a similar association [20]. Valenzuela et al. found an association between a high level of mental activity and a reduced rate of hippocampal atrophy and suggested that neuroprotection in medial temporal lobe may be one mechanism underlying the link between mental activity and lower rates of dementia observed in population-based studies [21]. It stands to reason that activities that seem to be neuroprotective in non-demented populations would be beneficial to people with already compromised cognitive abilities.

In the late 1980's, when I began working with my mother, I could only find two published articles about treatment studies for Alzheimer's persons with dementia that mentioned language activities [22,23]. Neither included description of the activities sufficient to permit replication. However, in the 1990's, speech pathologists began focusing attention on the study, assessment, and treatment of the language disorders of dementia.

In 1990, Michelle Bourgeois began publishing articles on useful and replicable techniques for enhancing communications skills of Alzheimer persons with dementia, such as memory wallets and memory books [24, 25, and 26].

In 1993, Bayles and Tomoeda published the Arizona Battery for Communication Disorders of Dementia, a comprehensive language assessment battery [27]. Other speech pathologists focused on the study and analysis of specific types of discourse production by dementia (Delete word in red.) persons with dementia, such as proverb interpretation [17].

A comprehensive literature review of cognitive interventions with aging and demented populations was published by Acevedo and Loewenstein in 2007 [29]. The section on interventions with older adults with Alzheimer's disease reviewed 37 articles. Most of those dealt with individual cognitive processes, were short-term, cross-sectional, theoretical or laboratory-based, rather than clinical in orientation, or were reviews of past studies. Several techniques based on past research they reviewed have been applied in clinical practice. The spaced retrieval technique, first described by Landauer and Bjork in 1978 [30] (and used, in fixed interval form, in my memory training method) has been applied by Camp and colleagues to aid in recall of practical information [31]. Relatively preserved procedural memory abilities have been tapped by Zanetti et al. [32,33], Farina et al. [34,35], Lowenstein et al. [36] and Spector et al. [37], for teaching functional activities of daily living, dance steps [38] and use of a mobile phone [39]. The authors also cite several promising multimodal cognitive rehabilitation models, such as the Quayhagens' caregiver-implemented programs [40, 41] and a review of such programs [42].

In conclusion, they point out that most of the studies are limited in that they deal with single cognitive processes and simple ADLs, whereas most real-world tasks are complex. They also cite the need for inclusion of compensatory strategies and the training of family members or caregivers who can continue interventions when a research study is completed.

AD Rehab took a broad and longitudinal approach to cognitive-linguistic interventions and assessment and provided the compensatory aids and caregiver involvement which Acevedo and Loewenstein recommend. Fourteen different conversation- and memory-stimulating strategies were employed. Students solicited their partners 'opinions on adult and controversial topics that tapped into preserved value systems rather than depending on weakened episodic memory. Participants were also involved in "real-world" tasks through their supervised volunteer experiences and regular workouts in a fitness center that served medical students, university hospital employees and post-surgery patients, as well as persons with dementia. Family members were trained to supervise one physical fitness workout per week, but enjoyed respite from care giving during the two student-supervised treatment sessions per week. Most significant, participants were able to remain in the program for as long as they were able to take part (within the four funded operational years).

In addition to doing annual assessment using a battery of standardized neuropsychological, mood, and fitness tests, discourse on a variety of topics was systematically elicited and analyzed for up to four years on some persons with dementia. Seven participants received training on customized biographical memory tapes. All participants had memory books created by one of their student partners. Certificates of achievement and award ribbons were presented to all participants at a special luncheon at the conclusion of each semester that was attended by student partners and family members.

Rational for Physical Exercise

While the general benefits of exercise for reducing the negative effects of aging [43] and its benefits in the prevention of specific illnesses such as cardio-vascular disease [44] and diabetes [45] have been widely publicized, the AD Rehab program had already ended when articles began appearing that associated physical activity in early- and mid-life with a reduced risk of dementia in later life.

The Canadian Study of Health and Aging studied more than 6400 individuals aged 65 years or over for 5 years and found that high levels of physical activity in earlier life correlated with reduced risks of dementia [46]. A study of 6000 women over age 65 which tracked their physical activity habits for eight years found that women who walked the most were least likely to show cognitive decline[47] Two 2004 studies published in JAMA, involving more than 18,000 elderly women [48] and 2257 men [49] replicated that study's results.

Animal researchers have found several possible explanations for the cognitive benefits of exercise. One study found that running fostered neurogenesis and learning in mice [50]. Another found that wheel-running mice had an increase in brain-derived neurotrophic factor (BDNF), a molecule that fosters learning and protects neurons against degeneration that leads to cognitive decline [51]. Other researchers have found that people who experience "silent strokes" have twice the risk of developing dementia, so that exercise that increases blood flow to the brain can reduce the risk of developing Alzheimer's [52].

A 2005 study by Adlard et al. found that providing an enriched environment (i.e. toys, running wheels) for transgenic mice with AD-like brain amyloidosis reduced amyloid deposition and beta amyloid levels [53].

In 2006, Colcombe and colleagues reported that non-demented volunteers aged 60-79 who participated in six months of aerobic exercise showed a significant increase in brain volume [54].

An exhaustive review of English language studies on the relation of physical activity to Alzheimer's disease was published in 2008 in the Journal of the American Medical Directors Association [55]. Citing 160 published papers: epidemiological studies, short-term randomized clinical trials in non-demented persons, and animal research, the authors concluded:

> Regular physical activity is a key component of successful aging. In addition to its convincing multiple benefits, increasing evidence suggests that an active life has a protective effect on brain functioning in the elderly population. Physical activity may also slow down the course of AD. p.401.

Most of the intervention studies reviewed were on frail, severely demented nursing home populations, were of short duration, and did not report standardized measures of physical fitness or multiple cognitive measures before and after intervention.

Spanish researchers Perez and Cancela Carral published a review and analysis in 2008 of eight clinically relevant exercise intervention studies with Alzheimer's persons with dementia, including the AD Rehab study [56]. Four of the studies, (by Rolland et al. [57], Williams and Tappen [58], Namazi et al. [59], and another by Rolland et al. [60], were conducted in nursing homes, presumably on moderate to severe stage persons with dementia. Two (by Teri et al. [61,62], and the AD Rehab study), were with community dwelling and, presumably, mild to moderate persons with dementia, and one, by Palleschi [63], did not specify participants' residential status. The two outpatient studies by Teri and associates provided aerobic and strength and flexibility exercises and resulted in improved mood and behavior. Palleschi's study, which utilized an arms only bicycle, resulted in improved attention, verbal, and cognitive performance after three months of thrice-weekly exercise. The other study by Rolland et al. [60] utilized seven weeks of daily aerobic exercise only and reported improved cognitive and behavioral test performance. The nursing home study by Williams and Tappen found the group that had a combination of walking plus strength and flexibility exercises had better mood outcomes than groups that had just walking or unstructured conversation as interventions.

The AD Rehab study's improved fitness and mood outcomes were reported, but the review did not cite the previously published AD Rehab positive cognitive, memory and discourse outcomes [3,10,14]. These will be republished in the AD Rehab outcomes sections of the present chapter.

The authors concluded that regimens that combine aerobics with strength and flexibility exercises are more beneficial than single modality interventions. As neither of the reviews cited multi-year exercise intervention studies and their effects on fitness. mood, or cognition, the AD Rehab study remains the only one to document significant fitness improvement on standardized measures and non-decline on multiple neurospsychological tests for persons with Alzheimer's disease who exercised regularly from one to four years.

A step by step description of an exercise routine that was successfully used with a nursing home population to reduce adverse behaviors may be found in the article by Namazi and associates [59]. A copy of the exercise protocol used by AD Rehab and which is suitable for mild to moderate stage dementia persons with dementia as well as normal elderly, may be seen at the project's website [1].

Rationale for Partnered Volunteering

The inevitable change in status from worker/homemaker/care provider to care recipient after the onset of dementia creates a vacuum. Opportunities to be useful disappear, along with the positive feedback that the making of social contributions elicit. The status of patient or care recipient engenders feelings of uselessness, depression, and lowered self-esteem and reduced self-confidence.

Such individuals tend to withdraw socially and avoid conversations where their memory and language difficulties may become evident. The Volunteers in Partnership (VIP) Program at the University of Arizona was created to address this situation [16]. That program was the precursor to the subsequent Alzheimer (AD) Rehab by Students program, (often referred to as Elder Rehab to avoid tagging participants with an Alzheimer label).

The idea for supervised volunteer work came from observing that my mother remembered responsibilities towards others better than she remembered personal events, and that she and other persons with dementia got great satisfaction from helping others. During Bee's moderate stage, she'd forget she had visitors the moment after they left, but wouldn't forget to call for her frail and confused friend Billie and escort her to the dining room of their assisted living residence at mealtime.

Bee also remembered to water her plants and happily helped prepare fruit platters with the help of middle school volunteers for her residence's dinner buffet well into her moderate stage. Dick, a physically strong 60 year old with severe visual-spatial and orientation problems, pushed my mother around in a wheelchair during a visit to a zoo that required more walking than she could handle. Dick was given a videotape of that outing. His wife reported that he glowed proudly every time he saw himself pushing Bee around in that chair. When

Dick progressed to the severe stage, his wife was able to keep him calm and occupied by scattering the same bag of leaves on the front lawn for him to rake up each day.

In developing the rationale portion of the grant proposal that resulted in the funding of the Elder Rehab program, I searched the literature for justification of the volunteering component of the program. There was a substantial body of literature which documented the physical and mental health benefits of work [63,64], volunteer work [65], work therapy [66], and socially involving activity [67], for older adults and the mentally ill. Many nursing homes and residential treatment centers employ "work therapy" as key elements of their programs [68,69]. No literature was found that reported cognitive or language improvements as a result of work activities.

In preparation for this article, I again searched the literature using search terms such as volunteer work, work therapy, occupational therapy, work and mental health, work and elderly linked with Alzheimer's and/or dementia. Three references to volunteering among Alzheimer persons with dementia, other than for mention of their being volunteers in drug studies, were found. One was an online article describing a group in England, the Alzheimer's Society's Living with Dementia Working Group, in which early stage persons with dementia participate in planning and conducting educational and supportive activities for people with dementia and their caregivers [70]. Another described an outpatient program of the Rush Alzheimer's Family Care Center in Chicago, no longer in operation, in which small groups of mild to moderate stage persons with dementia were supervised by a social worker in doing volunteer work at a child daycare center [71]. The program was discontinued because of lack of transportation. In 2008, Alzheimer researcher Peter Whitehouse reported the successful use of persons with early stage dementia as reading coaches in a school directed by his wife. [72].

The positive quality-of-life effects of that activity has been documented in the not-yet-published doctoral dissertation of Whitehouse collaborator Danny George, now a faculty member at Penn State university. The award-winning "Buddy" program in Chicago that creates one-to-one relationships between medical student volunteers and persons with Alzheimer type dementia is creative and beneficial, but students, not persons with dementia, are doing the volunteering. That program has been replicated at the Boston University Alzheimer's Center and clearly benefits both medical students and persons with dementia [73].

Several reports of therapeutic work programs with other mental health populations were found. The Veterans' Administration conducted a randomized clinical trial of compensated work therapy among homeless drug-addicted veterans and found that those in the program had fewer drug and alcohol related problems, fewer drug-use related physical problems, fewer episodes of homelessness and incarceration and were more likely to initiate addiction treatment than a control group [74].

A program in Hartford, Connecticut provides one hour of free psychotherapy in exchange for 4 hours of volunteer work [75]. According to the project director, persons in the program have previously shuttled in and out of mental hospitals and suffered the loss of self-esteem that such hospitalization entails. The program "gets them into situations where they are helping others and are being thanked and rewarded with the approval of coworkers."

The National Alliance of the Mentally Ill, a U.S. advocacy group, makes the point eloquently:

Work is at the very core of contemporary life for most people, providing financial security, personal identity, and an opportunity to make meaningful contributions to community life [76].

AD Rehab: Program Operations

Student partners for study participants were recruited, at first, through presentations in speech and hearing sciences classes, later, in freshman chemistry classes (pre-requisite course for all health science majors) and via a listserv for honors students.

Volunteer activities the student-patient teams engaged in included reading to children at child daycare centers, grooming and walking dogs at an animal shelter, bagging beans and rice at a community food bank, stuffing envelopes at a non-profit agency, stamping in new books at a school library, taking a patient's dog to visit a nursing home, picking up trash in public parks, and pushing wheelchair-bound nursing home residents to and from activities and for rides around the grounds.

The students' duties included driving their partner in their (the student's) personal car to and from all activities, supervising and logging their exercise routines, administering memory- and language-stimulation exercises and recording patient responses, transcribing tape-recorded discourse samples, making photo-illustrated "this is your life" memory books, and creating personalized biographical memory tapes for their partners. They also attended a series of instructional seminars and wrote weekly reports about their partner's activities and papers about assigned readings.

Students participated for one semester. Persons with dementia stayed in the program as long as they were able until the four funded years ended. During the four years, 24 individuals completed at least 1 year (2 or 3 semesters), 13 of them completed 2 years (4 or 5 semesters), 8 completed 3 years (6 or 7 semesters), and 4 completed 4 years (8 semesters).

A treatment year consisted of two semesters, each consisting of ten weeks of three 1½-2 hour treatment sessions per week. One physical exercise session plus memory and language exercises and one volunteer work session plus a brisk walk were supervised by a student each week; a second weekly physical exercise session without cognitive activities was supervised by a family member.

Many students cited their VIP or AD Rehab participation in the personal statements they wrote as part of graduate school applications, referring to it as the most significant or meaningful experience in their undergraduate career. Informal follow-up with 15 students I was able to locate 3 or 4 years after their graduation found 11 of them in graduate school or jobs relating to health care or work with the elderly. Close friendships were formed between the students and their partners and with their partners' family members. Caregivers looked upon the students as important sources of support and information about their care recipients' behavior, needs, and accomplishments – an esteem- building role for young people vis-à-vis adults old enough to be their parents or grandparents.

RESULTS: AD REHAB OUTCOMES

The outcome sections of this article are reproduced from a prior publication with permission from Sage Publications [3].

Tests were administered at the end of semesters 2, 4, 6, and 8. Results are reported according to length of participation, with persons completing a given number of years regarded as a cohort, irrespective of when they entered. Physical illness and termination of the program were the main reasons for discontinuance of participation.

As will be seen, effects on global and cognitive functioning were most positive (no significant between year decline on five or six tests) after two or more semesters of participation.

Fitness

AD Rehab participants achieved highly significant fitness gains (p<.001) as measured by a six minute walk test, upper and lower body strength tests using MedX chest press and leg press machines, and in duration of aerobic exercise. Detailed descriptions of the exercise protocol, outcome measures, and results have been previously published [2].

Mood

Mood, as measured by the Geriatric Depression scale (GDS) [77], improved significantly for participants who completed two, three, and four years [2].

Cognitive and Language Outcomes

Paired t-tests were done to derive between-semester change scores for eight of the standardized cognitive tests administered: MMSE, CDR and Sum of Boxes [78,79], Verbal Fluency (Animals) and the 15-Item Boston Naming from the CERAD Neuropsychological Battery [80], ABCD, and the WAIS-R Comprehension and Similarities subtests [81]. Significant annual decline in mental status, as measured by the MMSE, occurred for all cohorts except the four year completers; however the decline, after the first year, was less than that of a similar CERAD group. (See section on AD Rehab and CERAD comparisons.) The mean annual decline in scores on the MMSE was

2.9 points for the one year completers
2.5 for the two-year completers;
2.0 for the three-year completers; and
1.0 for the four- year completers.

Maintenance of function, i.e., no significant between-year decline, on five or six of the cognitive and language measures occurred with cohorts that completed two or more years of participation.

The one-year completers (n=24) had no decline on only two measures: Verbal Fluency (Animals) and WAIS-R Similarities, between baseline and end-of-year one testing. The two-year completers (n=13) showed no decline on five measures: the CDR, Sum of Boxes, Verbal Fluency, Boston Naming, and WAIS-R Similarities between end-of-year one and end-of-year two testing.

The three-year completers (n=8) showed no decline on six measures: the CDR, Sum of Boxes, Boston Naming, ABCD, WAIS-R Similarities, and WAIS-R Comprehension between end-of-year two and end-of-year three testing.

The four year completers (n=4) showed a significant *improvement* on Sum of Boxes between end-of-year three and end-of-year four testing and no decline on five measures: MMSE, CDR. Verbal Fluency, Boston Naming, and WAIS-R Comprehension. It is noteworthy that the four year completers showed no significant mean decline from baseline to end of year 4 on six measures: CDR, Sum of Boxes, Verbal Fluency, Boston Naming, WAIS-R Comprehension, and WAIS-R Similarities. Though there was a steep dip in performance on Similarities (abstract reasoning) in year 3, the group recovered to baseline level at the 4th year testing session.

Global Functioning

The multi-year completer groups showed no significant between-year changes on the CDR (stage of dementia).

All four of the 4-year completers were at the same CDR stage of dementia at the end of treatment as they were 4 years previously, 3 at CDR 1 (mild); 1 at CDR 2 (moderate). One 3-year completer went from a baseline CDR of 0.5 (questionable dementia) to a 1; another who completed 6 semesters remained a 2 for the three years – this despite a hospitalization for a broken hip (not project-related) in her 5th semester; she was 90 years old when the program ended. Of the other two 3-year completers, one started and remained a CDR 1, but had to drop out because of physical illness after her third year. The other started as a CDR 2, with an MMSE of only 15, was rated a CDR 3 (severe stage) at the end of year 1, yet completed two more years of participation. She was finally terminated from our standard treatment because of her severe aphasia and incontinence. However, she continued to receive individual therapeutic services at her residence from a student volunteer, and enthusiastically attended all of the program's social activities during its fourth year.

Discourse Outcomes

Responses to eight prompt questions were analyzed and scored for four measures: the ratio of substantive on-topic statements to total statements, ratio of different nouns to total nouns, ratio of vague nouns to total nouns and ratio of negative statements to total statements. (Statements coded as negative included repetitious, off-topic, confabulatory, factually erroneous, incomplete and "meaning unclear" utterances.) The other discourse measures were the previously described proverb interpretation and picture description.

Of the four 4-year completers, 2 maintained or improved performance on 5 of the 6 discourse measures: the other 2 maintained or improved on 3 or 4 of the measures. The first eleven one-year completers showed no decline on all five of the discourse measures administered. (Negative utterances were not counted for this first group.)

The prompts and stimulus questions that were used may be seen in Appendix B.

Details of the data analysis system and the outcomes of the two sub-groups studied have been published [14,15].

Student Learning Gains

Six cohorts of students (n=69) were given an updated version of the AD Knowledge Test [82], before and after their participation. Mean score improved from 54% correct answers to 84%; change was very significant, $p < .001$. Highly positive course evaluations, personal letters of thanks to the project director, the prominence of this experience as described in students' graduate school and job applications and reflected in future career plans, and post-program involvement of students with their former partners are further evidence of the positive impact of the program on student participants. Follow-up phone calls and emails to former student participants in the spring of 2004 revealed that eleven of the 15 contacted were in or had completed medical, nursing, physical therapy or speech pathology graduate programs.

Caregiver Reactions

Sixteen caregivers responded to an evaluation questionnaire after the program's first year. Most frequently endorsed program benefit was opportunities to socialize (14 respondents). Other frequently endorsed benefit items were: improvement in mood/morale, feelings of usefulness, energy level, general quality of life (10 respondents each); connectedness to others (nine respondents); and conversation quality (eight respondents). Of the four program components, exercise was ranked the highest, in terms of perceived benefit to participants, followed by volunteer work, conversation stimulation, and memory training.

AD Rehab Outcomes Compared to CERAD Outcomes

The CERAD study tracked cognitive change in untreated AD persons with dementia from 1986 to 1994 [83]. Data from the 245 individuals in the CERAD database who most closely matched the 24-person Elder Rehab sample on diagnosis, age (54 to 59 and 73 to 88), race (white), and MMSE score at enrollment (15-29) were used as a comparison group. These two groups were compared at enrollment and those remaining in the CERAD sample at first, second, third, and fourth year followup testing were compared with the comparable AD Rehab cohorts on the following measures: MMSE, CDR, Sum of Boxes, Boston Naming, and Verbal Fluency.

Data were analyzed using a (Groups x Time) mixed analysis of variance (ANOVA). Results of post hoc comparison of test scores on the MMSE, CDR, Verbal fluency, CERAD 15-Item Boston Naming showed no difference between groups during the first year and both groups declined significantly ($p < 0.001$). However, analyses of data from subsequent years of the projects suggest that the groups began to diverge after the first year. For example, the CERAD group declined an average of four points on the MMSE from Year 1 to Year 2 ($p < 0.001$), while the AD Rehab group declined just two points during the same time period ($p = 0.02$). From Year 2 to Year 3, the CERAD group declined by three points ($p < 0.001$), AD Rehab by two ($p = 0.02$). The difference was most striking between Year 3 and Year 4, when the CERAD group declined by three ($p < 0.001$) and AD Rehab by just one ($p > 0.05$).

In the AD Rehab group ($n = 24$), 50% of the group had an average annual rate of decline during their participation in the project of less than three points. In the CERAD group ($n = 245$), only 42% of the group had an average rate of decline of less than three points. A binomial test comparing the two proportions indicated that the 8% difference was statistically significant, $p = 0.02$. Results of analysis of the Verbal Fluency, Boston Naming, CDR, and Sum of Boxes tests mirrored that of the MMSE.

CONCLUSION

Most research articles end by providing apologies for the study's limitations. This is followed by calls for ambitious goals such as future research to test the intervention or hypothesis in a randomized controlled trial, identification of the most salient element (in successful multi-component studies), replication of the study on large multi-site populations, inclusion of ethnically diverse populations among study subjects, extension of the intervention period to facilitate longitudinal data collection, and use of more ecologically valid environments for intervention, etc. In a perfect world, governments, corporations, and philanthropists would be generously granting funding to researchers to accomplish these worthy goals. However, the reality is that grant money is scarce and becoming even scarcer as the economic crisis, natural disasters, wars, environmental pollution, and public health emergencies eat up more and more of the world's resources.

Randomized controlled trials of multi-component interventions with proven benefits to experimental subjects mean the *withholding* of beneficial interventions to control subjects. Not only is this unethical, but imagine the reaction of persons and family members of persons assigned to a passive control activity after having been attracted to apply for a program advertising longterm exercise, cognitive, and work therapy or other socially-involving activities. Wait list control designs involving persons with a progressive dementia are only suitable when the waiting period is brief. Yet the benefits of multi-component intervention are robust only when they are of long duration.

Teasing out the "salient" element of a successful multi-component program would involve incurring far greater costs to find a huge pool of potentially eligible subjects to be recruited, screened, tested and randomly assigned, and a large staff of persons to design and supervise the individual program elements and analyze the results. Doing this on a multi-year basis would be prohibitive in cost and would probably require multiple sites with duplicate administrative costs. Random assignment could easily result in persons who would love to exercise being assigned to a sedentary cognitive intervention or persons who would love working with children or animals being sent to an exercise group. Treatment groups large enough to power such a study would be difficult to find and hugely expensive to recruit, test, and supervise. The beauty of multi-component programs is that participants, if they have been motivated to apply, are attracted to at least one of the components and are exposed to one or two others, to their ultimate benefit.

A major cost of research studies are the expenses involved in scientific selection and testing of subjects, design and provision of plausible, but supposedly inert control interventions, quality control of interventions to assure adherence to strict research criteria, and huge outlays to university sponsors of research for "indirect costs" to support research infrastructures. Why waste scarce resources on researching minutiae when they could be spent providing proven beneficial services?

Engaging ethnically-underserved populations in community-based, non-research-oriented programs should not be difficult. The disproportionate prevalence of diabetes, hypertension and other lifestyle-influenced diseases which are associated with dementia among low income and minority populations has been well-documented [84]. There is a tradition of inter-generational and extended family caregiving among Hispanic, African-American, native American, Asian, and other ethnic groups in the the U.S. [85]. We have seen evidence of programs that have successfully trained caregivers to supervise exercise and cognitive interventions. Why not make this type of training available to minority caregivers? Surely, each ethnic community has its own church, service, and/or health care organizations that could provide volunteer opportunities for supervised dementia (delete word in red)persons with dementia and help with outreach efforts.

We have also seen how undergraduate students and medical students can have their academic training enriched by one-to-one involvement with a person with dementia. Furthermore, we have seen how the lives of persons with Alzheimer's dementiapersons with are given new meaning by their roles as volunteers providing useful community service, such service also providing benefit to the agencies receiving their services, valuable experience to their student partners, and respite to family caregivers. The time to act is NOW. There is more than enough evidence to support the provision of multi-component life-enhancing, socially-involving, health-, mood- and behavior-improving activities for persons with dementia The use of students to deliver these interventions makes these treatments universally affordable.

Happily, this has finally been recognized. A U.S. Administration on Aging grant program has included the Elder Rehab model, along with a program by the editor of this journal, Elisabetta Farina and colleagues, in a list of seven evidence-based interventions for persons with dementia which applicants can select for replication.[88] The State of Wisconsin has selected the Elder Rehab model for their application, the deadline for which is May 15, 2010.

Post Script. Reference to the University of Arizona AD (Elder) Rehab website, where the exercise and language protocols are presented, has already been made. A convincing rationale for exercise as an intervention for potential participants and their caregivers may be found in a web monograph on the website of the National Center for Physical Activity and Disability, *Alzheimer's and Exercise,* at www.ncpad.org/disability (Alzheimer link). Two one-hour continuing education videos (now DVDs), produced originally for speech pathologists, but suitable for any would-be program planners, are available from the University of Arizona Board of Regents: one on the memory, language, and volunteer work [86] interventions in the VIP program and one on the language and exercise components of the AD Rehab program

[87]. Excerpts from these films may be seen on YouTube. One titled Alzheimer Exercise Treatment is usually at the top of the first page when those descriptive terms are entered. That video provides links to videos on Alzheimer volunteer work treatment, Alzheimer memory training, and Alzheimer video therapy by clicking on arkinaz. Anyone wishing further information or assistance, or copies of any of my published articles can contact me at arkinaz@earthlink.net.

APPENDIX A

Format for a Memory Tape Script

(Questions preceded by * were not known by subject at baseline. Script should contain 12-15 known and 12-15 not known facts.)

Hello Dorothy. This is Sharon Arkin speaking to you by tape recorder. *Can you repeat my name?* (5 sec. pause)_____ Again, my name Sharon Arkin.

The purpose of this tape is to help you relearn some things you may have forgotten about your life and to help you keep remembering the things you do remember. First I will give you some information. Then I will ask you questions about it. If you don't know the answer, don't worry, I'll give you the correct answer right away. Eventually, you should learn most of the information.

Before we begin, let me repeat my name. My name is *Sharon Arkin. Say my name if you can* (5 sec. pause)_____ *Sharon Arkin. (*2 sec. pause) Ready? Let's begin.

I spoke with your husband, Paul and he told me a little bit about you and your family. Let's see if I have it right. You were born in Detroit, Michigan on May 30, 1922. *What was the date and year of your birth?* (5 sec. pause)_____ *May 30, 1922.* (2 sec. pause) Your father's name was Lester Campbell and he was born in Glasgow, Scotland.. *Where was your father born?* (5 sec. pause)_____ *Glasgow, Scotland.* (2 sec. pause) Your father worked as a welder for General Motors. **What company did your father work for?* (5 sec. pause)_____ *General Motors.* (2 sec. pause) Your mother was a homemaker. Her maiden name was Martha Edmonds *What was your mother's maiden name? (5 sec. pause)_____ *Martha Edmonds.* (2 sec. pause) Your mother had six children, three boys and three girls.. You were child number 5. *What was your birth position in your family?*_____ (5 sec. pause) *Number 5.* (2 sec. pause)

Now for some review questions. First question

1.   On what date and year were you born? (5 second pause)_____
The correct answer is *May 30, 1922..* (2 sec. pause) Next question

2.   Where was your father born? (5 second pause)_____
The correct answer is *Glasgow, Scotland.* (2 sec. pause) Next question

3.   * What company did your father work for? (5 second pause)_____

The correct answer is *General Motors.* (2 sec. pause) Next question

4.   * What was your mother's maiden name? (5 second pause)_____
The correct answer is *Martha Edmonds.* (2 sec. pause) Next question

5.   * What was your birth position in your family? (5 second pause)_____
The correct answer is *Number 5.* (2 second pause)

Continue with additional 5-fact narratives and questions.

AD Rehab Discourse Prompts*

1. Tell me what you know about John F. Kennedy and his family.
Anything else you can tell me about John F. Kennedy and his family?
(Also assesses episodic memory.)

2. Tell me what you know about Alzheimer's Disease.
Tell me whether Alzheimer's Disease has affected your family in any way. If no elaboration, give one prompt. How has Alzheimer's Disease affected your family?
(Also used to assess insight.)

3. Tell me about your usual routine. The things you do nearly every day.

4 What are some things you enjoy doing once in a while?

5. What childhood memories does the word play remind you of?

6. What adult memories does the word play remind you of?

7. Tell me what you'd do if you had to plan and prepare a picnic for your family or some friends. Tell me what you'd do about food and drinks.
(Assesses procedural memory).

8. Suppose a thirteen year old daughter of a friend or a neighbor told you that she was pregnant and was afraid to tell her mother. What would you do?
What are the different ways a family could handle that situation?
(Also assesses problem-solving abilitiy)

Grocery Store picture (from the Aphasia Diagnostic Profiles by Nancy Helm-Estabrooks (1992) Riverside Publishing Company.) Participant is asked to describe what is seen in the picture. Only non-specific prompts are given, e.g., What else do you see? Information units and their ratio to total words, total nouns, different nouns, vague nouns counted.

Proverbs/Sayings. (From Delis, Kramer, and Kaplan (1984). California Proverb Test - Unpublished protocol.) Scored on a continuum from concreteness to abstractness. If concrete response is given, participant is asked for a more general or abstract response. Best answer is scored.

1. They see eye to eye.
2. Too many cooks spoil the both
3. Don't count your chickens before they are hatched.
4. Rome wasn't built in a day
5. You can't tell a book by its cover.

*Reproduced from a previously published article [3] with minor changes, with permission from Sage Publications, copyright March 2007

REFERENCES

[1]   www.u.arizona.edu/~sarkin/elderrehab.html. Website describing the AD Rehab by Students program at the University of Arizona.
[2]   Arkin, S: Student-led exercise sessions yield significant fitness gains for Alzheimer's patients. *American Journal of Alzheimer's Disease.* 2003; 18: 159-170.
[3]   Arkin, S: Alzheimer memory training: Students replicate learning successes. *American Journal of Alzheimer's Disease.* 2000; 15: 152-162.
[4]   Bourgeois M: *The Making of a Memory Book* (VHS) Pittsburh, PA: WQED.
[5]   Arkin, S: *Language-enriched Exercise for Clients with Alzheimer's Disease.* Tucson, AZ: Desert Southwest Fitness, 2005.
[6]   Arkin, S: Audio-assisted memory training with early Alzheimer's patients: Two single subject experiments. *Clinical Gerontologist.* 1992; 12: 77-96.
[7]   Arkin, S: Alzheimer memory training: Positive results replicated. *American Journal of Alzheimer's Disease.* 1998; 13:102-104.
[8]   Arkin, S: Alzheimer memory training: Students replicate learning successes. *American Journal of Alzheimer's Disease.* 2000; 15: 152-162.
[9]   Arkin, S: Alzheimer memory training: Addendum on long term retention. *American Journal of Alzheimer's Disease.* 2000; 15: 314-315.
[10]   Arkin, S; Rose, C; Hopper T: Implicit and explicit learning gains in Alzheimer's patients: Effects of naming and information retrieval training. *Aphasiology.* 2000; 14:723-742.
[11]   Mahendra, N; Arkin, S; Kim ES: Individuals with Alzheimer's disease achieve implicit and explicit learning: Previous success replicated with different stimuli. *Aphasiology.* 2007; 21(2):187-207.
[12]   Folstein, MF; Folstein, SE; McHugh PR: Mini-Mental State: A practical method for grading the cognitive state of patients for the clinician. *Journal of Psychiatric Research.* 1975: 12:189-198.
[13]   Arkin, S: Volunteers in Partnership: An Alzheimer's rehabilitation program delivered by students. *American Journal of Alzheimer's Disease.* 1996; 11:12-22.
[14]   Arkin, S; Mahendra, N: Discourse analysis of Alzheimer's patients before and after intervention: Methodology and outcomes. *Aphasiology.* 2001; 15:533-569.

[15] Mahendra, N; Arkin, S: Effects of four years of exercise, language, and social interventions on Alzheimer discourse. *Journal of Communication Disorders.* 2003; 36(5):395-422.

[16] Helm-Estabrooks, *N: Aphasia Diagnostic Profiles.* New York: Riverside Publishing, 1992.

[17] Chapman, S; Ulatowska, HK; Franklin, LR, et al.: Proverb interpretation in fluent aphasia and Alzheimer's disease: Implications beyond abstract thinking. *Aphasiology.* 1997; 11(4-5):337-350.

[18] ACSM (American College of Sports Medicine): Exercise Management for Persons with Chronic Diseases and Disabilities. Champaign, IL: *Human Kinetics,* 1998.

[19] Verghese, J; Lipton, RB; Katz, MJ, et al.: Leisure activities and the risk of dementia in the elderly. *New England Journal of Medicine.* 2003; 348:2508-2516.

[20] Wilson, RS; Bennett, DA; Bienias, JL, et al.: Cognitive activity and incident AD in a population-based sample of older persons. *Neurology.* 2002;59:1910-1914.

[21] Valenzuela, M; Brodaty, H; Wen, W, et al.: Lifespan mental activity predicts diminished rate of hippocampal atrophy. *Alzheimers' and Dementia.* 2008; 4 Suppl. 1: IC-02-03 T5-T5. Available online 23 July 2008.

[22] Quayhagen, MP; Quayhagen, M: Differential effects of family-based strategies on Alzheimer's disease. *The Gerontologist,* 1989;29:150-155.

[23] McEvoy, CL; Patterson, RL: Behavioral treatment of deficit skills in dementia patients. *The Gerontologist* 1986; 26:475-478.

[24] Bourgeois, MS: Enhancing conversational skills in patients with Alzheimer's disease using a prosthetic memory aid. *Journal of Applied Behavioral Analysis.* 1990; 23:31-64.

[25] Bourgeois, MS: Communication treatment for adults with dementia. *Journal of Speech and Hearing Research,* 1991; 34:831-844.

[26] Bourgeois, MS; Mason LA: Memory wallet intervention in an adult day-care setting. *Behavioral Interventions,* 1996; 11:3-18.

[27] Bayles KA; Tomoeda, C*K: Arizona Battery for Communication Disorders of Dementia (ABCD).* PRO-ED, Austin, TX, 1993.

[28] Bayles, KA; Kim, ES: Improving the functioning of individuals with Alzheimer's disease: Emergence of behavioral interventions. *Clinics in Communication Disorders.* 2003; 36(5):327-43.

[29] Acevedo, A; Loewenstein, DA: Nonpharmacological cognitive interventions in aging and dementia. *Journal of Geriatric Psychiatry and Neurology.* 2007; 20:239-249.

[30] Landauer, TK; Bjork, RA: Optimal rehearsal patterns and name learning. In: Gruneberg MM, Harris PE, Sykes RN, eds. *Practical Aspects of Memory.* New York, NY:Academic Press; 1978:625-632.

[31] Camp, CJ; Stevens, AB: Spaced-retrieval: A memory intervention for dementia of the Alzheimer's type. *Clinical Gerontologist.* 1990; 10:58-60.

[32] Zanetti, O; Rozzini, ME, Bianchetti, A; et al.: Procedural memory stimulation in Alzheimer's disease: Impact of a training programme. *Acta Neurologica Scandinavica.* 1997; 95:152-157.

[33] Zanetti, O; Zanieri, G; DiGiovanni, G; et al.: Effectiveness of procedural memory stimulation in mild Alzheimer's disease patients: A controlled study. *Neuropsychological Rehabilitation.* 2001; 11:263-272.

[34] Farina, E; Fioravanti, R; Chiavari, L; et al.: Comparing two programs of cognitive training in Alzheimer's disease; a pilot study. *Acta Neurologica Scandinavica.* 2002; 105:365-371.

[35] Farina, E; Mantovani, F; Fioravanti, R; et al.: Efficacy of recreational and occupational activities associated to psychologic support in mild to moderate Alzheimer's disease: A multicenter controlled study. *Alzheimer's Disease and Associated Disorders.* 2006; 20:275-282.

[36] Loewenstein, DA; Acevado, A; Czaja, SL; et al.: Cognitive rehabilitation of mildly impaired Alzheimer's disease patients on cholinesterase inhibitors. *American Journal of Geriatric Psychiatry.* 2004; 12:395-402.

[37] Spector, A, Thorgrimsen, L; Woods, B, et al.: Efficacy of an evidence-based cognitive stimulation therapy programme for people with dementia: Randomized controlled trial. *British Journal of Psychiatry.* 2003; 198:248-254.

[38] Rosler, A; Seifritz, E; Krauchi, K; et al.: Skill learning in patients with moderate Alzheimer's disease: A prospective pilot study of waltz lessons. *International Journal of Geriatric Psychiatry.* 2002; 17:1155-1156.

[39] Lekeu, F; Wojtasik, V; Van der Linden, M; et al.: Training early Alzheimer's patients to use a mobile phone. *Acta Neurologica Belgica.* 2002:102:114-121.

[40] Quayagen, MP; Quayhagen, M: Differential effects of family-based strategies on Alzheimer's disease. *Gerontologist.* 1989; 29:150-155.

[41] Quayhagen, MP; Quayhagen, M: Testing of a cognitive stimulation intervention for dementia caregiver dyads. In: Clare L, Woods RT, eds. *Cognitive Rehabilitation in Dementia.* New York, NY: Psychology Press Ltd; 2001:319-332.

[42] Clare, L; Woods, RT: Cognitive training and cognitive rehabilitation for people with early-stage Alzheimer's disease: A review. *Neuropsychological Rehabilitation.* 2004;14:385-406.

[43] Evans, W; Rosenberg, IH: *Biomarkers: The Ten Determinants of Aging You Can Control.* New York: Simon and Schuster, 1991.

[44] Miller, TD; Balady, GJ; Gletcher, GF: Exercise and its role in the prevention and rehabilitation of cardio-vascular disease. *Annals of Behavioral Medicine*; 1997 Summer; 19:220-229

[45] American Diabetes Association: Physical activity/exercise and diabetes. *Diabetes Care.* 2003;26:S73-S77

[46] Laurin, D; Verreault; R, Lindsay, J; et al.: Physical activity and risk of cognitive impairment and dementia in elderly persons. *Archives of Neurology.* 2001; 58:498-504.

[47] Yaffee, K; Barnes, D; Nevitt, M, et al.: A prospective study of physical activity and cognitive decline in elderly women: Women who walk. *Archives of Internal Medicine.* 2001; 161:1703-1708.

[48] Weuve, J; Kang, JH; Manson, JE; et al.: Physical activity, including walking, and cognitive function in older women. *JAMA.* 2004; 292:1454-1461.

[49] Abbott, RD; White, LR; Ross, W; et al.: Walking and dementia in elderly men. *JAMA.* 2004; 292:1447-1453.

[50] Van Praag, H; Kemperman, G; Gage, FH: Running increases cell proliferation and neurogenesis in the adult mouse dentate gyrus. *Nature Neuroscience.* 1999: 2:266-270.

[51] Cotman, C; Engesser-Cesar, C: Exercise enhances and protects brain function. *Exercise and Sport Science*. 2002; 30:266-270.

[52] Vermeer, SE; Den Heijer, T; Prins, ND; et al.; Silent brain infarcts and the risk of dementia and cognitive decline: The Rotterdam Scan Study. *New England Journal of Medicine*. 2003; 348:1215-1222.

[53] Adlard, PA; Perreau, VM; Pop, V; et al.: Voluntary exercise decreases amyloid load in a transgenic model of Alzheimer's disease. *Journal of Neuroscience*. 2005; 25;4217-4221.

[54] Colcombe, SJ; Erickson, KI; Scalf, PE; et al.: Aerobic exercise training increases brain volume in aging humans. *Journal of Gerontology A. Biological Science/Medical Science*. 2006; 61:1166-1170.

[55] Rolland, Y; Abellan van Kan, G, Vellas, B: Physical actdivity and Alzheimer's disease: From prevention to therapeutic perspectives. JAMDA (Journal of American Medical Directors Association). 2008; 9:390-405.

[56] Perez, CA; Cancel Carral, JM: Benefits of physical exercise for older adults with Alzheimer's disease. Geriatric Nursing. 2008; 29(6): 384-391.

[57] Rolland, Y; Pillard, F; Klapouszczak, A; et al.: Exercise program for nursing home residents with Alzheimer's disease: A one-year randomized, controlled trial. *Journal of the American Geriatric Society*. 200i7; 55:158-165.

[58] Williams, CL; Tappen, RM. Effect of exercise on mood in nursing home residents with Alzheimer's disease. *American Journal of Alzheimer's Disease and Other Dementias*. 2007; 22:389-397.

[59] Namazi, KH; Gwinnup, PB; Zadorozny, CA. A low intensity exercise/movement program for patients with Alzheimer's disease: The TEMP-AD protocol. *Journal of Aging and Physical Activity*. 1994(2); 2:80-02.

[60] Rolland, Y; Rival, L; Lafont, C, et al.: Feasibility of regular physical exercise for patients with moderate to severe Alzheimer disease. *Journal of Nutrition Health and Aging*. 2000; 4:109-13.

[61] Teri, L; McCurry, S; Buchner, D; et al.: Exercise and activity level in Alzheimer's disease: A potential treatment focus. *Journal of Rehabilitation Research and Development*. 1998:135:411-419.

[62] Ter,i L; Gibbons, I; McCurry, S; et al.: Exercise plus behavior management in patients with Alzheimer's disease: A randomized controlled trial. *JAMA*. 2003; 290:2015-1022.

[63] Abramson, JH; Ritter, M; Gofin, J; et al.: Work-health relationships in middle-oaged and eldery residents of Jerusalem. *Social Science and Medicine*. 1942; 34:747-755.

[64] Soumeri, SB; Avorn, J: Perceived health, life satisfaction, and activity in urban elderly: A controlled study of the impact of part-time work. *Journal of Gerontology*. 1983: 38:356-362.

[65] Keys, LM. Former patients as volunteers in community agencies: A model work program. *Hospital and Community Psychiatry*. 1982; 33:1017-1018.

[66] Griffin, RM; Mouheb, F. Work therapy as a treatment modality for the elderly patient with dementia. *Physical and Occupational Therapy in Geriatrics*. 1987; 5:67-82.

[67] Hughes, M. *Enhancing the Self-Esteem of the Nursing Home Resident*. LaGrange, TX: M and H Publishing, 1991.

[68] Butin, DN; Heaney, C. Program planning in geriatric psychiatry: A model for psychosocial rehabilitation. In Taira ED (ed.). *The Mentally Impaired: Strategies and Interventions to Maintain Function*. New York: Haworth, 1991.

[69] Mace, NL. Principles of activities for persons with dementia. *Physical and Occupational Therapy in Geriatrics*. 1987; 5:13-27.

[70] Alzheimer's Society Living with Dementia Working Group. http://alzheimers.org.uk/site/scripts/documents_info.php?documentID=468

[71] Stansell, J: Volunteerism: contributions by people with dementia. In PB Harris (Ed.) *The person with Alzheimer's Disease: Understanding the Experience*. Baltimore: Johns Hopkins University Press, 2002.

[72] Shapiro, J: Back to school may help those with Alzheimer's: Interview with Peter Whitehouse. National Public Radio. Morning Edition: June 12, 2009. www.npr.org/templates/story/story.php?storyId=91402614

[73] FSM Newsletter. Buddy Program reveals human side of disease. Feinberg School of Medicine. July 2008. Available online at www.brain.northwestern.edu/pdfs/buddy/FSM_NewsletterJuly08.pdf.

[74] Kushner, TM; Rosenheck, R; Campinell, AB; et al.: Impact of work therapy on health status of homeless substance-dependent veterans: A randomized controlled trial. *Archives of General Psychiatry*. 2002: 59(10):938-944.

[75] Whitaker, R: Cash, check or volunteer work: A new way to pay for therapy. Psychology Today online: www.Psychologytoday.com/print/24287.

[76] NAMI (National Alliance on Mental Illness) Fact Sheet. August 1999. Cited in WHO. Mental Health and Work. Available online at: www.who.int/mental_health/media/en/712.pdf

[77] Yesavage, J; Brink, T; Rose, T; et al.: Development and validation of a geriatric depression screening scale: A preliminary report. *Journal of Psychiatric Research*. 1983; 17:37-49.

[78] Berg, L: Clinical Dementia Rating (CDR). *Psychopharmacology Bulletin*. 1988; 24:637-663.

[79] Morris, JC: Clinical Dementia Rating (CDR). Current version and scoring rules. *Neurology*. 1994; 43:2412-2414.

[80] Morris, JC; Heyman, A; Mohs, RC; et al.: The Consortium to Establish a Registry for Alzeimer's Disease (CERAD). Part I. Clinical and neuropsychological assessment of Alzheimer's disease. Neurology. 1989; 39:1159-1165.

[81] Wechsler, D: *Manual for the WAIS-R. San Antonio*, TX: Psychological Corporation, 1981.

[82] Dieckman, L; Zarit, S; Gatz, M: Alzheimer's Disease Knowledge Test. *Gerontologist*. 1988; 28:402-406.

[83] Heyman, A; Fillenbaum, G; Nash, F (eds.): Consortium to Establish a Registry for Alzeimer's Disease: The CERAD experience. *Neurology*. 1997; 49(suppl 3, whole issue).

[84] Manton, KG; Stallard, E. Health and Disability Differences Among Racial and Ethnic Groups. Washington, DC: National Research Council, 1997.

[85] Valle, R. Caregiving Across Cultures: Working with Dementing Illness and Ethnicity. New York, NY: Routledge/Taylor Francis Group, 1998.

[86] Arkin, S: Volunteers in Partnership: A Rehabilitation Program for Alzheimer Patients. Telerounds #26. One hour video produced by the University of Arizona Board of Regents, 1996. Available from cherylt@email.arizona.edu

[87] Arkin, S: Effects of Exercise and Cognitive Stimulation on the Progression of Alzheimer's Disease. Telerounds #64. One hour video produced by the University of Arizona Board of Regents, 2002. Available from cherylt@email.

[88] Alzheimer Disease Supportive Service Program: Evidence-based Programs to Better Serve People with Alzheimer's Disease and Related Disorders (OMB Approval No. 0985-0018).

In: Dementia: Non-Pharmacological Therapies
Editor: Elisabetta Farina, pp. 119-135

ISBN: 978-1-61470-736-3
© 2012 Nova Science Publishers, Inc.

EFFECT OF PERSONALIZATION OF PRIVATE SPACES IN SPECIAL CARE UNITS ON INSTITUTIONALIZED ELDERLY WITH DEMENTIA OF THE ALZHEIMER TYPE

Kevin Charras[*,1], *John Zeisel*[2], *Joel Belmin*[3],
Olivier Drunat[4], *Melanie Sebbagh*[4],
Genevieve Gridel[4] *and Frederic Bahon*[4]

[1] Fondation Médéric Alzheimer, Paris, France.
[2] Hearthstone Alzheimer Care, Woburn, MA, U.S.A.
[3] Hôpital Charles-Foix, Ivry-sur-Seine, France.
[4] Hôpital Bretonneau, Paris, France.

ABSTRACT

This study is based on the general finding that non-pharmacological factors such as interior design and architectural characteristics of environments can help reduce symptoms of Dementia of the Alzheimer Type (DAT). The research presented here is the result of an experimental study of the effects of environmental personalization on behavioral disorders of people with DAT in a French special care unit (SCU). Based on a review of earlier studies we expected to find that increased personalization would lead to positive behavioral outcomes – reduced agitation and aggression – and to improved quality of life. A randomized controlled trial design was employed involving four special care units on the same floor of a French hospital. Cognitive, behavioral and physiological variables were measured. The hypotheses were partially confirmed and unexpected outcomes were observed. Results of the study are discussed according to the behavioral and psychological issues, as well as to quality of life outcomes of architectural design.

Keywords: Alzheimer's disease; environment-behavior (E-B), personalization, quality of life, Special Care Unit (SCU), non-pharmacological.

[*] Corresponding author: Kevin Charras, Ph.D, Psychosocial Interventions Program Manager, Fondation Médéric Alzheimer, 30 rue de Prony, 75017 Paris, France, e-mail : charras@med-alz.org. Kevin Charras benefited from the 2005 doctoral grant from the Fondation Médéric Alzheimer (Paris, France) for this study.

INTRODUCTION

Environment and Behavioural Health of People with Dementia of the Alzheimer Type

This study is based on the general finding that non-pharmacological factors such as interior design and architectural characteristics of environments can help reduce symptoms of Dementia of the Alzheimer Type (DAT) (Zeisel, Silverstein, Hyde, Levkoff, Lawton and Holmes, 2003). Zeisel *et al.*'s research with 427 participants of American origin identifies associations between characteristics of the architectural environment in fifteen special care units (SCU) and symptoms of agitation, aggression, depression, social withdrawal, as well as psychotic symptoms.

A thorough literature review (Zeisel *et al.*, 2003) demonstrates that proximal physical environmental characteristics of long-term care facilities significantly influence certain behaviors: (1) camouflaged exits reduce elopement attempts (Dickinson and McLain-Kark, 1998); (2) privacy reduces aggression and agitation and improves sleep (Morgan and Stewart, 1998); (3) common spaces with a unique non-institutional character are associated with reduced social withdrawal (Gotestam and Melin, 1987); (4) walking paths with multisensory activity nodes decrease exit seeking, improve mood, and engage family members (Cohen-Mansfield and Werner, 1998); (5) residential character is associated with reduced social withdrawal, greater independence, improved sleep, and more family visits (Minde, Haynes, and Rodenburg, 1990); (6) sensory comprehension reduces verbal agitation (Burgio, Scilley, Hardin, Hsu, and Yancey, 1996; Cohen-Mansfield and Werner, 1997); (7) therapeutic garden access reduces elopement attempts and improves sleep (Stewart, 1995); (8) increased safety leads to greater independence (Sloane *et al.*, 1991), which in turn is associated with fewer falls (Capezuti, Strumpf, Evans, Grisso, and Maislin, 1998).

To systematize and quantify these results and highlight the behaviors associated with environmental factors of their environment-behavior (E-B) model, Zeisel *et al.* (2003) conducted a study using a statistical methodology recommended by Teresi (1994)—hierarchical linear modeling.

According to Zeisel *et al.* (2003), environmental factors with particular effects on the mental health of people with DAT, include: effective design strategies to control exits reduce symptoms of depression; social withdrawal is related to the variability of common spaces; residential characteristics of SCUs and sensory comprehension reduce aggressive behaviors; and private spaces are correlated with reductions in behavioral agitation and aggression as measured by the Cohen-Mansfield agitation inventory. One explanation for these results might be that the environments studied attenuated cognitive pressure on and stress of residents with DAT, thus reducing their anxiety and aggression. Another explanatory hypothesis is that the environmental design features allow residents increased control over their own lives and therefore reduce their tendencies to withdraw or eventually to become depressed. Two environmental design features that research has shown lessen behavioral symptoms are sensory comprehension and the degree of intimacy and personalization provided by private spaces (Zeisel *et al.*, 1994; Zeisel *et al.*, 2003). These factors show significant negative correlations with *Cohen-Mansfield Agitation Inventory* scores and according to the authors, this can be explained by familiarity and sense of security that personalized environments provide.

Since the environment cannot be considered independent of the culture in which it evolves (Moser, 2003), we wanted to test these latter results in a French cultural context. We focused on the private space of SCUs to avoid the difficulties of operationalizing sensory comprehension.

Privacy and Personalization

According to Zeisel *et al.* (2003), the degree of privacy/personalization in SCUs is negatively associated with scores of patients on the Cohen-Mansfield agitation inventory. Compared to residents that did not live in such conditions, residents living in facilities with more privacy – more individual rooms and more personalization – had lower scores on this scale as well as reduced anxiety and aggression.

Day and Calkins (2002) also observed that residential and non-institutional features in care environments had positive therapeutic effects for people with DAT, such as improved communication skills, autonomy, social abilities, mobility, emotional responses, behavioral disorders, motor activity, apathy and hallucinations. Maslow's hierarchy of needs (1954) can help explain these outcomes as follows: We can assume that the reduced level of anxiety and agitation observed by Zeisel *et al.* (2003) derives from the sense of security that personalization of private spaces provides. This meets Maslow's hypothesis (1954), further developed by Zeisel and Raia (2000), that the basic need for shelter, like nutrition and primary physiological needs, serves as a prerequisite to access more complex needs at higher levels of the hierarchy, such as social belonging, self-assertion and emotions.

Hall (1966) points out that personalization is subjective and requires taking into account the perception of the individual in respect to his/her cultural origins. Brawley (1997) emphasizes that social context, experience, age and social position explain why the same spatial conditions are often perceived differently and result in different reactions. Day and Cohen (2000) conclude that cultural heritage is an essential aspect of identity for elderly people with or without DAT. According to Valle (1989) how individuals acculturate can be seen as a continuum (Figure 1). At the *traditional* end of the continuum, individuals retain beliefs and behaviors of their culture of origin. At the intermediate, or *bicultural*, level of the continuum individuals share the attributes of their culture of origin with those of the dominant culture they live in. People at the opposite end of the continuum, the *assimilation level*, adopt the values and behaviors of the dominant culture.

As individuals with dementia decline cognitively, it is likely that they tend to return to the traditional end of the continuum (Valle, 1989), suggesting that people with DAT function at their highest capacity when their environments, caregivers and families are adapted to specific cultural patterns corresponding to their decline. Day *et al.* (2000) suggest that architectural design interventions based on culture have a therapeutic value when integrated with interactions or activities requiring simple and comprehensible cognitive tasks.

The aim of the study presented here is to identify the effects of personalization of private spaces on behavioral disorders of people with DAT in a French SCU, one of the two dimensions that make up the "private space" factor in Zeisel *et al's* (1994) E-B model. Based on review of the various studies cited in this introduction we expected to find that increased personalization leads to positive behavioral outcomes -- reduced agitation and aggression – and to improved quality of life.

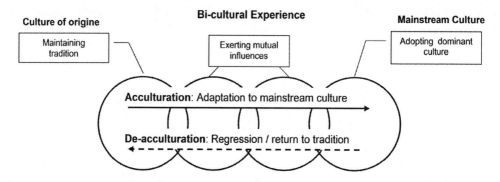

Figure 1. Cultural embeddedness according to Valle (1989, *in* Day and Cohen, 2000).

METHOD

Experimental Design

Four special care units for people with DAT all on the same floor of the Bretonneau hospital (Paris, France), each with 15 residents, served as the study setting. The architectural and organizational environments in the four units were comparable, allowing us to assume that there was no bias due to differences in the architecture or organization of care. To avoid selection bias, two of the four units randomly selected as controls did not receive any experimental treatment (control group) while the other two received experimental treatment (experimental group).

The study employed a double-blind controlled randomized experimental design. People who completed the questionnaires, although they were aware of the study – environmental modifications being difficult to hide – were not aware what impacts the interventions and assessments were designed to determine. Medical doctors conducting the experiment presented the assessments to participating staff as a part of data collection for patients' medical records. The same assessments were administered before the intervention and six months after living with the environmental modifications, to allow long enough exposure to the intervention.

Description of the Intervention

Decorating each resident's room with the assistance of the resident, the family carer and a member of the hospital staff represented the experimental intervention. A letter was initially sent to families in the experimental units inviting them to select and bring a range of personal effects belonging to their resident family member. The letter mentioned wall decorations, ornaments, pictures, towels, and any other object that may be considered personalization. The letter requested of the family carer that the selected decorative objects should be recognized by the participant as belonging to him/her, and if possible that the objects had belonged to the resident for a long time to counter the possibility of what Piolino *et al.* call a *reversed temporal gradient* (Piolino, Desgranges, Belliard, Matuszewski, Lalevée, De La Sayette and Eustache, 2003). After the objects were at the hospital, family members and staff carers were asked to make a final selection of objects together with the resident and to arrange the decoration in the resident's room. We suggested that the main selection criterion for suitable decorations should be the degree to which the resident expressed emotions and memories when looking at the object.

Personalizing one's space is extremely subjective and its meaning different for each person (Figure 2). Some residents were more comfortable with few personal elements, while others preferred more decoration.

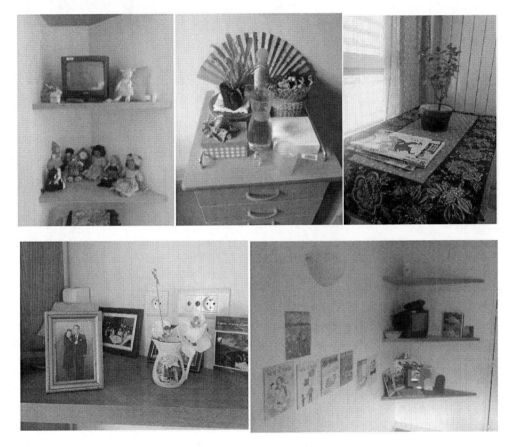

Figure 2. Examples of personalized rooms.

We observed that personalization seldom took place at once, but rather was a gradual process that evolved during the six months of experimentation. A time adjustment was necessary to enable participants to get used to their personalized environment. The process of personalization itself was subject to change depending what personalizing elements were available and on the evolution of participant tastes. The experimenters undertook no process of personalization in the private spaces of the control group (Figure 3). However, if families and residents decided to add decorative elements in the room on their own, we did not intervene for obvious ethical reasons but did continue to include them in the control group since their actions were not done at our recommendation.

In order to identify the experimenters and differentiate them from visitors in the hospital, the medical staff suggested that the experimenters wear MD white jackets. Residents as well as their legal guardians were asked to formally consent to be part of the experiment.

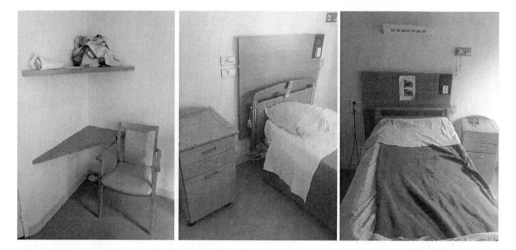

Figure 3. Examples of rooms of the control group.

Measures

The *Mini Mental Status Examination* (MMSE; *Folstein, Folstein and McHugh, 1975)* scale was administered to each participating resident in order to establish a descriptive overview of the stage of cognitive impairment of study participants.

The *Neuropsychiatric Inventory* (NPI; Cummings, Mega, Gray, Rosenberg-Thompson, Carusi and Gornbein, 1994) was administered to assess the presence, frequency and severity of 12 behavioral disturbances that occur commonly among dementia patients: delusions, hallucinations, dysphoria, anxiety, agitation/aggression, euphoria, disinhibition, irritability/lability, apathy, aberrant motor activity, sleep disorders and eating disorders.

In addition to these cognitive and behavioral measures we wanted to include one pre-post measure of residents' quality of life. Because no quality of life measure had been validated in French for people with DAT at the time of our study, we decided to use weight as our quality of life indicator. Others have argued that this physiological variable is a good indicator of quality of life (Martin, Kayser-Jones, Stott, *et al.*, 2007; Nijs, de Graaf, Kok and van Staveren, 2006; Brocker, Benhamidat, Benoit, *et al.*, 2003), particularly because malnutrition is considered a recurrent factor that often occurs in DAT (Belmin, Pequignot, Konrat and Pariel Madjlessi, 2007).

Participants

At the beginning of the study, 58 participant families gave consent for study participation, 30 in experimental units and 28 in control units (23 men and 35 women in total). The mean age for men was 80.41 years ($SD = 7.3$) and 85.1 years ($SD = 9.5$) for women. Mean length of stay at the hospital was 28.76 months ($SD = 18.68$). Fifty-five of the 58 participants (94.8%) were formally diagnosed with dementia, including 29 (50%) with dementia of Alzheimer type, 14 (24.1%) with mixed dementia, 5 (8.6%) with vascular dementia, 3 (5.2%) with dementia associated with Parkinson's disease, 2 (3.4%) with a fronto-temporal dementia, and 2 (3.4%) with dementia with Lewy bodies. Out of the 3 (5.2%) participants who had not received a dementia diagnosis, 2 (3.4%) presented a cognitive impairment consequent to a diagnosis of chronic hallucinatory psychosis and 1 (1.7%) had severe behavioral disorders. Among all participants, 26 had psychiatric antecedents not considered a reaction to their current illness (depressive syndrome, acute delirious episode, alcoholism syndrome...), 20 did not have any psychiatric antecedents, and for 11 no antecedents were specified. More than half of the participants had no academic diploma ($n = 37$; 63.8%), 10 (17.2%) had a degree equivalent to or below the baccalaureate, 9 (15.5%) had higher education, and for 2 of them, education was not specified. All MMSE scores were below 10, indicating severe cognitive impairments.

Studies of people with dementia face significant numbers of dropouts. This study was no exception. Among the 58 participants, 14 died during the experimental period and one moved away, reducing the final number of study participants to 43 (18 men and 25 women, see table 1 for the distribution in each group). The 15 dropouts were distributed fairly homogeneously in both control and experimental groups, although only one control unit and one experimental unit were particularly affected. Thus, although mortality was evenly distributed between the control and experimental conditions it was not evenly distributed between the four SCUs.

Table 1. Distribution of male and female participants according to the different experimental conditions (experimental mortality considered)

	Males	Females
Experimental group	9	14
Control group	9	11

Table 2. Mean (SD) values according to the experimental conditions

	Experimental group	Control group
Age	83,9 (9)	81,6 (10,19)
MMSE	3,47 (2,15)	3,65 (1,96)
Weight	66,82 (17,19)	61,82 (12,58)

Table 3. Mean weight (SD) of the two weighing (kg) by sex and experimental condition

	Experimental group	Control group	Mean values
Male	71,19 (20,58)	67,8 (8,91)	69,49 (15,48)
Female	62,45 (13,6)	55,84 (12,61)	59,14 (13,2)
Mean values	66,82 (17,19)	61,82 (12,58)	--

**Table 4. Mean weight in kg (SD) according to
gender and time of evaluation**

	Weight 1	Weight 2
Male	69,07 (15,03)	69,92 (16,19)
Female	59,54 (12,89)	58,75 (13,75)

No significant differences were observed between the control and experimental subjects with regard to age, average weight at the first weighing, or MMSE scores (Table 2). These analyses allow us to consider our groups as homogeneous.

One descriptive measure – gender – was related to the dependent variable of weight in our study. As one might imagine, men (M=69,5 kg) are on average significantly heavier than women (M=59,14 kg ; $F_{1,41}$=6,00; p<,0187 ; Table 3). Because this relationship continued to hold in the second evaluation as it did in the first (M_f= -0,88, M_m=0,86 ; $F_{1,41}$=2,10; p<,1544 ; Table 4), our analysis of this variable does not differentiate between male and female participants.

Statistical Analysis

In order to compare scores between and within each condition and each measure, for both the experimental and control groups, statistics employed in this study included analysis of variance (ANOVA) with repeated measures, using student's 't' test and Fisher's test. Correlation analysis was also used in order to study possible links between variables.

RESULTS

Effect of Personalization on Weight of Participants

As explained above, weight is employed as the study indicator for quality of life. The data indicate that while the weight curves for the four SCU groups were significantly different ($F_{3,39}$=3.14; p<.0359 ; Figure 4), participants in the experimental group tended to gain weight (M_{pre}= 65.87, M_{post}= 66.9), while weight decreased for the control group (M_{pre}= 61.12, M_{post}= 59.9; $F_{1,41}$=3.61, p<.06 ; Figure 5).

Analyzing the two SCUs that experienced several deaths, the experimental SCU showed less weight loss than the control SCU. More precisely, the experimental SCU experiencing deaths had neither weight loss nor weight gain (experimental group 2; M_{pre}= 65.76, M_{post}= 65.55) while residents of the equivalent control SCU decreased in average weight (control group 1; M_{pre}=60.86, M_{post}= 57.93). Similarly, participants' mean weight increased in the experimental SCU with no deaths (experimental group 1; M_{pre}= 65.94, M_{post}= 67.8) while average weight in the equivalent control SCU neither increased nor decreased (control group 2; M_{pre}= 61.31, M_{post}= 61.46).

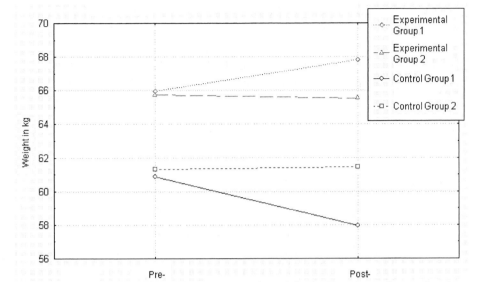

Note: Control Group 1and experimental group 2: experienced deaths; Experimental group 1 and control group 2: experienced no death.

Figure 4. Mean weight per unit of care before and after personalization.

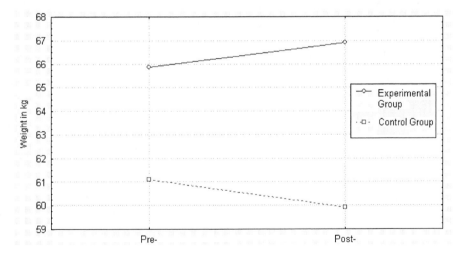

Figure 5. Mean weights pre- and post-intervention according to the experimental conditions.

Effects of Personalization on NPI Behavioral Items

Employing analysis of variance (Fisher's "F") we find no significant interaction effect between the global mean NPI scores and the experimental conditions (Table 5). Nevertheless, employing student's t test for smaller numbers, we observe a significant increase in the global control group mean score ($M= 11.63$; $t= 2.49$, $p<.03$) but not in the experimental group global mean score ($M= 7.11$; $t= 2.11$, ns).

Single item NPI scores result from multiplying an item's frequency by its severity. Two items – depression and disinhibition – achieve significance at $p<.03$ and one – apathy – shows a trend at $p<.07$.

Disinhibition or impulsivity decreased significantly in the experimental group pre- and post-personalization ($M_{pre}= 1.94$; $M_{post}= 0.78$). In the control group disinhibition/impulsivity pre- and post-personalization increased significantly ($M_{pre}= 0.55$ Vs. $M_{post}= 1.27$; $F_{1,27}=4.77$, $p<.03$).

Dysphoria or depression score shifts indicate an increase in depression in the experimental group pre- ($M_{pre}= 0.33$) and post-experimental intervention ($M_{post}= 2.28$), whereas scores decrease significantly for the control group ($M_{pre}= 3.91$ Vs. $M_{post}= 3.09$; $F_{1,27}=5.09, p<.03$).

Table 5. Mean scores NPI items according to the experimental conditions and the time of evaluation

	Experimental group pre-intervention	Experimental group post-intervention	Control group pre-intervention	Control group post-intervention	Interaction Effects
Delusion	1,17	2,44	1,64	4,36	*Ns*
Hallucination	2,56	2,06	0,00	1,91	*Ns*
Agitation	3,44	4,22	2,82	4,09	*Ns*
Dysphoria/Depression	*0,33*	*2,28*	*3,91*	*3,09*	*$F_{1,27}=5.09, p<.03$*
Anxiety	2,67	5,22	2,64	3,82	*Ns*
Euphoria	0,00	0,33	0,00	1,82	*Ns*
Apathy/Indifference	5,83	3,89	3,09	3,09	*$F_{1,27}=3.4, p<.07$*
Disinhibition/Impulsivity	*1,94*	*0,78*	*0,55*	*1,27*	*$F_{1,27}=4.77, p<.03$*
Irritability	0,33	2,17	1,09	3,27	*Ns*
Aberrant motor activity	2,06	2,33	4,36	2,18	*Ns*
Night-time behaviour disturbances	0,67	2,94	0,55	2,27	*Ns*
Appetite	2,33	1,78	0,91	2,00	*Ns*
Total score	23,33	30,44	21,55	33,18	*Ns*

Although apathy or indifference did not achieve the same level of significance as the previous two variables, there is a tendency for apathy to decrease in the experimental group pre- and post personalization ($M_{pre}= 5.83$ Vs. $M_{post}= 3.89$), while for the control group the average score remain stable ($M_{pre}= 3.09$ Vs. $M_{post}= 3.09$; $F_{1,27}=3.4, p<.07$).

Both agitation and irritation as measured by the NPI remained stable pre- and post-personalization for the experimental and control groups with no significant differences (agitation : $F_{1,27}=,05$; $p<,8226$; irritation : $F_{1,27}=,07$; $p<,7953$).

Relations between Weight and NPI Scores

Because weight is the study indicator for life quality, we examined the relationship between average weight and average NPI single item scores (Table 6). We found significant negative correlations between weight and the global NPI score ($r= -.39$, $t= -2.14$, $p<.04$), as well as the agitation sub-score (r= -.49, t= -2.87, p<.008). We found no significant correlation between weight and either depression or apathy. We therefore consider these two items to be independent of weight.

Table 6. Correlations between weight and NPI scores

NPI / Weight	r
Delusion	-0,24
Hallucination	-0,26
Agitation	-0,49*
Dysphoria/Depression	-0,18
Anxiety	0,28
Euphoria	-0,07
Apathy/Indifference	0,07
Dis-inhibition/Impulsivity	0,31
Irritability	-0,23
Aberrant motor activity	-0,25
Night-time behavior disturbances	-0,28
Appetite	0,00
Total score	-0,39**

*Significant p<.04 .

** Significant p<.008.

DISCUSSION

The central hypothesis of this study is that private space personalization would contribute to reducing agitation in persons with DAT. While we found no effect of private space personalization on agitation as measured by the NPI, we did find reductions of other behavioral problems in the experimental group compared to participants in the control condition as well as increased weight.

The lack of observed effect on agitation is most likely linked to the severity of cognitive impairment in our study population, which was quite severe. According to Steinberg *et al.* discussing the place of intra-individual variables such as gender and severity of dementia, agitation is a high frequency behavior in severe dementia (Steinberg, Corcoran, Tschanz, Huber, Welsh-Bohmer, Norton, Zandi, Breitner, Lyketsos and Steffens, 2006). Thus, the ceiling effect for this item in the case of severe dementia could partly explain why this variable does not appear to be affected by private space personalization in our study.

Another explanation could be that this study focused on only one of the two secondary dimensions – privacy and personalization – of the environmental factor Zeisel *et al.* define as "privacy" in their E-B model (2003). Personalization on its own does not preserve the privacy of residents. The combination of these two secondary dimensions might well reduce symptoms such as agitation, although this study does not shed light on that question.

Induced Equilibrium through Personalization

The effect of personalizing bedrooms on the global NPI score as well as on the "disinhibition" sub-score appears consistent with data from Zeisel *et al.* (2003) concerning the privacy/personalization factor. Disinibition does not seem to be biased by a ceiling effect according to the severity of the disease, indicating greater sensitivity and better discrimination (Steinberg *et al.*, 2006).

This result is consistent with Benoit *et al.*'s results in their study of NPI symptoms comparing institutionalized people living with DAT and people with DAT living at home (Benoit, Robert, Staccini, Brocker, Guerin, Lechowski and Vellas, 2005). These authors found that people living in institutions compared to those living at home, had lower MMSE scores and higher scores for agitation and disinhibition. These results support the hypothesis and findings from other studies quoted above that environments with more residential appearance contribute to decreases in some psycho-behavioral symptoms. These findings also reinforce our assertion that agitation as measured by the NPI may be biased by severity of the illness and institutionalization.

"Apathy" NPI scores decreased among those whose rooms were personalized compared to those with no personalization in their rooms. Because apathy is often associated with slower cognitive and executive functions (Bullock and Lane, 2007), we conclude that personal objects that belonged to residents for a long time including family pictures, paintings and ornaments stimulate mnesic, cognitive and affective functions associated with a kind of reminiscence when used to personalize rooms.

Reminiscence therapies aimed at facilitating recall of past experiences improve intra- and interpersonal processes as well as quality of life (Teri, Logsdon, Peskind *et al.* 2000; Goldwasser, Auerbach and Harkins, 1987). Moreover, material Woods (1992) describes useful for reminiscence therapy are similar to the objects families and residents employed to personalize participants' rooms (photos, letters, maps, music, etc.). This link makes it even more probable that the objects benefited those in the experimental group.

Further support for our conclusions is found in Spaull, Leach and Frampton's study (1998) indicating that sensory stimulation tends to improve processing as well as adaptive behaviors among people with DAT.

Personalization and Quality of Life

The weight of participants in our study showed a significant negative correlation with participants' global NPI score. Banerjee *et al.*'s study supports these quality of life findings. Their study found that quality of life, measured by the DEMQOL scale, correlated positively with participants' global NPI scores as well as several NPI sub-scores including agitation (Banerjee, Smith, Lamping, Harwood, Foley, Smith, Murray, Prince, Levin, Mann and Knapp, 2006).

The case for weight as an indicator of quality of life and support for our interpretation of these data is also found in Brocker *et al.* (2003) and Léger *et al.* (2000). Our findings that weight is negatively associated with agitation are consistent with the results of Léger *et al.* (2000) on the somatic effects of agitation behaviors of people living with DAT.

Facilitating Environmental Changes

The differences between participants in the two SCUs in which more patients died and participants in the two more stable SCUs are also constructive. Although the experimental group in both pairs had better average weight profiles than the control groups, both of the groups in which deaths occurred had less weight gain than the other two groups. We hypothesize therefore that personalization provides familiarity and reassurance that patients rely on to cope with distressing situations, better enabling them to compensate for otherwise disturbing changes in the SCU. Familiarity, represented in our study by personalization of the environment, has been shown clearly to be linked to specific areas of the brain and therefore to be important in understanding DAT. Neuroscience studies demonstrate that the rhinal and peri-rhinal cortex and other brain areas involved in environmental exploration are particularly sensitive to familiarity of environmental stimuli (Ranganath, Yonelinas, Cohen, Dyb, Tomb and D'Esposito, 2003) and are defective in people living with DAT. Indeed, the rhinal cortex is an area severely affected by neurofibrilary degeneration processes at the earliest stage of DAT (Blaizot, Meguro, Millien, Chavoix and Baron, 2002).

Among those who faced many deaths between the two sets of measures, we observed that the weight in the intervention groups remained stable during the experiment, while it decreased for the controls. We hypothesize therefore that participants who benefited from the intervention were able to deal more effectively with the changes imposed by these deaths, than those who did not benefit from the personalization intervention.

From Psychotic to Neurotic Processes

Although, according to Steinberg *et al.* (2006), depression shows a ceiling effect among people with severe dementia as does agitation, depression also seems to be sensitive to room personalization, but in an unexpected direction. Although depression scores on the NPI decreased only marginally in the control group, they increased significantly in the experimental group. Teri *et al.* (1999) in their study of comorbidity among people with Alzheimer's found that over 50% of their sample had both anxiety and depression symptoms. One possible explanation therefore is that environmentally induced stimulation through personalization revives psychological and identity processes, making those participants who are more aware of their actual present situation more anxious and more depressed. A clinical explanation would posit that the decrease of apathy among participants – associated according to some authors with psychotic processes (Jolley *et al.*, 2006; Rapoport *et al.*, 2001) – was supplanted by neurotic processes characterized by anxiety and depression.

The relationship between personalization and depression clearly merits future study in greater depth employing more specific measures than the NPI. One fruitful approach is likely to be the inclusion of measures of social support because as Moser (2003) points out the interaction between social and physical environments can significantly affect the impact of both.

Limitations of the Study

Despite the strength of our findings, possible limits to the analysis must not be overlooked. The small size of our samples may have lead to our over-estimating the magnitude of the results. Deaths experienced and drop outs among participants, although not linked to our experimental treatment, may have influenced results in ways we are not aware. The lack of a validated French quality of life scale at the time of our study resulted in our using weight as a proxy-measure. Perhaps using a validated quality of life scale would have influenced results. Finally, the study would clearly have benefitted from inclusion of the secondary "privacy" factor *intimacy*. This would have enabled us to replicate the results found by Zeisel *et al.* (2003) for the entire *privacy* dimension of the E-B model.

CONCLUSIONS

These experimental results provide insight into possible health and behavioral outcomes linked to environmental personalization and more specifically the personalization of private spaces of people living with DAT in an institutional setting. The results suggest that future studies might fruitfully study the effects of such a protocol on the social environment of the person with DAT – on caregivers and relatives of participants. Personalized environments necessarily provide information to others about personal and autobiographical characteristics of the person who lives there (Zeisel *et al.*, 1994), enabling both institutional and family caregivers to become more familiar with the persons living with DAT. This characteristic of physical environment thus fully reflects the structural triangulation between persons living with DAT in institutional settings, the institutional caregiver and the family caregiver (Colombo, Vitali, Molla, Cioia and Milani, 1998). The results of this study emphatically make clear the importance of including environment among the significant nonpharmacological treatments available for institutionalized people living with DAT.

ACKNOWLEDGMENT

The authors wish to thank the participants of this study as well as their families.

REFERENCES

Banerjee, S., Smith, S., Lamping, D., Harwood, R., Foley, B., Smith, P., Murray, J., Prince, M., Levin, E., Mann, A., Knapp, M. (2006). Quality of life in dementia - more than cognition. An analysis of associations with quality of life in dementia. *Journal of Neurology, Neurosurgery and Psychiatry*, 77, 146-148.
Belmin, J., Péquignot, R., Konrat, C., Pariel-Madjlessi, S. (2007). Troubles cognitifs et démences: une priorité de santé publiques. *La Presse médicale*, *36*(10), 1500-1510.
Benoit, M., Robert, Ph., Staccini, P., Brocker, P., Guerin, O., Lechowski, L., Vellas, B., REAL.FR Group (2005). One-year longitudinal evaluation of neuropsychiatric symptoms

in Alzheimer's disease. The REAL.FR study. *The Journal of Nutrition, Health et Aging*, *9*(2), 95-99.

Blaizot, X., Meguro, K., Millien, I., Baron, J.C., Chavoix, C. (2002). Correlations between visual recognition memory and neocortical and hippocampal glucose metabolism. *J Neurosci, 22*, 9166-9170.

Brawley, E.C. (1997). *Designing for Alzheimer's disease: Strategies for creating better care environments*. New York: John Wiley et Sons, Inc.

Brocker, P., Benhamidat, T., Benoit, M., Staccini, P., Bertogliati, C., Guerin, O., Lechowski, L., Robert, Ph. (2003). Etat nutritionnel et maladie d'Alzheimer: résultats préliminaires de l'étude REAL.FR. *Revue de Médecine Interne. Suppl 3*, 314s-318s.

Bullock, R., Lane, R. (2007). Executive dyscontrol in dementia, with emphasis on subcortical pathology and the role of butyrylcholinesterase. *Curr Alzheimer Res, 4*(3): 277-93.

Burgio, L., Scilley, K., Hardin, M.J., Hsu, C., Yancey, J. (1996). Environmental "white noise": an intervention for verbally agitated nursing homer residents. *J. Gerontol., 51*B: 364-73.

Capezuti, E., Strumpf, N.E., Evans, L.K., Grisso, J.A., Maislin, G. (1998). The relationship between physical restraint removal and falls and injuries among nursing home residents. *J Gerontol, 53*A: M47-M52.

Cohen-Mansfield, J., Werner, P. (1997). Management of verbally disruptive behaviors in nursing home residents. *J Gerontol, 52*A: M369-M377.

Cohen-Mansfield, J., Werner, P. (1998). The effects of an enhanced environment on nursing home residents who pace. *Gerontologist*; *38*: 199-208.

Colombo, M., Vitali, S., Molla, G., Gioia, P., Milani, M. (1998). The home environment modification program in the care of demented elderly: Some examples. *Archives of Gerontology and Geriatrics, 26*, 83–90.

Cummings J.L., Mega M., Gray K., Rosenberg-Thompson S., Carusi D.A., Gornbein J. (1994). The Neuropsychiatric Inventory: comprehensive assessment of psychopathology in dementia. *Neurology, 44*(12): 2308-14.

Day, K., Calkins, P. (2002). Design and dementia. In R.B. Bechtel et A. Churchmann. (Eds.), *Handbook of Environmental Psychology*. New York : John Wiley et sons, Inc.

Day, K., Cohen, U. (2000). The Role of Culture in Designing Environments for People with Dementia: A Study of Russian Jewish Immigrants. *Environment and Behavior, 32*, 361-399.

Dickinson, J.I., McLain-Kark, J. (1998). Wandering behavior and attempted exits among residents diagnosed with dementia-related illnesses: a qualitative approach. *Journal of Women and Aging*; *10*, 23-35.

Folstein, M.F., Folstein, S.E., McHugh, P.R. (1975). Mini-mental state. A practical method for grading the cognitive state of patients for the clinician. *Journal of psychiatric research 12*(3), 189-98.

Goldwasser, A.N., Auerbach, S.M., Harkins, S.W. (1987). Cognitive, affective and behavioural effects of reminiscence group therapy on demented elderly. *Inter G Ag and Hum Develop, 25*: 209–222.

Gotestam, K.G., Melin, L. (1987).Improving well-being for patients with senile dementia by minor changes in the ward environment. In: L.Levi (ed.). *Society, stress, and disease* (pp.295-297). Oxford: Oxford University Press.

Hall, E.T. (1966). *La dimension cachée*. Paris : Le Seuil, 1978.

Jolley, S., Garety, P.A., Ellett, L., Kuipers, E., Freeman, D., Bebbington, P.E., Fowler, D.G., Dunn, G. (2006). A validation of a new measure of activity in psychosis. *Schizophr Res, 85*(1-3): 288-95.

Leger, J.M., Moulias, R., Vellas, B., Monfort, J.C., Chapuy, P., Robert, P., Knellese, S., Gerard, D. (2000). Causes et retentissements des états d'agitation et d'agressivité du sujet âgé. *L'Encéphale, XXVI* ; 32-43.

Martin, C.T., Kayser-Jones, J., Stotts, N.A., Porter, C., Froelicher, E.S. (2007). Risk for low weight in community- dwelling, older adults. *Clin Nurse Spec, 21*(4), 203-11.

Maslow, A. (1954). *Motivation and Personality* New York: Harper and Row.

Minde, R., Haynes, E., Rodenburg, M. (1990). The ward milieu and its effect on the behaviour of psychogeriatric patients. *Can J Psychiatry, 35*: 133-38.

Morgan, D.G., Stewart, M.J. (1998). Multiple occupancy versus private rooms on dementia care units. *Environment and Behavior, 30*; 487-504.

Moser, G. (2003). Questionner, analyser et améliorer les relations à l'environnement. In Moser, G., Weiss, K. (Eds.), *Espaces de vie: Aspects de la relation homme-environnement*. Paris: A.Colin.

Nijs, K.A., de Graaf, C., Kok, F.J., van Staveren, W.A. (2006). Effect of family style mealtimes on quality of life, physical performance, and body weight of nursing home residents: cluster randomised controlled trial. *British Medical Journal, 332*(7551), 1180-4.

Piolino, P., Desgranges, B., Belliard, S., Matuszewski, V., Lalevée, C., De La Sayette, V., Eustache, F. (2003). Autobiographical memory and autonoetic consciousness: triple dissociation in neurodegenerative diseases. *Brain, 126*(10): 2203-19.

Ranganath, C., Yonelinas, A.P., Cohen, M.X., Dy, C.J., Tom, S.M., D'Esposito, M. (2004). Dissociable correlates of recollection and familiarity within the medial temporal lobes. *Neuropsychologia, 42*(1), 2-13.

Rapoport, M.J., van Reekum, R., Freedman, M., Streiner, D., Simard, M., Clarke, D., Cohen, T., Conn, D. (2001). Relationship of psychosis to aggression, apathy and function in dementia. *International Journal of Geriatric Psychiatry, 1*, 123-30.

Spaull, D., Leach, C., Frampton, I. (1998). The effects of sensory stimulation for older adults who have a dementia. *Behavioural and Cognitive Psychotherapy, 26*, 57-68.

Steinberg, M., Corcoran, C., Tschanz, J.T., Huber, C., Welsh-Bohmer, K., Norton, M.C., Zandi, P., Breitner, J.C., Steffens, D.C., Lyketsos, C.G. (2006). Risk factors for neuropsychiatric symptoms in dementia: the Cache County Study. *Int J Geriatr Psychiatry, 21*, 824-830.

Stewart, J.T. (1995). Management of behavior problems in the demented patient. *Am Fam Phys, 52*: 2311-20.

Teresi, J. (1994). Overview of methodological issues in the study of chronic care populations. *Alzheimer Dis Assoc Disord, 8* (Suppl. 1), S247-273.

Teri, L., Logsdon, R. G., Peskind, E., Raskind, M., Weiner, M. F., Tractenberg, R. E., et al. (*2000*). Treatment of agitation in Alzheimer's disease: a randomized , placebo-controlled clinical trial. *Neurology, 55*(9):1271-1278.

Teri, L., Ferretti, L.E., Gibbons, L.E., Logsdon, R.G., McCurry, S.M., Kukull, W.A., McCormick, W.C., Bowen, J.D. and Larson, E.B. (1999) Anxiety in Alzheimer's disease: Prevalence and Comorbidity. *Journals of Gerontology: Medical Sciences*, 54A(7), M348–M352.

Valle, R. (1989). Cultural and ethnic issues in Alzheimer's disease family research. In E.Light et B.D.Lebowitz (Eds.), *Alzheimer's disease treatment and family stress: Directions for research* (pp.112-154). Rockville, MD: Department of Health and Human Services.

Woods, A. (1992). What can be learned from studies on reality orientation? In G.M.M. Jones, B.L. Miesen (eds). *Care Giving in Dementia: Research and Application* (pp. 121–136). Tavistock/Routledge: New York.

Zeisel, J., Hyde, J., Levkoff, S. (1994). Best practices: An environment-behavior (E-B) model for Alzheimer special care units. *American Journal of Alzheimer's Care and Related Disorders and Research, 9*, 4-21.

Zeisel, J., Raia, P. (2000). Non pharmacological treatment for Alzheimer disease: A mind-brain approach. *American Journal of Alzheimer's Disease and Other Dementias, 15 (6)*, 331-340.

Zeisel, J., Silverstein, N.M., Hyde, J., Levkoff, S., Lawton, M.P., Holmes, W. (2003). Environmental correlates to Behavioral Health Outcomes in Alzheimer's Special Care Units. *The Gerontologist, 43*(5), 697-711.

In: Dementia: Non-Pharmacological Therapies
Editor: Elisabetta Farina, pp. 137-159

ISBN: 978-1-61470-736-3
© 2012 Nova Science Publishers, Inc.

FOCUS AND EFFECTIVENESS OF PSYCHOSOCIAL INTERVENTIONS FOR PEOPLE WITH DEMENTIA IN INSTITUTIONAL CARE SETTINGS FROM THE PERSPECTIVE OF COPING WITH THE DISEASE[*]

R. M. Dröes[#,1,2], L. D. van Mierlo[1], H. G. van der Roest[2] and F. J. M. Meiland[1,2]

[1] Dept of Psychiatry.
[2] Dept. of Nursing home Medicine,
EMGO institute for Health and Care Research,
VU University medical center, Amsterdam, The Netherlands.

ABSTRACT

Introduction: The care for persons with dementia with chronic diseases has changed much in the past decades. This counts for the care for people with dementia as well. The care presently offered is not merely aimed at improving or stabilizing the medical condition of the person, but also at improving their quality of life by supporting the person in accepting his disease and coping with the consequences of it. Based on this perspective, many psychosocial interventions were developed in the past decades. The aim of this study was to get insight in the effectiveness of these interventions in the different adaptation areas.

Method: Several literature reviews into psychosocial interventions offered in institutional care to people with dementia were analysed. The reviews covered the period from 1970 until 2007. The interventions were categorised according to their aim to support people in coping with one or more adaptive tasks, as described in the Adaptation-coping model (Dröes, 1991; Finnema et al., 2000).

Results: Most of the investigated psychosocial interventions were aimed at supporting people with dementia in Maintaining an emotional balance and Coping with disabilities. Regarding *Maintaining an emotional balance* psychomotor therapy, music

---

[*] This paper is an elaboration of a lecture that was presented at 'Non-pharmacological therapies in dementia: a theoretical-practical course - Synergy with pharmacological therapies'. Casa di Cura San Pio X, Milano 22-24 Oct. 2009, and the symposium "Dementia, the identity of an illness, meaning of the care", Università Cattolica del Sacre Cuore di Milano, 24 October 2009.

[#] Corresponding author: Prof. dr. Rose-Marie Dröes, Psychosocial care for people with dementia, Dept. of Nursing home medicine and Dept. of Psychiatry/Alzheimer center, EMGO institute for Health and Care Research, VU University medical center, Valeriusplein 9, 1075 BG Amsterdam, tel. +31-20-7885454. e-mail: r.droes@ggzingeest.nl

therapy, adapting the living environment, validation, snoezelen en pet therapy are most frequently investigated and have shown to be able to positively influence behaviour symptoms, such as: agression, apathy, restlessness, depressive and anxious behavior. In the area of *Coping with own disabilities* interventions such as reality orientation, activity groups, normalising living pattern and structuring daily activities have shown to be effective in improving cognitive functioning and conducting daily activities. Also relatively many studies are conducted into *Maintaining social relationships* and *Coping with the care environment* (e.g. homely environment with enough privacy and normal living pattern). Few studies investigated interventions to help people *Develop an adequate care relationship with professional carers* and to *Preserve a positive self-image.* No studies were found into interventions to help people *Cope with an uncertain future.* The most broad effects were found with pet therapy, snoezelen, psychomotor therapy, normal living pattern and creating a homely environment.

Conclusion: Psychosocial interventions can be utilised for adaptation problems in several areas. For each area several interventions are available. Choices for individual treatment need to be based on the individual needs, personal characteristics, preferences and goal behaviour of the person with dementia.

Future research should focus on better designed studies (RCT's) and predictors of effective psychosocial interventions for the treatment of different adaptation problems.

Keywords: psychosocial interventions, persons with dementia, Adaptation-coping model.

INTRODUCTION

The perspective on care for chronic persons with dementia, and therefore also the care for chronic *psychogeriatric* persons with dementia, such as people with Alzheimer's disease and other types of dementia, has changed profoundly over the last 40 years. Today, the emphasis is no longer only on medical-hygienic issues, but also on psychosocial aspects such as: guiding the person in accepting his disease, coping with the consequences of the disease, and ultimately on the quality of life. The setting of new goals in care has led to the development of a range of new care and treatment methods.

In this paper the different perspectives on care and treatment are outlined. The perspective of the person with dementia is addressed as well: what does dementia mean to him, what are the problems he encounters, and what does he have to do to maintain a certain balance. Subsequently it is examined what psychosocial treatment methods are used to support people with dementia in coping with the consequences of dementia (in order to maintain a balance in mood and behaviour), and what results these methods have had so far. And finally, some conclusions are drawn and recommendations are made.

Changing Insights into Care and Treatment

Until fourty years ago aid to people with dementia was based almost exclusively on the *medical model* (see Figure 1; Dröes, 1991). The aid from this medical perspective focuses on treating, and if possible curing the disease, and so for a long time there was a therapeutic nihilism regarding people with dementia. For as long as the cause of dementia was unknown, and as long as the degeneration of the brain tissue could not be influenced, the dementia process could not be turned around or brought to a halt. The treatment of people with dementia therefore consisted mainly, apart from professional care, of symptomatic and social measures (like psychopharmacological therapy and occupational therapy).

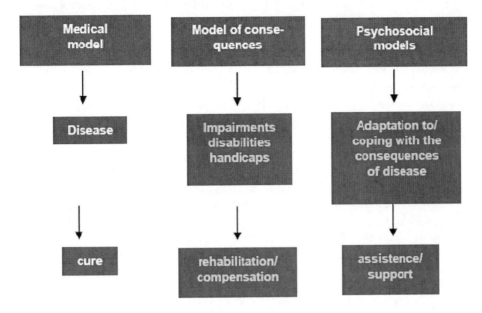

Figure 1. Perspectives in care and treatment.

Starting from about 1970 the emphasis in the treatment shifts to reactivation, partly because of the development of the rehabilitation function in the nursing home where people with dementia often reside. The objective of the treatment at that time is (apart from nursing, care and if necessary medical assistance) the reactivation of the patient to the maximum attainable level of physical, psychological, and social functioning. Not the disease, but the *consequences* of disease (impairments, disabilities, handicaps; ICIDH, 1980), are central in the rehabilitation model. This is why this model is also referred to as the *Model of consequences* (Bangma, 1988). For the person with dementia this meant that the treatment was aimed at preventing, or slowing down the further deterioration of his level of functioning. The emphasis was on *(re)activating* cognitive functions (for example memory training and reality orientation training (ROT)), and on *functional compensation* (for example signposts in the corridors of the nursing home, a photograph of the resident near his own bedroom, and functional colours, each department or functional service or door having its own colour). In this context the term *prosthetic environment* is frequently used.

As a result of this shift in interest from 'disease' to 'the consequences of disease' over the course of the 1980s, there is a gradual increase in interest in the *psychosocial* consequences of dementia. Attention gradually shifts from *functional thinking* to *the experiences* of the person with dementia (Dröes, 1991). Do the cognitive activation strategies actually benefit this person psychologically? Do they enhance the quality of life? Memory training has not yielded the anticipated or hoped-for effect. In some cases the confrontation with their own disabilities actually prove to *de*motivate rather than stimulate the person with dementia. Gradually the care sector is becoming more sensitive to the emotions and experiences of the person with dementia, and develops more understanding for his behaviour, and also how this behaviour is affected by the interaction with the environment (Dröes, 2007). Based on this understanding the sector has endeavoured, since the 1990s, to develop and offer *emotion-oriented care*: care that is actually in line with the emotional world, experiences and the needs of individuals (APA, 1997; Van der Kooij, 2003).

The theoretical models used to describe and explain the experiences, behaviour and mood of psychogeriatric residents, originate in clinical psychology, developmental psychology, social psychology and psychiatry. We call them *emotion-oriented or psychosocial models* because they focus on the emotions and experiences of the person with dementia and the psychosocial consequences of the disease. Examples of these models are:

-    The Developmental Stage Model of Erikson (1963). This model was applied for the first time in the psychogeriatric field by Naomi Feil (1989), founder of the Validation approach. Erikson distinguished various stages in human development, and the last stage before death is: finding ego integrity. During this final stage conflicts of the past are thought to be resolved through reminiscing. According to Feil this final stage is difficult to successfully complete if you are suffering from dementia, because of the cognitive disorders. However, elderly people with dementia will also sometimes be troubled by unresolved conflicts from the past. By giving them the opportunity to express their feelings they also, according to Feil, can experience a certain degree of relief, which she calls 'resolution'.
-    The Dialectical Frame work of Kitwood (1992): Kitwood, an English social psychologist, viewed the behaviour of people with dementia and the process of dementia not merely as the consequence of increasing neurological damage, but as the result of the interplay of many factors, such as: personality, life history, physical health, and the social-psychological environment. He points specifically at the impact (both positive and negative) that the *environment* can have on people with dementia. Kitwood has strongly influenced dementia care in the United Kingdom, especially with the method he developed called 'Dementia Care Mapping'. This is a method of observing the (positive and negative) behaviour of nursing home residents and how this relates with the behaviour of the (professional) caregiver.
-    The Attachment Theory of Bowlby (1969, 1973,1980): This theory was introduced in the psychogeriatric field in the Netherlands by Bère Miesen (1990). According to Miesen a part of the behaviour of elderly people with dementia (namely their being fixated on their own parents, thinking they are alive, and feeling the constant need to be near them) can be explained by the absence of attachment figures in the immediate environment, e.g. in the nursing home, and the anxiety this induces. The person with dementia will only feel safe again when he starts to attach to the new environment and the persons in it. Miesen tested the attachment theory in a study among psychogeriatric nursing home residents (N=40) and found that two thirds of these residents showed parent-fixation. The degree and the way in which parent fixation existed appeared to be related to the stage of dementia. It was especially exhibited by people with dementia who had a low level of cognitive functioning.
-    The Adaptation-coping model (Dröes, 1991; Finnema et al, 2000a): This model, that is based on the stress-appraisal-coping model of Lazarus en Folkman (1984) and the crisis model of Moos and Tsu (1977), is a conceptual explanation model to

understand the behaviour of people with dementia and the adaptation and coping processes people with dementia go through. Central in the model are a set of adaptive tasks that people with dementia encounter as a consequence of their illness (such as 'coping with own disabilities' and 'preserving an emotional balance'; see Psychosocial treatment). The degree to which each adaptive task is experienced as stressfull depends on the individual cognitive appraisal of the task. According to the model behaviour and mood disregulations in people with dementia can be partly explained as difficulties people have with coping with these adaptive tasks. The model is also intended as a broad framework based on which all aspects of the psychosocial care can be organized (see Psychosocial treatment). The model was tested and validated in research into the effectiveness of Psychomotor therapy in nursing home residents with probable Alzheimer's disease in which a confirmatory factor analysis on the applied outcome instruments showed outcome clusters that could be identified as outcomes on different adaptive tasks (Dröes, 1991) and by means of qualitative observational research in nursing homes, in which observation data were collected in four of the adaptive tasks areas, which resulted in operationalization of the behaviour in each of these areas; De Lange, 2004). The usefulness of the model was also tested in care practice as a base for a comprehensive support programme for people with dementia and their carers, the Meeting Centers Support Programme (MCSP). To support people in coping with the different adaptive tasks, in the MCSP different treatment strategies are applied (reactivation, resocialization, optimizing emotional functioning) and support activities offered (e.g. recreational activities, a social club, discussion groups and psychomotor therapy) (Dröes et al., 2000, 2004; Finnema et al., 2000a)

Other examples of stress-coping models are the Progressively Lowered Stress Threshold model (Hall and Buckwalter, 1987; Smith et al., 2004) that shows that the threshold at which people with dementia experience stress becomes lower when the dementia progresses and the Hagberg Psychodynamic model (1997), which is based on coping in a life span perspective.

The development of new, emotion-oriented models naturally does not mean that the medical model and the Model of Consequences have become worthless. In general one could say that the use of a particular theoretical framework must be guided by the patient's care request or needs. For many requests for assistance a combination of the various perspectives will be preferable. In psychosocial care the starting point is a psychosocial request for assistance, or expressed or observed need.

THE PSYCHOSOCIAL AID REQUEST: THE PERSPECTIVE OF THE PERSON WITH DEMENTIA

What are the requests for assistance and needs of people with dementia? Apart from the cognitive impairments that occur in dementia, that can be viewed as direct consequences of the degeneration of the brain, making people more or less dependent in activities of daily living, we also almost always see in people with dementia *other* types of disregulation in mental functioning, behaviour and mood. Examples are depressed, anxious, aggressive and rebellious behaviour, agitation, wandering, suspicious behaviour, delusions and hallucinations.

In the past these behaviour and mood disorders were viewed as resulting more or less directly from the brain degeneration. Today the prevailing view is that, in addition to organic or biological factors, psychological and social factors can play an important role in the disruption of the balance.

For example it is very possible that a person with dementia becomes disregulated partly because he has difficulty coping with the changes he goes through in the dementia process (Cohen, 1991; Dröes, 1991; Cotrell and Schulz, 1993; Cotrell and Lein, 1993; Reisberg, 1996; Hagberg, 1997; Clare et al., 2002; Dröes et al., 2006; De Boer et al., 2007). These, usually far-reaching, changes, from 'not knowing your way home when you leave the supermarket' up to and including 'admission into a nursing home' can lead to huge stress. The individual tries to cope with this, consciously or subconsciously. In this way, it is thought, he attempts to regain a sense of control and balance. This adaptation process is not equally smooth and adequate in all cases, mainly because of differences in specific cognitive impairments, in the personality of individuals and their interaction with the environment.

The fact that people with dementia experience a lot of stress is also well known from neuro-biological research: different stress-regulating systems in the brain are shown to be highly activated in Alzheimer's Disease (Hoogendijk et al., 1999). Intervention studies, in which group discussions are conducted with people with dementia, also confirm the stress-coping concept (Labarge and Trtanj, 1995; Moore, 1997): the problems people with dementia reported experiencing were linked on the one hand to their own cognitive decline and the disabling consequences this has for their everyday functioning, on the other hand with the emotionally challenging adaptation demands the disease brings for them and for their environment (Cohen, 1991; Dröes, 1991; Kiyak and Borson, 1992; Cotrell and Schulz, 1993; Cotrell and Lein, 1993; Clare, 2002). We are also increasingly hearing similar testimonies in the Alzheimer's Cafes (Miesen and Jones, 1997) and Meeting Centres for people with dementia and their primary carers (Dröes et al, 2003). Recent research among people with dementia and informal carers by Van der Roest et al. (2009) shows that some 30% of community dwelling people with dementia experience psychological distress.

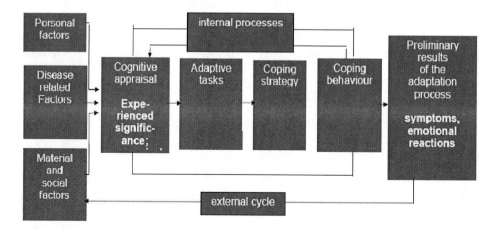

Figure 2. The adaptation-coping model (Dröes, 1991; Finnema et al., 2000).

In the past fourty years a range of psychosocial treatment methods have been developed that aim to reduce these problems and that have also partly proven effective (Dröes, 1997; Finnema et al, 2000b; Smits et al., 2007; Moniz-Cook and Manthorpe, 2008). Before describing the areas on which those treatments were targeted and their effects, a definition of 'psychosocial treatment' is presented.

Psychosocial Treatment

Psychosocial treatment can be described as the aid or care that is offered to reduce or prevent the mental and behavioural problems that occur in the process of adaptation to the consequences of dementia. In other words, offering assistance in coping with various consequences of dementia. From a theoretical perspective psychosocial aid must be viewed as the action that results from the psychosocial models, for instance the Adaptation-coping model (Dröes, 1991, 1996; Finnema et al., 2000a; see Figure 2). The essence of this model is that dementia causes changes in the life of the person with dementia that he will have to cope with in order to preserve a balance. In other words, an adaptation process takes place. The individual is faced with disability, this threatens his emotional balance, interaction with friends changes, etcetera. Coping with these indirect consequences of the dementia is operationalized in this model with the term *adaptive tasks* or assignments. The way in which the individual copes with the different adaptive tasks is influenced by his own life history, his mental and physical health, and his social and material circumstances (on the left of the model). What we ultimately see is the result of the adaptation process, namely the behaviour, emotional reactions and symptoms (on the right of the model).

The adaptation-coping model distinguishes seven general adaptive tasks, following Moos and Tsu's crisis model (1977):

- coping with one's own disability
- preserving an emotional balance
- preserving a positive self-image
- preparing for an uncertain future
- dealing with the day care, the care home or nursing home environment and procedures
- developing an adequate care relationship with staff
- developing and maintaining social relations.

If a person with dementia develops behavioural problems, for example very passive, restless or aggressive behaviour, then according to the model this may indicate he or she has problems with one or more of the listed adaptive tasks. In addition the way in which the person with dementia copes with the different adaptive tasks may be influenced by the way in which he is treated by his environment. Does this environment, for example, show understanding for the emotions of the person with dementia and does it actually offer security, social contact and practical assistance? Or does the environment confront the individual with his disability and lack attention for the emotions this causes?

These are the questions that are asked in psychosocial care and that form the starting point for the treatment. The key is to gain insight into the experiences of the person with dementia (as far as possible) and the way in which he/she, in interaction with his/her environment, copes with the consequences of his/her dementia, and subsequently to offer assistance to help him/her.

Examples of psychosocial treatment methods that have been applied in psychogeriatric care in the past 40 years, and are still used today (see e.g. Dröes, 1997; Finnema et al., 2000b; Moniz-Cook and Manthorpe, 2008), are:

- Supportive psychotherapy
- Psychomotor therapy
- Behaviour therapy
- Normalising living pattern and living environment
- Activity groups
- Reality orientation
- Music therapy
- Reminiscence
- Validation
- Integrated emotion-oriented care
- Snoezelen
- Aroma therapy
- Simulated presence therapy,
- Pet therapy.

Focus and Effects of Psychosocial Treatment Methods in Institutional Care Settings: An Analysis of the Literature

Based on three previous literature reviews (Dröes, 1991; Dröes et al., 1997; Finnema et al., 2000b) and a recent literature study into the relationship between personal characteristics of people with dementia and effectiveness of psychosocial treatment (Van Mierlo et al., 2009), we analysed the literature on psychosocial intervention studies with positive outcomes from 1970-2007 to get insight in their focus and effects in the different adaptation areas as defined in the Adaptation-coping model.

METHODS

For this analysis we used the following inclusion criteria: We included all studies that were reported on in the four mentioned reviews of Dröes (1991), Dröes et al. (1997), Finnema et al. (2000b) and Van Mierlo et al. (2009), that investigated the effect of psychosocial treatment methods in people with the diagnosis Alzheimer's Disease and Dementia (not otherwise specified) residing in institutional care settings, and that reported positive treatment outcomes. We made no restrictions regarding study design. Studies with no positive effect(s) were excluded from our analysis. In the mentioned reviews used for this analyses the following databases and key words were used in the literature searches:

- Dröes (1991) and Dröes et al (1997) searched the following electronic databases in the period of 1970-1996: Social Science Citation Index, International bibliography of Alzheimers Disease and senile dementia (Biosciences Information Services), Dissertation Abstracts on line, Exerpta Medica, Mental Health Abstracts, Sociological Abstracts, Index Medicus, Psychological Abstract and a series of professional journals in the field of Aging, Psychiatry, Psychology, Gerontology, Physical activity and Rehabilitation. They used the following keywords: aging, movements, psychogeriatric, psychomotor, psychosocial, therapy, dementia, effect(s), elderly, evaluation, SDAT, senile dementia, behavio(u)r therapy/treatment, movement therapy, activity therapy, psychotherapy, group therapy, dance therapy, music therapy, occupational therapy, play therapy, drama therapy, validation therapy, reminiscence, and reality orientation training.
- Finnema et al. (2000b), that focused their review on psychosocial methods that could be integrated in 24-hour care, searched the following electronic databases in the period of 1990-1998: Medline, PsycLit, Embase, Sociofile and Current Contents. In the search the terms dementia and Alzheimer's Disease were coupled separately with the following search terms: emotion-oriented, validation (therapy), sensory integration/sensory stimulation/snoezelen/multi-sensory environment/multi-sensory enhancement, simulated presence therapy and reminiscence (therapy)/life review. The snowball effect furthermore enabled the researchers to retrieve other publications based on the references in the publications initially found.
- In the literature study of Van Mierlo et al. (2009) the search was performed through the electronic databases of PubMed, PsycINFO and Cinahl (from January 1990 to February 2008). The aim of this search was to find studies in which psychosocial interventions had been proven to be effective for subgroups of people with dementia. To structure the literature search, firstly reviews were searched on three key categories: "dementia", "person with dementia", and "effective care and support". Within each category, a search strategy was made, based on keywords (Mesh, Thesaurus and Tree) and free text words (intervention studies, outcome studies). The reviews were analyzed for studies that met the inclusion criteria (effects reported on subgroups of people with dementia, such as Alzheimer dementia and female participants), as well as on living situation (at home or in an institutional care setting)

We found 92 studies in these reviews in which positive effects were reported. To get insight in the areas in which the psychosocial treatments have been effective and the type of effects found, we categorized all studies and outcomes based on the earlier mentioned adaptive tasks (see Table 1). We furthermore inventoried for each treatment method in which adaptation area and in which stage(s) of dementia they had reported positive outcomes (see Table 2).

**Table 1. Psychosocial treatments and positive outcomes categorized
into adaptive task areas on which the treatments focused**

Adaptive task	a. Publication reference / total number of publications b.Outcomes
Coping with one's own disability Treatments focused on maintaining functional abilities by activating and decreasing excess disabilities	a. Arkin, 2003; Bergert and Jacobson, 1976; Biernacki and Barrat, 2001; Casby and Holm, 1994; Edwards and Beck, 2002; Francese et al., 1997; Friedman and Tappen, 1991; Gerdner et al., 1993; Gerdner, 2000; Gibson, 1994b; Gorissen, 1985; Greene et al., 1983; Gustafsson, 1976; Hanley et al, 1981; Hanley and Lusty, 1984; Hopman-Rock et al., 1999; Karlsson et al., 1985; Lord and Garner, 1993; Lund et al., 1995; Mayers and Griffin, 1990; Melin and Götestam, 1981; Namazi and Hayes, 1994; Namazi and Johnson, 1992a,b; Nooren-Staal et al., 1995; Norberg, 1986; Reeve and Ivison, 1985; Rogers et al., 1991; Tabourne, 1995; Williams et al., 1987; Yesavage, 1981. Total 31
	b. (+) Improved cognition: memory performace, orientation, recall, recognition of names and faces, learning abilities, attention span, language, communication, attention, biographical knowledge; improved awareness, improved ability to stay engaged in activities; improved functioning on ADL, selfcare, independent dressing, improved eating behaviour, increased appetite, increased physical strength. (-) less incontinence.
Preserving an emotional balance Treatments frequently focused on improving affective functioning and decreasing e.g. apathetic, paranoid, aggressive, agitated and disruptive behaviour, and anxiety	a. Arno and Frank, 1994; Arkin, 2003; Bellelli et al., 1998; Bianchetti et al., 1997; Birchmore and Clague, 1983; Buettner et al., 1996; Camberg et al., 1999; Casby and Holm, 1994; Churchill et al., 1999; Clark et al., 1998; Cleary et al., 1988; DeYoung et al., 2002; Dröes et al., 1991, 1996; Edwards and Beck, 2002; Fine and Rouse-Bane, 1995; Finnema et al., 2005; Gerdner and Swanson, 1993; Gibson, 1994a,b; Goddaer and Abraham, 1994; Greene et al., 1983; Haffmans et al, 2001; Holm et al.; 1999; Holmberg et al, 1997; Holtkamp et al., 1997; Karlsson et al., 1985; Kim and Bushmann, 1999; Lord and Garner, 1993; Lovell et al., 1995; Lund et al., 1995; McCabe et al. 2002; McCallion et al., 1999; McMinn and Hinton, 2000; Mishima et al., 1994; Moffat et al, 1993; Namazi and Hayes, 1994; Namazi et al., 1994; Norberg et al., 1986; Okawa et al., 1991; Opie et al., 2002; Pinkston and Linsk, 1988; Rasneskog et al., 1996a,b; Romero and Wenz, 2001; Rovner et al., 1996; Spaull and Leach, 1998; Toseland et al., 1997; Van Weert et al., 2005 ; Volicer et al., 1994; Watson, 1998; Welden and Yesavage, 1982; Whall et al., 1997; Witucki and Twibell, 1997; Woods and Ashley, 1995. Total 54
	b. (+) Improved mood, cheerfulness, affect, happy facial expression, lively, expression of emotions, improved sleeping. (-) decreased depression, agitation, screaming, aggression, anxiety, restless behaviour, repetitive behaviour, rebellious behaviour, hyperactivity, restlesness at night, apathy, boredom, discomfort, hallucinations; less physical restraints; less behavioural problems, less disruptive vocalisations, paranoid expressions, less fidgeting; less dangerous behaviour, less psychotropic drugs, less antipsychotics, less antianxiety agents.

Adaptive task	a. Publication reference / total number of publications b. Outcomes
Developing and maintaining social relations Treatment focused on developing or maintaining social contacts and decreasing symptoms caused by social isolation	a. ArnoandFrank, 1994; Ballard et al., 2002; Camberg et al., 1999; Churchill et al., 1999; Dröes, 1991, 1996; Gibson, 1994a; Gustafsson, 1976; Head et al., 1990; Lord and Garner, 1993; Hopman-Rock et al., 1999; McCabe et al., 2002; Melin and Götestam, 1981; Morton and Bleathman, 1991; Moss et al., 2002; Okawa et al., 1991; Olderog-Millard and Smith, 1989; Pollack and Namazi, 1992; Rovner et al., 1996; Sloane et al., 2004; Spaull and Leach, 1998; Tabourne, 1995; Van Weert et al., 2005 ; Williams et al., 1987; Woods and McKiernan, 1995. Total 24
	b. (+) Improved communication, social contacts, social interaction, speech, verbal and nonverbal expression, word fluency, discourse pattern, interest, group cohesion, touching each other. (-) less social inappropriate behaviour, less talking to oneself, less withdrawn behaviour.
Dealing with day care, care home or nursing home environment Treatment focused at promoting meaningful daytime activities and feeling at home	a. Burton, 1980 ; Churchill et al., 1999; Edwards and Beck, 2002; Götestam, 1987; Götestam and Melin, 1990; Greene and Jamieson, 1979; Groene, 1993; Gustafsson, 1976; Hanley, 1981(report of two studies); Hanley et al., 1981; Hussian, 1988; Jenkins, 1977; Reeve and Ivison, 1985; Rovner et al, 1996; Sloane et al., 2004; Williams et al., 1987. Total 17
	b. (+) Increased activity level, orientation in place, participation in activities, appetite; (-) decreased sleeping during day time, less passive behaviour, disruptive behaviour, screaming, physical aggression, wandering.
Developing an adequate care relationship with staff Treatment focused on promoting desired autonomy and decreasing excessive dependent behaviour	a. Blackman, 1979; Clark et al., 1998; De Lange, 2004; Haffmans et al, 2001; Sandman, 1988 Total 5
	b. (+) Improved eating behaviour, initiative and social behaviour during meals, cooperative behaviour, more adequate care relationship (wanted dependency and desired autonomy); (-) decreased rebellious behaviour, aggression
Preserving a positive self-image Treatment focused at promoting self esteem and life satisfaction	a. Dröes, 1991, 1996; Camberg et al., 1999, Finnema et al, 2005; Van Weert et al., 2005 ; Woods and Ashley, 1995 Total 5
	b. Increased satisfaction, self confidence, self esteem, improved decorum
Preparing for an uncertain future Treatment focused at dealing with feelings about the uncertain future and questions on the meaning of life	a. no publications found Total 0
	b. --

RESULTS

Looking at the different adaptive tasks (see Table 1) we found that in the past decades studies focused especially on methods that in one way or another attempted to assist the person with dementia in *preserving an emotional balance* and in *coping with one's own disability*. In the last fifteen years in particular there has been a considerable increase in research in this field. Regarding 'preserving an emotional balance', psychomotor therapy, music therapy, adapting the living environment, validation, snoezelen and animal-assisted or pet therapy were investigated most frequently and they proved to have a positive effect on emotional behavioural symptoms, such as: aggression, apathy, restlessness, depressive, agitated and anxious behaviour.

The studies of methods in support of *coping with the own disability* generally concerned the stimulation of the use of the residual cognitive abilities and acting (e.g. reality orientation, activities groups, normalization of living pattern and structuring activities). Here one can see besides an improved cognition (e.g. memory, orientation, attention span, biographical knowledge) also improved ability to stay engaged in activities, improved functioning on selfcare, and increased physical strength.

Methods for the *improvement of social relationships* and support for *dealing with the nursing home environment* have also been studied relatively often, unlike methods to stimulate an adequate *care relationship with staff*. Remarkable, positive effects have been achieved in the latter two areas with the behavioural therapy approach and reality orientation training. As far as dealing with the living environment is concerned positive outcomes have been achieved by normalisation of the living environment (a homely environment with sufficient privacy and a recognizable living pattern), such as a positive effect on the orientation, social behaviour, and activity level of people with dementia. To date, few studies have addressed methods in support of *preserving a positive self-image*. And finally, no studies were found into methods to address problems with *preparing for an uncertain future*.

Table 2(a). Treatment effects of the different psychosocial interventions categorized into the seven adaptive tasks areas. For each treatment method it is indicated in what stages of dementia it can be applied (L=Light/mild; M=Moderate; MS=Moderate severe; S=Severe; VS=Very severe)

Treatment method severity (number of effect areas)		Adaptive task						
		1 disability	2 emot	3 self image	4 future	5 environm	6 staff	7 relations
Psychomotor therapy	M-MS (5)	X	X	X			X	X
Normal living pattern	M-MS (4)	X	X			X		X
Behaviour therapy	M-S (4)	X	X			X	X	
Activity groups	M-MS (4)	X	X			X		X
Music therapy	M-VS (4)		X	X			X	X
Reality orientation/CS	M-MS (4)	X	X			X		X
Reminiscence	M-MS (3)	X	X					X
Integrated emotion-oriented	MS-S (3)		X	X			X	
Pet therapy	M-MS (3)		X			X		X
Snoezelen	M-VS (3)	X	X	X				
A.G.E. Dementia Care Program	L-S (3)		X			X		X

Most methods showed some efficacy in more than one adaptation area (e.g. psychomotor therapy in 5 areas and reminiscence in 3 areas)(see Table 2). However, it must be underlined that some methods are aimed at people with mild to moderate severe dementia and others at people with severe and very severe dementia. Some methods are mainly aimed at one specific adaptive area, such as supportive psychotherapy (coping with own disabilities) and bright light therapy (maintaining an emotional balance).

Table 2(b). Treatment effects of the different psychosocial interventions categorized into the seven adaptive tasks areas. For each treatment method it is indicated in what stages of dementia it was investigated (L=Light/mild; M=Moderate; MS=Moderate severe; S=Severe; VS=Very severe)

Treatment method Severity (number of effect areas)	Adaptive task						
	1 disability	2 emot	3 selfimage	4 future	5 environm	6 staff	7 relations
Education family visit MS-S (2)		X					X
Simulated presence therapy S-VS (2)		X					X
Alzheimer Rehab by students L-M (2)	X	X					
Validation M-S (2)		X					X
Person centered showering S-VS (2)		X				X	
Supportive psychotherapy L-M (1)	X						
Structuring activities M-S (1)	X						
Dementia Special Care Unit S-VS (1)		X					
Expressive physical touch M-VS (1)		X					
Nutritional Program L-S (1)	X						
Bright light therapy M-S (1)		X					
Behavioral management unit L-S (1)		X					
Aroma therapy S-VS (1)							X

CONCLUSION

Based on the analysis of the literature we can conclude that in the last four decades the focus of psychosocial intervention studies in institutionalised care settings has been mainly on interventions that aim to support people with dementia to find an *emotional balance* (thus trying to prevent or reduce psychological and behavioural disregulations), and to help them *cope with their disabilities* by stimulating the use of residual cognitive abilities (thus trying to prevent excess disabilities). Much less attention was given to the other areas, such as maintaining social contacts, preserving a positive self-image, coping with the nursing home environment and developing an adequate care relationship with the staff.

Positive outcomes achieved by normalisation of the livng environment, such as better orientation, improved social behaviour and activity level of people with dementia, is an argument in favour of letting people with dementia stay in their own familiar living environment as long as possible. That is to say, if this is not experienced as too taxing by the person with dementia and his environment.

Based on the intervention outcomes we may also conclude that the large majority of psychosocial methods applied to people with dementia living in institutions seems to be effective for more than one adaptive task or area and specific behaviour or mood problem. According to our review of the scientific literature, methods on which the most comprehensive effects regarding 3 or more adaptive tasks were reported, are: *psychomotor therapy* (Norberg et al., 1986; Mayers and Griffin, 1990; Arno and Frank, 1994; Dröes and Van Tilburg, 1997; Francese et al, 1997; Holmberg, 1997; Warson, 1998; Hopman-Rock et al., 1999), *behaviour therapy* (Jenkins, 1977; Blackman, 1979; Burton, 1980; Hussian, 1980; Birchmore and Clague, 1983; Pinkston and Linsk, 1988; Sandman et al., 1988; Götestam and Melin, 1990), *normalising living pattern and living environment* (Gustafsson, 1976; Melin and Götestam, 1981; Cleary, 1988), *activity groups* Panella et al., 1984; Karlsson et al, 1985), *music therapy* (Gerdner and Swanson, 1993; Lord and Garner, 1993; Casby and Holm, 1994; Goddaer and Abraham, 1994; Rasneskog et al., 1996; Clark et al, 1998; Gerdner, 2000), *reminiscence* (Head et al., 1990; Morton and Bleathman, 1991; Gibson, 1994a,b; Namazi and Hayes, 1994, Tabourne, 1995; Woods and McKiernan, 1995), *reality orientaton* (Bergert and Jacobson, 1976; Hanley et al., 1981; Greene et al., 1983; Hanley and Lusty, 1984; Gorissen, 1985; Reeve and Ivison, 1985; Williams et al., 1987; Götestam, 1987), *integrated emotion-oriented care* (Finnema et al., 2005), *pet therapy* (Churchill et al., 1999; McGabe et al, 2002; Edwards and Beck, 2002), *snoezelen* (Arno and Frank, 1994; Holtkamp et al., 1997; Witucki and Twibell, 1997; Spaull and Leach, 1998; Van Weert et al, 2005) and the *A.G.E. Dementia Care Program* (Rovner et al., 1996). This large array of treatments implies that psychosocial treatment methods are widely applicable (for problems in several adaptation areas), though not all methods are applicable in all stages of dementia. This means that the choice of which treatment method to use for which individual depends on the aid question, need(s) or adaptation problem(s), the severity of dementia, person-related factors, preferences and target behaviour. This is important to keep in mind when selecting therapy methods for individual people with dementia.

We would like to emphasize that the distinction we made into the seven adaptive tasks or areas was made from a theoretical perspective with the purpose to get insight into the focus of research in the field of psychosocial interventions in the past decades. This does not mean that the original studies were designed with these specific aims regarding adaptation and coping.

Though the results of the effect studies on psychosocial interventions are very promising, it must be mentioned that the quality of many studies in the past 40 years was quite moderate. Despite the fact that there is a growing tendency to apply stronger research designs in the last two decades, we therefore have to be cautious generalizing the results of individual studies. In future studies better designed, controlled, and preferably randomized clinical trials (RCT), are needed to draw firm conclusions on the effectiveness of the different treatment methods. Comparative research into psychosocial methods for different adaptive tasks is also needed, as well as research into the determinants of effective methods to be able to get answers to the question: for whom and for which problem works what best? (see also Smits et al, 2007; Van Mierlo et al, 2009).

More research is needed as well in the areas in which very little research was done to date, such as interventions aiming to support institutionalized people with dementia to develop an adequate care relationship with care professionals, to preserve a positive self-image, to maintain social relationships and to prepare for an uncertain future. These adaptation areas seem directly linked to important aspects of quality of life as mentioned by people with mild to moderate severe dementia in day care and meeting centers and in nursing homes (Dröes et al., 2006), such as autonomy and freedom, self esteem and feeling useful, and spirituality. They definitively deserve more attention in research than they received in the past. Types of interventions that in institutionalized care are used in the mild to moderate stages of dementia for these targets are, for example: Integrated emotion-oriented care in which the offered care and activities are person-centered and well attuned to the abilities, experiences and preferences of the person with dementia (Van der Kooij, 2003; Finnema et al. 2005; De Lange, 2004), reminiscence (Gibson, 1994a,b; Tabourne, 1995), pet therapy (Churchill et al., 1999; McCabe et al., 2002) and Validation (individually or in groups; Bleathman and Morton, 1992; Toseland, 1997). Recently also discussion groups are set up to help people get into contact and discuss their experiences with peers, and to support them in their coping with the changes they go through in their life and the uncertain future (Manthorpe and Moniz-Cook, 2009; Cheston, 2009). More research is needed into these type of interventions. In the more severe stages for instance music therapy and snoezelen are applied to add quality to life. However, further research is recommended here as well (Sherratt et al., 2004; Van Weert et al., 2005).

With the growing number of people with dementia, savings in health care and the expected shortage of care personnel in the coming decades psychosocial care in institutional settings comes highly under pressure. We would like to conclude with the statement that our study shows that there are enough arguments to recommend that in future research and care practice substantial attention should be given to the further development and application of psychosocial methods in dementia care. Only this will ensure that there will be less need to rely on psychopharmacotherapy to control behavioural and psychological symptoms in dementia and will accomplish that persons with dementia, at home and in institutions, in all stages of the disease really feel supported in finding and maintaining an emotional balance in the process of coping with the consequences of the disease.

REFERENCES

APA (1997). American Psychogeriatric Association: Practice Guideline for the Treatment of Patients with Alzheimer's Disease and other dementias of late life. Work group on Alzheimer's Disease and related dementias and Steering Committee on practice guidelines. *Am. J. Psychiatry* 145 (suppl 5), 1-39.

Arkin, S.M. (2003). Student-led exercise sessions yield significant fitness gains for Alzheimer's patients. *Am. J. Alzheimers Dis. Other Dementias*, 18, 159-170.

Arno, S., Frank, D.I. (1994). A group for "wandering" institutionalized clients with primary degenerative dementia. *Perspect Psychiatr Care*, 30, 13-16.

Ballard, C., O'Brien, J., James, I., Mynt, P., Lana, M., Potkins, D., Reichelt, K., Lee, L., Swann, A. and Fossey, J. (2001). Quality of life for people with dementia living in residential and nursing home care: the impact of performance on activities of daily living, behavioral and psychological symptoms, language skills, and psychotropic drugs. *Int. Psychogeriatr,* 13, 93-106.

Bangma, B.D. and Kap, A. (1988). Inleiding revalidatiegeneeskunde; patiëntgericht hulpverlenen. Van Gorcum, Assen/Maastricht.

Bellelli, G., Frisoni, G.B., Bianchetti, A., Boffelli, S., Guerrini, G.B., Scotuzzi, A., Ranieri, P., Ritondale, G., Guglielmi, L., Fusari, A., Raggi, G., Gasparotti, A., Gheza, A., Nobili,

G. and Trabucchi, M. (1998). Special care units for demented patients: a multicenter study. *Gerontologist,* 38, 456-462.

Bergert, L. and Jacobson, E. (1976). Träning av realitetsorientering hos en grupp patienter med senil demens. *Nordisk Tidskrift för Beteendeterapi,* 5, 191-200.

Bianchetti, A., Benvenuti, P., Ghisla, K.M., Frisoni, G.B. and Trabucchi, M. (1997). An Italian model of dementia special care unit: results of a pilot study. *Alzheimer Dis. Assoc Disord,* 11, 53-56.

Biernacki, C. and Barrat, J. (2001). Improving the nutritional status of people with dementia. *Br. J. Nurs.,* 10, 1104-1114.

Birchmore, T. and Clague, S. A behavioral approach to reduce shouting. *Nursing Times,* 79, 1983 (4) 37-39.

Blackman, D.K., Gehle, C. and Pinkston, E.M. (1979). Modifying eating habits of the institutionalized elderly. *Social Work Research and Abstracts,* 18-24.

Bleathman, C. and Morton, I. (1992). Validation therapy: extracts from 20 groups with dementia sufferers. *Journal of Advanced Nursing,* 17, 658-666.

Bowlby, J. *Attachment and Loss.* Vol. 1: Attachment, Vol 2: Seperation, Vol 3: Loss. London: Hogarth Press, 1969, 1973,1980.

Buettner, L., Lundegren, H., Lago, D., Farrel, P., and Smith R. (1996). Therapeutic recreation as an intervention for persons with dementia and agitation: An efficacy study. *Am. J. Alzheimers Dis. Other Dementias,* 11, 4-12.

Burton, M.A. (1980). Evaluation and change *in a psychogeriatric ward through direct observation and feedback.* Br. J. of Psychiatry, 137(4), 566-571.

Camberg, L., Woods, P., Ooi, W.L., Hurley, A., Volicer, L., Ashley, J., Odenheimer, G. and McIntyre, K. (1999). Evaluation of Simulated Presence: a personalized approach to enhance well-being in persons with Alzheimer's disease. *J. Am. Geriatr. Soc.,* 47, 446-452.

Casby, J.A. and Holm, M.B. (1994). The effect of music on repetitive disruptive vocalizations of persons with dementia. *American J. Occupational Therapy,* 48 (10), 883-889.

Cheston, R. (2009). Group psychotherapy for people with early dementia. In: Moniz-Cook, E., Manthorpe, J. (eds.) (2009). *Psychosocial interventions in early stage dementia; a European evidence-based text* (INTERDEM-network), London, UK: Jessica Kingsley Publishers.

Churchill, M., Safaoui, J., McCabe, B.W. and Baun, MM. (1999). Using a therapy dog to alleviate the agitation and desocialization of people with Alzheimer's disease. *J. Psychosoc. Nurs. Ment. Health Serv.,* 37, 16-22.

Clare, L. (2002). We'll fight it as long as we can: coping with the onset of Alzheimer's disease. *Aging and Mental Health,* 6(2), 139-148.

Clark, M.E., Lipe, A.W. and Bilbrey, M. (1998). Use of music to decrease aggressive behaviors in people with dementia. *J. Gerontol. Nurs,* 24, 10-17.

Cleary, T.A., Clamon, C. Price, M. and Shullaw, G. (1988). A reduced stimulation unit: effects on patients with Alzheimer's Disease and related disorders. *The Gerontologist,* 28 (4), 511-514.

Cohen, D. (1991). The subjective experience of Alzheimer's disease: The anatomy of an illness as perceived by patients and families. *The American Journal of Alzheimer's Care and Related Disorders and Research,* 6-11.

Cotrell, V. and Lein, L. (1993). Awareness and denial in the Alzheimer's Disease victim. *Journal of Gerontological Social Work*, 19(3/4), 115-132.

Cotrell, V. and Schulz, R. (1993). The perspective of the patient with Alzheimer's Disease: A neglected dimension of Dementia research. *The Gerontologist*, 33 (2), 205-211.

De Boer, M.E., Hertogh, C.M.P.M., Dröes, R.M., Riphagen, I.I., Jonker, C. and Eefsting, J.A. (2007). Suffering from dementia: the patient's perspective; An overview of the literature. *International Psychoger*iatrics, 19(6), 1021-1039. Epub Aug 30.

De Lange, J. (2004). Omgaan met dementie; het effect van geïntegreerde belevingsgerichte zorg op adaptatie en coping van mensen met dementie in verpleeghuizen; een kwalitatief onderzoek binnen een gerandomiseerd experiment. [Dealing with dementia; effects of integrated emotion-oriented care on adaptation and coping of people ith demetia in nursing homes; a qualitative study as part of a randomized clinical trial.] Academic thesis, Erasmus Universiteit Rotterdam.

DeYoung, S., Just, G. and Harrison, R. (2002). Decreasing aggressive, agitated or disruptive behavior: participation in a behavior management unit. *J. Gerontol. Nurs.* 28, 22-31.

Dröes, R.M. (1991). In Beweging; *over psychosociale hulpverlening aan demente ouderen.* [In Movement; on psychosocial care for people with dementia. Academic Thesis Vrije Universiteit, Amsterdam. Intro, Nijkerk.

Dröes, R.M. (1997). Psychosocial treatment for demented patients; methods and effects. In B. Miesen and G. Jones (Eds.), *Care-giving in dementia* II. (pp. 127-148). UK: Routledge,.

Dröes, R.M. Insight in coping with dementia; listening to the voice of those who suffer from it. *Aging and Mental Health*, 2007; 11(2):115-118.

Dröes, R.M., Breebaart, E., Tilburg, W. van and G.J. Mellenbergh The effect of integrated family support versus day care only on behavior and mood of patients with dementia. *International Psychogeriatrics*, 2000, 12(1), 99-116.

Dröes, R.M., Meiland, F.J.M., Schmitz, M. and Tilburg, W. van Effect of combined support for people with dementia and carers versus regular day care on behaviour and mood of persons with dementia: results from a multi-centre implementation study. *International Journal of Geriatric Psychiatry*, 2004,19, 1-12.

Dröes, R.M. and Tilburg, W. van (1996). Amélioration du comportement agressif par des activités psychomotrices. *L'Année Gérontologique*, 10, 471-482.

Dröes, R.M., Meiland, F.J.M., Schmitz, M.J., Vernooij-Dassen, M.J.F.J., Lange, J. de, Derksen, E., Boerema, I., Grol, R.P.T.M. Grol and Tilburg, W. van (2003). Implementatie Model Ontmoetingscentra; een onderzoek naar de voorwaarden voor succesvolle landelijke implementatie van ontmoetingscentra voor mensen met dementie en hun verzorgers. Eindrapport maart 2003. Amsterdam, The Netherlands: Vrije Universiteit.

Dröes, R.M., Boelens-Van der Knoop, E.C.C., Bos, J., Meihuizen, L., Ettema, T.P., Gerritsen, D.L., Hoogeveen, F., Lange, J. de and Schölzel-Dorenbos, C. (2006). Quality of life in dementia in perspective; an explorative study of variations in opinions among people with dementia and their professional caregivers, and in literature. *Dementia: The International Journal of Social Research and Practice*, 5(4), 533-558.

Edwards, N.E. and Beck, A.M. (2002). Animal-assisted therapy and Nutrition in Alzheimer's disease. *West J. Nurs. Res.* 24, 697-712.

Erikson, E.H. (1963). *Childhood and society.* New York: W.W. Norton and Company.

Feil N. (1989b). Validation: an empathic approach to the care of dementia. *Clin. Gerontol.*, 8(3), 89-94.

Fine, J.I., Rouse-Bane, S. (1995). Using Validation techniques to improve communication with cognitively impaired older adults. *Journal of Gerontological nursing*, 21(6),39-45.

Finnema, E., Dröes, R.M., Ribbe, M., Tilburg, W. van (2000a). A review of psychosocial models in psychogeriatrics; implications for care and research. *Alzheimer Disease and Associated Disorders*, 14(2), 68-80.

Finnema, E., Dröes, R.M., Ribbe, M. and Tilburg, W. van (2000b). The effects of emotion-oriented approaches in the care for persons suffering from dementia; a review of the literature. *International Journal of Geriatric Psychiatry*, 15(2),141-161.

Finnema, E., Dröes, R.M, Ettema, T.P., Ooms, M.E., Adèr, H., Ribbe, M.W. and Tilburg, W. van (2005). The effect of integrated emotion-oriented care versus usual care on elderly persons with dementia in the nursing home and on nursing assistants; a randomized clinical trial. *International Journal of Geriatric Psychiatry*, 20(4),330-43.

Francese, T., Sorrel, J., Butler, F. (1997). The effects of regular exercise on muscle strength and functional abilities of late stage Alzheimer's residents. *Am. J. Alzheimers Dis. Other Demen.*, 12, 122-127.

Friedman, R. and Tappen, R.M. (1991). The effect of planned walking on communication in Alzheimer's Disease. *JAGS*, 39, 650-654.

Gerdner, L.A. (2000). Effects of individualized versus classical "relaxation" music on the frequency of agitation in elderly persons with Alzheimer's disease and related disorders. *Int. Psychogeriatr*, 12, 49-65.

Gerdner, L.A. and Swanson, E.A. (1993). Effects of individualized music on confused and agitated elderly patients. *Archives of Psychiatric Nursing*, 7 (5), 284-291.

Gibson, F. (1994a,b).What can reminiscence contribute to people with dementia? In: *Reminiscence reviewed: Evaluations, archievements, perspectives.* Bornat J. (ed.). Buckingham, England: Open University Press.

Goddaer, J. and Abraham, I.L. (1994). Effects of relaxing music on agitation during meals among nursing home residents with severe cogitive impairment. *Archives of Psychiatric Nursing*, 8(3),150-158.

Gorissen, J.P. (1985). Een onderzoek naar het effect van realiteitsoriëntatie-training op een groep psychogeriatrische patiënten. T. *Gerontologie and Geriatrie*, 16, 235-239.

Götestam, K.G. (1987). Learning versus environmental support for increasing reality orientation in senile demented patients. *Europian Journal of Psychiatry*, 1, 7-12.

Götestam, K.G. and Melin, L. (1990). The effect of prompting and reinforcement of activity in elderly demented inpatients. *Scandinavian J. of Psychology*, 31, 2-8.

Greene, J.G. and Jamieson, M. (1979). Reality Orientation with psychogeriatric patients. *Behav. Res. and Therapy*, Vol. 17, 615-618.

Greene, J.G., Timbury, G.C., Smith, R. and Gardiner, M. (1983). Reality orientation with elderly patients in the community: An empirical evaluation. *Age and Aging*, 12, 38-43.

Groene, R.W. (1993). Effectiveness of music therapy 1:1 intervention with individuals having Senile Dementia of the Alzheimer's Type. *Journal of Music Therapy*, 30 (3), 138-157.

Gustafsson, R. (1976). Miljötherapi pa en avdeling för patienter med senil demenz. *Scandinavian J. of Behavior therapy*, Vol. 5 (1), 27-37.

Haffmans, P. M., Sival, R. C., Lucius, S. A., Cats, Q. and van Gelder, L. (2001). Bright light therapy and melatonin in motor restless behaviour in dementia: a placebo-controlled study. *Int. J. Geriatr. Psychiatry*, 16: 106–110.

Hagberg, B. (1997). The dementias in a psychodynamic perspective. In B. Miessen and G. Jones (Eds.) *Caregiving in Dementia:Research and Applications* (pp. 14-35).London, UK: Routledge,.

Hall, G. R., and Buckwalter, K. C. (1987). Progressively lowered stress threshold: A conceptual model for care of adults with Alzheimer's disease. *Archives of Psychiatric Nursing*, 1(6), 399-406.

Hanley, I.G. (1981). The use of signposts and active training to modify ward disorientation in elderly patients. *J. Behav. Therapy and Exp. Psychiatry*, 12, 241-247.

Hanley, I.G. and Lusty, K. (1984). Memory aids in Reality Orientation: a single-case study. *Behav. Res. and Therapy,*. 22(6), 709-712.

Hanley, I.G., McGuire, R.J. and Boyd, W.D. (1981). Reality orientation and dementia: A controlled trial of two approaches. *Br. J. Psychiatry*, 138, 10-14.

Head, D.M., Portnoy, S. and Woods, R.T. (1990). The impact of reminiscence groups in two different settings. *Int. Journal of Geriatric Psychiatry*, 5, 295-302.

Holm, A., Michel, M., Stern, G.A., Hung, T.M., Klein, T., Flaherty, L., Michel, S. and Maletta, G. (1999). The outcomes of an inpatient treatment program for geriatric patients with dementia and dysfunctional behaviors. *Gerontologist* 39, 668-676.

Holmberg, S.K. (1997). A walking program for wanderers: volunteer training and development of an evening walker's group. *Geriatr Nurs* 18, 160-165.

Holtkamp, C.C., Kragt, K., van Dongen, M.C., van RE, Salentijn, C. (1997). Effect of snoezelen on the behavior of demented elderly. *Tijdschr Gerontol Geriatr* 28, 124-128.

Hoogendijk, W.J.G., Feenstra, .M.G., Botterblom, M.H., Gilhuis, J., Sommer, I.E., Kamphorst, W., Eikelenboom, P. and Swaab, D.F. (1999). Increased activity of surviving locus ceruleus neurons in Alzheimer's disease. A*nn. Neurol.*, Jan;45(1),82-91.

Hopman-Rock, M., Staats, P.G., Tak, E.C. and Dröes, R.M. (1999). The effects of a psychomotor activation programme for use in groups of cognitively impaired people in homes for the elderly. *Int. J. Geriatr. P*sychiatry, 14, 633-642.

Hussian, R.A. (1988). Modification of behaviors in dementia via stimulus manipulation. *Clinical Gerontologist*, 8(1), 37-43.

ICIDH (1980). International Classification of Impairments, Disabilities and Handicaps. *WHO*, Geneva, 1980.

Jenkins, J., Felce, D., Lunt, B. and Powell, L. (1977). Increasing engagement in activity of residents in old people's homes by providing recreational materials. *Behavior Research and Therapy*, 15,429-434.

Karlsson, I. Båne, G., Melin, E., Nuth, A.L. e.a. (1985). *Mental activation - Brain plasticity. Normal Aging, Alzheimer's Disease and senile dementia*. Gottfries, C.G (Ed.), Editions de l'Université de Bruxelles.

Kitwood, T. and Bredin K. (1992). Towards a theory of dementia care: personhood and well-being. *Ageing and Society* , 12,269-87.

Kim, E.J. and Buschmann, M.T. (1999). The effect of expressive physical touch on patients with dementia. *Int. J. Nurs. Stud.*, 36, 235-243.

Kiyak, H. and Borson, S. (1992). Coping with chronic illness and disability. In: Ory MG, Abeles RP, Lipman PD (eds.) *Aging, health, and behavior* (pp. 141-173). Newbury Park CA: Sage Publications, Inc..

Kooij, C.H. van der Gewoon lief zijn? (2003). Het maieutisch zorgconcept en het invoeren van Geintegreerde belevingsgerichte zorg op psychogeriatrische verpleeghuisafdelingen. Academic thesis, Vrije Universiteit, Amsterdam.

LaBarge, E. and Trtanj, F. (1995). A support group for people in the early stages of dementia of the Alzheimer-type. *Journal of Applied Gerontology*, 14 (3), 289-301.

Lazarus, R.S. and Folkman, S. (1984). *Stress, appraisal, and coping*. New York: Springer Publ. Comp..

Lord TR, Garner JE. 1993. Effects of music on Alzheimer patients. *Percept Mot Skills*, 76, 451-455.

Lovell, B.B., Ancoli-Israel, S., Gevirtz, R. (1995). Effect of bright light treatment on agitated behavior in institutionalized elderly subjects. *Psychiatry Res.*, 57, 7-12.

Lund, D.A, Hill, R.D., Caserta, M.S. and Wright, S.D. (1995). Video Respite: an innovative resource for family, professional caregivers, and persons with dementia. *Gerontologist*, 35, 683-687.

Manthorpe, J. and Moniz-Cook, E. (2009). Developing group support for men with mild cognitive difficulties and early dementia. In: Moniz-Cook, E., Manthorpe, J. (eds.) (2008). *Psychosocial interventions in early stage dementia*; a European evidence-based text (INTERDEM-network). London, UK : Jessica Kingsley Publishers.

Mayers, K.M. and Griffin, M. (1990). The play project; use of stimulus objects with demented patients. *J. of Gerontological Nursing*, 16 (1), 32-37.

McCabe, B.W., Baun, M.M., Speich, D. and Agrawal, S. (2002). Resident dog in the Alzheimer's special care unit. *West J. Nurs. Res.* 24, 684-696.

McCallion, P., Toseland, R.W., Freeman, K. (1999). An evaluation of a family visit education program. *J. Am. Geriatr. Soc.*, 47(2), 203-14.

McMinn, B.G. and Hinton, L. (2000). Confined to barracks: The effects of indoor confinement on aggressive behavior among inpatients of an acute psychogeriatric unit *Am. J. Alzheimers Dis. Other Demen.* 15: 36 - 41.

Melin, L. and Götestam, K.G. (1981). The effects of rearranging ward routines on communication and eating behaviors of psychogeriatric patients. *J. of Applied Behavior Analysis,* Vol. 14(1), 47-51.

Miesen, B. (1990) *Gehechtheid en dementie*. Versluys Uitg. BV, Almere.

Miesen, B. and Jones, G. (1997). The Alzheimer Café Concept: A Response to the Trauma, Drama and Tragedy of Dementia. In: Miesen, B., Jones, G. (eds.), *Care-giving in Dementia: Research and applications*. Vol. 3. (pp. 307-333). London, UK: Routledge.

Mishima, K., Okawa, M., Hishikawa, Y., Hozumi, S., Hori, H., Takahashi, K. 1994. Morning bright light therapy for sleep and behavior disorders in elderly patients with dementia. *Acta Psychiatr. Scand*, 89, 1-7.

Moffat, N., Parker, P., Pinkney, L., et al. (1993*). Snoezelen - An experience for people with dementia*. Chesterfield: ROMPA.

Moniz-Cook, E. and Manthorpe, J. (eds.) (2009). *Psychosocial interventions in early stage dementia; a European evidence-based text* (INTERDEM-network). London, UK: Jessica Kingsley Publishers.

Moore, I. (1997). Living with Alzheimer's: Understanding the family's and patient's perspective. *Geriatrics*, 2, S33-S36.

Moos, R.H. and Tsu, V.D. (1977). The crisis of physical illness: An overview. In: R.H. Moos (Ed.), *Coping with physical illness*. New York/London: Plenum Medical Book Company,.

Morton, I. and Bleathman, C. (1991). The effectiveness of Validation therapy in dementia; a pilot study. *Int. Journal of Geriatric Psychiatry*, 6, 327-330.

Moss, S.E., Polignano, E., White, C.L., Minichiello, M.D., Sunderland, T. (2002). Reminisence group activities and discourse interaction in Alzheimer's disease. *J. Gerontol. Nurs.*, 28, 36-44.

Namazi, K.H., Hayes, S.R.. 1994. Sensory stimuli reminiscence for patients ith Alzheimer's disease: relevance and implications. *Clinical Gerontologist*, 14, 29-46.

Namazi, K.H. and Johnson, B.D. (1992a). Dressing independently: a closet modification model for Alzheimer's disease patients. *Am. J. Alzheimers Dis. Other Demen*, 7, 22-28.

Namazi, K.H. and Johnson, B.D. (1992b). The effects of environmental barriers on the attention span of Alzheimer's disease patients. *Am. J. Alzheimers Dis. Other Dementias*, 7, 9-15.

Namazi, K.H., Gwinnup, P.B., Zadorozny, CA. (1994). Low Intensity Exercise/Movement Program for Patients With Alzheimer's Disease: The TEMP-AD Protocol. *J. Aging Phys. Ac*, 2, 80-92.

Namazi, K.H., Zadorozny, C.A. and Gwinnup, P.A. (1995). The influences of physical activity on patterns of sleep behavior of patients with Alzheimer's Disease. *Int. J. Aging and Human Development*, 40 (2),45-153.

Nooren-Staal W.H.C. van, Frederiks, C.M.A. and Wierik, M.J.M. te (1995). Validation: effecten bij bewoners en personeel in een verzorgingshuis. *T. voor Gerontologie en Geriatrie*, 26, 117-121.

Norberg, A., Melin, E. and Asplund, K. (1986). Reactions to music, touch and object presentation in the final stage of dementia. *Int. J. of Nursing studies*, 23, 315-323.

Okawa, M., Mishima, K., Hishikawa, Y., Hozumi, S., Hori, H. and Takahashi, K. (1991). Circadian rhythm disorders in sleep-waking and body temperature in elderly patients with dementia and their treatment. *Sleep*, 14, 478-485.

Olderog-Millard, K.A. and Smith, J.M. (1989). The influence of group singing therapy on the behavior of Alzheimer's Disease patients. *J. of Nursing Therapy*, 26, 1989 (2), 58-70.

Opie, J., Doyle, C. and O'Connor, D.W. (2002). Challenging behaviors in nursing home residents with dementia: a randomized controlled trial of multidisciplinary interventions. *Int. J. Geriatr. Psychiatry*, 17, 6-13.

Pinkston, E.M. and Linsk, N.L. (1988). *Care of the elderly: A family approach*. Pergamom Press Inc., New York/Oxford.

Pollack, N.J. and Namazi, K.H. (1992). The effect of music participation on the social behavior of Alzheimer's disease patients. *Journal of Music Therapy*, 29 (1), 54-67.

Rasneskog, H. Bråne, G., Karlsson, I. and Kihlgren, M. (1996). Influence of diner music on food intake and symptoms common in dementia. *Scandinavian Journal of Caring Science*, 10(1),11-17.

Reeve, W. and Ivison, D. (1985). Use of environmental manipulation and classroom and modified informal reality orientation with institutionalized, confused elderly ppatients. *Age and Aging*, 14,119-121.

Reisberg, B. (1996). Behavioral intervention approaches to the treatment and management of Alzheimer's Disease: A research agenda. *Int. Psychogeriatrics*, 8(suppl. 1), 39-44.

Rogers J.C., Holm, M.B., Burgio, L.D, Granieri, E., Hsu, C., Hardin, J.M., McDowell B.J. (1999). Improving morning care routines of nursing home residents with dementia. *J. Am. Geriatr. Soc.*, 47, 1049-1057.

Romero, B. and Wenz, M. (2001). Self-maintenance therapy in Alzheimer's disease, *Neuropsychol Rehabil*, 11, 333-355.

Rovner, B.W., Steele, C.D., Shmuely, Y., Folstein M.F. (1996). A randomized trial of dementia care in nursing homes. *J. Am. Geriatr. Soc.*, 44, 7-13.

Sandman, P.O., Norberg, A. and Adolfsson, R. (1988). Verbal communication and behavior during meals in five institutionalized patients with Alzheimer-type dementia. *J. of Advanced Nursing*, 13(5), 571-578.

Sherratt, K., Thornton, A., Hatton, C. (2004). Music interventions for people with dementia: a review of the literature. *Aging and Mental Health*, 8(1), 3-12.

Sloane, P.D., Hoeffer, B., Mitchell, C.M., McKenzie, D.A., Barrick, A.L, Rader, J., Stewart, B.J., Talerico, K.A., Rasin, J.H., Zink, R.C., Koch, G.G. (2004). Effect of person-centered showering and the towel bath on bathing-associated aggression, agitation, and discomfort in nursing home residents with dementia: a randomized, controlled trial. *J. Am. Geriatr. Soc.*, 52, 1795-1804.

Smits, C.H., de Lange, J., Dröes, R.M., Meiland, F., Vernooij-Dassen, M., Pot, A.M. (2007). Effects of combined intervention programmes for people with dementia living at home and their caregivers: a systematic review. *Int. J. Geriatric Psychiatry*, 22, 1181-1193.

Smith, G.H. (1986) A comparison of the effects of three treatment interventions on cognitive functioning of Alzheimer patients. *Music Therapy*, 6A (1), 41-56.

Smith, M., Gerdner, L. A., Hall, G., and Buckwalter, K. C. (2004). The history, development, and future of the progressively lowered stress threshold model: A conceptual model for dementia care. *Journal of the American Geriatrics Society*, 52(10), 1755-1760.

Spaull, D. and Leach, C. (1998). An evaluation of the effects of sensory stimulation with people who have dementia. *Behavioural and Cognitive Psychotherapy*, 26(1), 77-86.

Tabourne, C.E.S. (1995). The effects of a life review program on disorientation, social interaction and self-esteem of nursing home residents. *Int. J. Aging Hum. Dev.*, 41(3), 251-66.

Teri, L. (1994) Behavioral treatment of depression in patients with dementia. *Alzheimer's Disease and Associated Disorders*, 8 (suppl. 3), 66-74.

Toseland, R.W., Diehl, M., Freeman, K., Manzanares, T., Naleppa, M. and McCallion, P. (1997). The Impact of Validation Group Therapy on Nursing Home Residents With Dementia. *J. Appl. Gerontol*, 16(1), 31-50.

Van der Roest, H.G., Meiland, F.J.M., Comijs, H.C., Derksen, E., Jansen, A., Hout, H. van, Jonker, C. and Dröes, R.M. What do community dwelling people with dementia need? A survey among those who are known by care and welfare services. *International Psychogeriatrics*, 2009 Oct;21(5),949-65. Epub 2009 Jul 15.

Van Mierlo, L.D., Van der Roest, H.G., Meiland, F.J.M. and Dröes, R.M. Personalized Dementia Care; proven effectiveness of psychosocial interventions in subgroups. *Aging Research Reviews*, 2009 Sep 23. [Epub ahead of print]

Van Weert, J.C., van Dulmen, A.M., Spreeuwenberg, P.M., Ribbe, M.W. and Bensing, J.M. (2005). Behavioral and mood effects of snoezelen integrated into 24-hour dementia care. *J. Am. Geriatr. Soc.*, 53, 24-33.

Volicer, L., Collard, A., Hurley, A., Bishop, C., Kern, D. and Karon, S. (1994). Impact of special care unit for patients with advanced Alzheimer's disease on patients' discomfort and costs. *J. Am. Geriatr. Soc.*, 42, 597-603.

Watson, N.M. (1998). Rocking chair therapy for dementia patients. Its effect on psychosocial well-bering and balance. *Am. J. of Alzheimers's Disease and Other Dementias*, 13(6), 296-308.

Welden, S. and Yesavage, J.A. Behavioral improvement with relaxation training in senile dementia. *Clinical Gerontologist*, Vol. 1, 1982 (1), 45-49.

Whall, A.L., Black, M.E., Groh, C.J., Yankou, D.J., Kupferschmid BJ, Foster NL. (1997).The effect of natural environments upon agitation and aggression in late stag dementia patients. *Am. J. Alzheimers Dis Other Dementias*, 12, 216-220.

Williams, R., Reeve, W., Ivison, D. and Kavanagh, D. (1987). Use of environmental manipulation and modified informal reality orientation with institutionalized, confused elderly subjects: a replication. *Age and Aging*, Vol. 16, 315-318.

Witucki, J.M. and Twibell, R.S. (1997). The effect of sensory stimulation activities on the psychological well being of patients with advanced Alzheimer's disease. *Am. J. Alzheimers Dis Other Dementias*, 12, 10-15.

Woods, P. and Ashley, J. (1995). Simulated Presence Therapy: using selected memories to manage problem behaviors in Alzheimer's disease patients. *Geriatric Nursing*, 16(1),9-14.

Woods, B., McKiernan, F. (1995). Evaluating the impact of reminiscence on older people with dementia. In: Haight, B.K. and Webster, J.D. (eds.) *The art and science of reminiscing: theory, research, methods and applications.* Washington DC, USA: Taylor and Francis, 233-242.

Yesavage, J.A. (1984). Relaxation and memory training in 39 elderly patients. *Amer. J. Psychiatry,* 141(6), 778-781.

In: Dementia: Non-Pharmacological Therapies
Editor: Elisabetta Farina, pp. 161-172

ISBN: 978-1-61470-736-3
© 2012 Nova Science Publishers, Inc.

ORIGINS OF MONTESSORI PROGRAMMING FOR DEMENTIA

Cameron J. Camp*

Hearthstone Alzheimer Care.

ABSTRACT

The focus of this article is on the evolution of the use of Montessori educational methods as the basis for creating interventions for persons with dementia. The account of this evolution is autobiographical, as the development of Montessori Programming for Dementia (MPD) initially was through the efforts of myself and my research associates. My initial exposure to Maria Montessori's work came as a result of my involvement with my own children's education. This exposure influenced ongoing research on development of cognitive interventions for persons with dementia. A brief description of Montessori's work with children and the educational methods she developed is followed by a description of how this approach can be translated into development of activities for persons with dementia. Assessment tools to document effects of MPD were created, focusing on observational tools to measure engagement and affect during individual and group activities programming for persons with dementia. Examples of the use of MPD by researchers, staff members, and family members are given, as well as examples of how persons with dementia can provide MPD to other persons with dementia or to children. Finally, examples of MPD's dissemination internationally and future directions for research are presented.

Keywords: Montessori method, cognitive rehabilitation, engagement, activity, "I'm still here" approach.

INTRODUCTION

Because of the personal nature of this article, it is largely written in the first person. I thank the many persons who, over many years, have worked with me and discussed this approach to the treatment of dementia.

---

* Preparation of this manuscript was supported, in part, by grant R34 MH075799 from the National Institute of Mental Health to Cameron Camp. For further information or question about the contents, please contact: Cameron J. Camp, Ph.D., Hearthstone Alzheimer Care; 23 Warren Ave., Suite 140; Woburn, Massachusetts, 01801, USA; camp@thehearth.org; 440-829-4927.

Recently, Beck, Levinson, and Irons (2009) traced the origins of J. B. Watson's famous experiment with "Little Albert," and their detective work led to the discovery of the person who probably was the infant in Watson's laboratory and shown in his films of conditioning experiments. In a similar manner, this article traces the origins of the use of Montessori educational techniques as interventions for persons with dementia. In my case, however, I have a distinct advantage over Beck, Levinson, and Irons. They had to make inferences and deductions based on records, circumstantial evidence, and the sometimes erroneous or conflicting evidence presented by the memories of persons associated with events that occurred almost 90 years ago. In my case, I only have to contend with omissions or false memories generated in my own mind over the course of the last 32 years of my life experiences. However, it is hoped that the reader will be indulgent, and that the tracing of the origins of this intervention will serve as an inspiration to younger researchers to be open to interruptions in their careers and to serendipity.

When I was a graduate student working on my doctoral degree in psychology at the University of Houston, I studied cognition and aging. However, when I started graduate school I was married and had a 2-year-old daughter, who was later diagnosed as learning disabled. I worked during semester breaks at child care centers to better understand normal child development. I also worked part time for a while at a school for children with emotional and learning disabilities, to better understand my daughter and her challenges.

While at that school I was introduced to teaching materials that were labeled "Montessori." That was my first introduction to the term, in 1977. I bought several toys at a department store that were labeled "Montessori teaching toys" for my daughter. I found them to be cleverly constructed, but did not examine them in great detail. They seemed to interest my daughter. In 1979 I graduated with a doctorate in experimental psychology, with a dissertation project that involved examining age differences in fact recall and inferential reasoning from world knowledge systems in normal younger and older adults (Camp, 1981). In fact, some of my sample consisted of members of a society of persons with high scores on intelligence tests. I was far away from the field of Alzheimer's disease or intervention development.

I began my academic career as an assistant professor at Fort Hays State University in Hays in western Kansas. There were no Montessori schools in the town, though my daughter attended an excellent school for children with developmental disabilities. My son and youngest daughter were born in Hays. While there I was recruited by my department chairperson to teach weekend seminars in memory improvement as a means of increasing student credit hour production for the department and university (Camp, 1996). This started an interest in developing memory interventions for normal older adults (c.f., Anschutz, Camp, Markley, and Kramer, 1985; 1987) as well as in examining what types of memory strategies were spontaneously utilized by normal younger and older adults (Camp, Markley, and Kramer, 1983a; b).

In 1983 we moved to New Orleans, where I was on the faculty of the psychology department of the University of New Orleans. My oldest daughter went to special education classes in public schools, but my son was able to enroll in a Montessori school. Three years later my youngest daughter enrolled in the same Montessori school. I began to examine the environment, teaching materials, and methods associated with Montessori education.

While my past research had focused on normal aging, once I moved to New Orleans I began to work with adult day health centers. In a New Orleans suburb one of the first adult day centers in the U.S. focused specifically on providing services to persons with dementia was opening. I began to work with this center and several others in the area, and so began a new direction of my research. This involved developing interventions for challenging behaviors associated with dementia.

I was struck by the potential of Montessori methods as interventions for persons with dementia, though initially this was only a theoretical interest. My research at the time focused on developing a memory improvement technique – spaced retrieval – as an intervention for persons with dementia (Camp, 1996; 2006a). This involves giving persons practice at successfully remembering information over successively increasing time intervals. Spaced retrieval is, in essence, the use of shaping from behavioral technology applied to memory (Bjork, 1988). There is evidence that spaced retrieval engages implicit memory in persons with dementia (Camp, 2006; Camp and Foss, 1997; Foss and Camp, 1994). It soon became clear that using interventions targeted at memory systems that were impaired in persons with dementia might not be as effective as working with systems that were either intact or less damaged.

I began to write about the use of memory interventions for normal older adults and persons with dementia that would target either explicit or implicit memory, using either external or internal storage of information (Camp et al., 1993). At that time, it also seemed to me as if Montessori materials were capable of accessing implicit or procedural learning systems very efficiently. For example, to teach the geography of the United States children are presented a puzzle with wooden pieces. Each piece is in the shape of a state, with a wooden peg attached that can be used to lift and place the puzzle piece. A template or map of the United States is provided, with an outline of each state available. Children place each puzzle piece on the corresponding shape outlined on the template. Once they become proficient with this task, they are presented the task again but without the outlined template. With practice, they learn where all of the states are located in relation to each other and to the United States as a whole. AND, the peg attached to each puzzle piece is located where the capitol of the state is located. For the state of Wyoming, the peg is in the lower right corner (where Cheyenne is located), and for the state of Oregon, in the upper left corner (where Salem is located). Unconsciously, automatically, and effortlessly these children learn the locations of the state capitols. Maria Montessori said "they will learn through their hands."

To teach children phonics (which can start at three years of age or even earlier), a letter from the alphabet is cut out of sandpaper and glued to a wooden square. A child is invited to learn a lesson regarding the square. For example, in the Roman alphabet a child would see a "t" on the square. The teacher would put two fingers on the sandpaper and trace the letter, pronouncing the phonetic sound of the letter at the same time. The child, after observing the demonstration, would imitate these actions. In so doing, the child "feels" the phonic, hears the phonetic sound of the letter, sees the phonic, and makes the movements of the kinesthetics necessary to draw the letter. In addition, however, there is a subtle lesson embedded in the materials themselves. The background color of paint on the wooden squares for all consonants is one color, and the background color for all vowels is a second, contrasting color. This fact is not pointed out by teachers, but by mere manipulation of these sandpaper letters a child unconsciously learns which ones are "special," i.e. are vowels.

In addition, my wife, Linda, began to study to become a Montessori pre-school teacher. I had the opportunity to type up her lesson plans for her training, which gave me a great deal more exposure to the Montessori method of education for children. Maria Montessori was the first woman M.D. in Italy. An advocate of women's rights, her first work was with children who were deemed "unteachable," often with mental retardation. Montessori developed training regimens based on rehabilitation techniques, and these "defective" children began to pass educational tests designed for normal children. Later, she was asked to work with 3- to 6-year old children in a housing project in the poor section of Rome. Given the janitor's daughter to train as a teacher, Montessori created the first "children's house" (Casa dei Bambini), as well as an educational system based on her earlier work and on systematic observation. She field tested her approach and materials, and continued to do so for 50 years in children's houses around the world. Lillard (2005) describes some key principles of the Montessori method, almost all of which apply to best care practices for dementia. Some of these include the need to include movement and motor learning in activities, providing freedom and choice within an ordered structure, providing contexts and activities that are of interest to the person, allowing learning from peers, embedding activity within a culturally relevant context, providing both empathy and high expectations, and providing a structured environment that provides the supports needed to facilitate success.

Later, I was asked to teach Child Development at the Montessori training center in New Orleans where my wife received her certification as a Montessori teacher of preschool children. I had been struck by the fact that Montessori's approach could be viewed as containing features of a number of different theoretical orientations. For final exams in my class, Montessori teachers-in-training had to present two activities from the perspective of a Montessori philosophy and approach. Then, they had to present the same lessons from the perspective of two other theoretical orientations. For example, a Montessori activity could be viewed as the creation of a "zone of proximal development" from the perspective of L.S. Vygotsky. The materials and procedures associated with the activity provide the assistance necessary to allow the individual to display abilities and behaviors beyond those which could be achieved without such assistance (Vygotsky, 1978). A Montessori activity might be viewed as a self-directed, individualized learning task from the point of view of B. F. Skinner, in which the materials guide learning, prevent error, and provide continuous feedback, with success providing reinforcement for the learner (Skinner, 1954).

In my own mind, I was beginning to see linkages between Montessori's approach and the translation of concepts in neuroscience into practical interventions for persons with dementia. And so, I suggested to a graduate student that he might examine the use of Montessori teaching materials with person living with dementia at the adult day center for persons with dementia as a master's thesis project. Shortly after this, I left New Orleans, though the student, David Vance, continued his study and published research based on his thesis (Vance and Porter, 2000).

In 1995 I left academia, literally and figuratively, and my family moved to Cleveland, Ohio, where I began work at the Myers Research Institute of Menorah Park Center for Senior Living. It was at this point that I decided to explore the use of Montessori techniques for persons with dementia in earnest, and began piloting the use of this intervention with the assistance of my wife. Menorah Park had an adult day health center, assisted living, skilled nursing facilities (including a special care unit for persons with dementia), and later a home health agency. My staff and I began to develop Montessori Programming for Dementia (MPD) within each of these programs.

The Montessori Method. The Montessori teaching method is used to train children in the areas of practical life (activities of daily living), sensorial experiences, language, math, engaging and maintaining the environment, science, and social skills. Developmentally and programmatically based, Montessori techniques seem well-suited for persons with dementia. Each lesson is first presented at its simplest level and each subsequent lesson, increasing in complexity, is a variation of previously mastered skills or concepts. Materials are taken from the everyday environment and are designed not to be "toys" but tools to practice independent living. Persons with dementia need structure and order in their environment and activities; changes in routine or physical surroundings may be upsetting (Vance et al., 1996). Maria Montessori said the same of her young students, and thus all activities involve a structure and order that comfort and allow attention to be focused. Activities involve immediate feedback, high probability of success, and repetition. Tasks are broken down into steps that can be mastered and then sequenced, an approach familiar to occupational therapists. Montessori-based programming makes use of a number of rehabilitation principles and techniques, including: task breakdown, guided repetition, task progression from simple to complex and concrete to abstract, etc. Such programming also takes advantage of principles for dementia interventions including extensive use of external cues, reliance on procedural / nondeclarative/implicit memory rather than declarative/explicit memory, etc. Persons with dementia demonstrate the ability to learn through procedural or nondeclarative memory, a phenomenon remarkably similar to what Montessori described as "unconscious learning" in her children (Vance et al., 1996).

MPD activities can be structured to be used in one-on-one, small group, or large group situations. As stated earlier, activities are chosen for individuals based on their abilities and interests. Examples include sorting pictures or words into categories such as "Fruits vs. Vegetables," which may be given to someone who enjoyed gardening, or "Cities in Europe vs. Cities not in Europe" for someone who enjoyed travel or geography. Fine motor tasks such as using scissors to cut out pictures to be used in the category sorting activities or using a screwdriver to help repair a faucet are activities that can provide practice in maintaining fine motor function while allowing individuals to create/produce items as a result of their practice, which is another key Montessori concept.

Other examples of Montessori-based activities involve the use of templates, or outlines of materials onto which the actual materials are placed. A template of a place setting at a meal would involve a piece of paper with the outline of a plate, knife, fork, spoon, and glass for what [delete "what"] liquid refreshment. Using this template as a guide, a person with dementia can set the table for himself or herself. A template of dentures could be placed on a table next to the bed, and the person with dementia could learn the habit of taking out dentures and putting them on a template when [change "when" to "before"] going to sleep.

We also use templates to help persons with HIV or with diabetes to take medications appropriately. For example, we worked with a man who was HIV+ and who had difficulty remembering which medications to place in his weekly pillbox. Cognitive deficits, including executive dysfunction and short term memory difficulties, are commonly seen in persons with HIV, especially if the disease has progressed to produce HIV-associated dementia (HAD). For this person, we created a template to use when filling his pillbox. The template was similar in size and dimensions to the weekly pillbox. Life size pictures of his pills were glued onto the template in columns (each column representing pills for one day of the week). His task was to match his actual pills to the pictures, and once all of the pictures had been matched, to place each column's pills into the appropriate container in his actual pill box. He improved in this task with practice, and we used spaced retrieval to train him to take out the template and use it at a consistent time (Sunday evenings). Both by the report of this person and that of his physician, this person with HIV was much better able to follow his medication regimen. Furthermore, the use of the template eliminated placing inappropriate medications into the pillbox (Skrajner et al., 2007). An important point to be made from this example is that even when pharmacologic interventions may be necessary, it is critical that nonpharmacologic interventions be included in the treatment regimen to insure that persons with cognitive deficits can adhere to medical regimens successfully. For more detailed description of MPD and its applications, the reader is referred to the following sources: (Camp, 1999; 2006b; Camp et al., 2006; Joltin, Camp, Noble, and Antenucci, 2005; Skrajner et al., 2007).

Initially, MPD was developed and implemented by researchers. We quickly determined that the effects produced by these activities often were profound, but did not easily map onto existing outcome measures. After careful observation and extensive discussion, it was decided that the most significant construct affected by MPD was that of engagement – connectedness with the social and physical environment. Further, we determined that engagement had different forms or aspects. As a result, we created the MPES – Menorah Park Engagement Scale. In its original form, engagement was defined as having four categories: Constructive Engagement (CE), which involved direct interaction – verbal or physical – between the person with dementia and the target activity. Examples would include speaking about the activity or to the activity director, holding or manipulating objects related to the activity, etc. Passive Engagement (PE) involved watching the activity but not directly taking part in it. Both CE and PE are considered positive forms of engagement, and persons with dementia sometimes need to simply watch an activity before they gain the confidence to begin to actively take part at a later time. Self-engagement (SE) was defined as engagement with oneself rather than the target activity, such as picking at one's clothes, talking to yourself, etc. Non-engagement (NE) was defined as sleeping or staring into space for 10 seconds or longer.

In an initial study (Judge, Camp, and Orsulic-Jeras 2000), 10-minute observations were taken of nine person living with dementia with dementia during Montessori-based programming and 10 person living with dementia with dementia during regular activities programming at an adult day health center, with the amount of time observed during each specific form of engagement recorded. In the MPES scoring, categories of engagement are mutually exclusive, so that if a person is talking about the target activity appropriately while picking at their blouse, the person would be coded as exhibiting constructive engagement. The purpose of the MPES is to record the highest level of engagement that the person with dementia is capable of displaying. Person living with dementia in Montessori-based programming showed significantly more constructive engagement and less passive engagement that person living with dementia in regular activities programming.

In a second study, we worked with sixteen residents of residents on an advanced dementia unit in a long-term care facility during standard activities programming and during MPD activities. In addition to using the MPES as before, we adopted the Affect Rating Scale (ARS), developed by Lawton, Van Haitsma, and Klapper (1996), a standardized and validated measure of pleasure, anger, anxiety/ fear and sadness. Type of affect observed was recorded during the same 10-minute observation session as when MPES data was being recorded. For the ARS, a five-point scale was used to record each affect observed: 1 = never observed; 2 =

less than 16 seconds; 3 = 16 – 59 seconds; 4 = 1 – 5 minutes; 5 = more than 5 minutes. Each data recording session focused on a single person.

These residents with advanced dementia showed significantly more constructive engagement and less passive engagement, as well as significantly more pleasure, while participating in Montessori-based activities than in regularly scheduled activities programming. Results being produced by such studies led to activities staff asking for training in the implementation of such programming. Engagement is now being recognized as an extremely important element of quality of life and of successful intervention for persons with dementia (e.g., Cohen-Mansfield, Dakheel-Ali, and Marx, 2009).

Our current version of the MPES has been simplified so that it can be used by staff in care settings for persons with dementia so that these staff members can document the effects being produced by MPD. Rather than recording specific amounts of time within an observation window, engagement categories are scored as "1 – never observed," "2 – observed up to half of the time," and "3 – observed more than half the time." Affect categories have been simplified to Pleasure and Anxiety/Sadness (i.e., positive and negative valence in affect), using the same 3-point scale as with engagement categories. We have found that MPD is still able to produce significant effects using this modified version of the MPES. (Copies of the MPES are available from the author on request; email: camp@thehearth.org).

Implementation of MPD by care staff. In a project funded by the U.S. National Institute of Mental Health (C. Camp, PI), it was demonstrated that staff could be trained to implement MPD "from the ground up" in a variety of care settings, including adult day health centers, assisted living facilities, and skilled nursing homes. In addition, MPD implemented by these trained staff produced significantly more positive engagement while decreasing forms of negative engagement in persons with dementia compared to standard activities programming (Skrajner et al., 2007). Home health workers also have been trained to implement MPD and have done so successfully (Gorzelle, Kaiser, and Camp, 2003).

Implementation of MPD by family members. Family members watching staff implement MPD requested training in this approach as a way of maximizing the quality of their visits with relatives who had dementia, and so we have trained family members to use such activities (Rose et al., 2003; Schneider and Camp, 2002). In a further study, we trained family members to engage persons with dementia at end of life in hospice care (Skrajner et al., 2007). For example, daughters worked with mothers on flower arranging, washing and drying dishes, matching samples of wall paper with different borders for wallpaper (for an older adult who was an interior designer), using maracas to keep time to favorite music, matching photos of food with the part of a meal they represented (dessert, main course, etc.), and working through finger mazes (mazes that sit on a table top and which have paths that are traced with a finger). All daughters reported that using these activities allowed better quality, more focused visits. Most daughters showed other visitors (husbands, grandchildren, friends, and staff) how to use the activities, as well.

Implementation of MPD by persons with dementia. We also have developed training techniques to allow persons with early, [delete comma after "early"] to moderate stage dementia to serve as small group activity leaders for persons with more advanced dementia in adult day care, assisted living, and long-term care (Camp and Skrajner, 2004; Camp, Skrajner, and Kelly, 2005; Skrajner and Camp, 2007). For example, we developed printed materials to facilitate creation of reading and discussion groups. The activity is known as Reading

Roundtable®, and the stories are designed to be age appropriate and interesting. Topics range from the invention of the game of basketball to stories of movie stars to stories of famous persons such as Leonardo da Vinci. Pages are printed only on one side, and participants take turns reading single pages aloud to the group while the rest of the participants follow along silently. Questions and discussion items follow the stories. Using the simplified MPES, we found that when persons with early to moderate dementia led reading and discussion groups of persons with dementia in adult day health care and in long-term care with more advanced dementia, significantly more constructive engagement and pleasure, and significantly less non-engagement were seen than were observed with these same group members during regular activities programming led by activities staff members (Skrajner and Camp, 2007).

In an interesting case study (Mattern and Kane, 2007), a resident at Menorah Park with Huntington's disease (HD) asked if she could do something to help residents with Alzheimer's disease. While her fine motor skills were severely impaired, and she had to use a walker to ambulate, she had good social skills and could still read. Focusing on her strengths, the Reading Roundtable® task was modified to allow her to lead it successfully. First, each page of a reading roundtable story was put onto a single slide of a PowerPoint presentation file. This file was loaded onto a tablet computer with touch screen capability, such that all one had to do to advance a PowerPoint slide was to touch the screen. The computer was attached to a large screen TV monitor.

The resident with HD would gather other residents who were members of the reading group and have them come to the room with the large screen TV monitor. Staff would have loaded the PowerPoint file into the computer beforehand. The first page of the story would be on the screen, and the woman with HD would read this aloud to the group. Then she would touch the screen of the computer to advance to the next page. She then would invite a member of the group to read the page aloud while the rest of the group followed along. This pattern continued through the reading of the story and discussion questions. Thus, focusing on her remaining cognitive, physical, and social abilities, we enabled this person to effectively fill the role of volunteer group leader.

These two examples illustrate another key element in MPD – the need to create meaningful social roles for persons with dementia. This not only produced [change "produced" to "produces"] positive effect [change "effect" to "affect"] for the individual, but it also contributes to the creation of communities, where persons with dementia not only live, but live well.

Intergenerational programming. MPD also has been used to enable persons with dementia to serves as mentors to young children by presenting activities to children as a teaching device (e.g., how to fold clothes, how to use tools, how to pronounce letters, how to count and add, etc.). Such programming has been shown to significantly increase positive forms of engagement and affect display in persons with dementia compared to standard activities programming in adult day health centers (Camp et al., 2004), as well as in long-term care facilities (Camp et al., 1997; Lee, Camp, and Malone, 2007). This type of intergenerational programming has been successfully implemented by other researchers (Gigliotti et al., 2005).

MPD as an assessment tool. A further use of MPD has been the use of such activities as an assessment tool for persons with moderate to advanced dementia (Camp, Koss, and Judge, 1999; Skrajner et al., 2007; Camp et al., in press).

International research. In Taiwan (Lin et al., 2009), MPD was shown to significantly reduce agitation and aggressive behaviors in long-term care residents with high levels of agitation (scores of ≥ 35 on the Cohen-Mansfield Agitation Index - long form), as well as significantly increase positive affect. Researchers in Australia, led by Dr. Daniel O'Connor, are now working to replicate these results (van der Ploeg et al., 2009). In Spain, researchers have created MPD interventions for the Spanish culture, and found that when used with persons with advanced dementia, increased engagement was produced. What was very interesting in their results was that persons with dementia taking part in MPD showed significant increases in mental status scores (MMSE), as well (Buiza, 2007; Etxeberria et al., 2006).

Training in the implementation of MPD has been conducted across the United States and Canada, as well as in Europe, Australia, and Asia. Training materials to allow implementation of this approach have been translated into Spanish, French, Greek, Japanese, Korean, and Mandarin. As this approach focuses on capturing the remaining strengths and capacities of persons with dementia, it can be used to personalize plans of care that can be integrated into programs, such as restorative nursing in long-term care settings, within a wide variety of care delivery settings and reimbursement systems.

In 2008 I left Menorah Park and began working with Hearthstone Alzheimer Care. With their seven assisted living residences in the United States, there is now an opportunity to test MPD on a system-wide level, in a variety of settings, and in a very real world context. MPD also fits nicely within the overall "I'm Still Here" approach (Zeisel, 2009) developed by the President of Hearthstone Alzheimer Care. In addition, with Hearthstone-affiliated facilities in the U.S. and other countries, there is the potential to conduct additional applied research with MPD on an international scale, which should add to the considerable and growing interest in MPD and the overall "I'm Still Here" approach around the world.

CONCLUSION

My oldest daughter is now in her mid-30s, and works at a part-time job while living at home with us. We use Montessori methods with her to enable my daughter to function more independently, to be engaged, and to focus on her strengths and abilities. We want her to live well, as I want persons with dementia to live well. I recently received a call from a former graduate student who is interested in adapting MPD for use with adults with developmental disabilities.

Thus, what began as an attempt to help my daughter and learn more about child development has evolved into an intervention system that is helping older adults with dementia around the world, and that may further develop into a system for helping adults like my daughter living with developmental disabilities. The cycle has come full circle.

It is my hope that this case history of the development of MPD will provide other researchers, especially those early in their careers, to be willing to explore new opportunities as they arise. While the outcome of straying away from the beaten path is less certain than staying on it, it also can be far more interesting and worthwhile.

REFERENCES

Anschutz, L., Camp, C. J., Markley, R. P., and Kramer, J. J. (1987). Remembering mnemonics: A 3-year follow-up on the effects of mnemonics training in elderly adults. *Experimental Aging Research, 13,* 141-143.

Anschutz, L., Camp, C. J., Markley, R. P. and Kramer, J. J. (1985). Maintenance and generalization of mnemonics for grocery shopping by older adults. *Experimental Aging Research, 11,* 157-160.

Beck, H. P., Levinson, S. and Irons, G. (2009). Finding little Albert: A journey to John B. Watson's infant laboratory. *American Psychologist, 64,* 605-614.

Bjork, R. A. (1988). Retrieval practice and the maintenance of knowledge. In Gruneberg, M. M., Morris, P., and Sykes, R. (Eds). *Practical Aspects of Memory, 2,* pp. 396-401. London: Academic Press.

Buiza, C. (2007). MBDP: An international perspective. Presented at the First International Montessori Based Dementia Programming Conference, Columbus, USA, Nov., 2007.

Camp, C. J. (2006a). Spaced retrieval: A case study in dissemination of a cognitive intervention for persons with dementia. In D. Koltai Attix and Kathleen A. Welsch-Bohmner (Eds.) *Geriatric neuropsychological assessment and intervention* (pp. 275-292). New York: The Guilford Press.

Camp, C. J. (2006b). Montessori-Based Dementia Programming™ in long-term care: A case study of disseminating an intervention for persons with dementia. In R. C. Intrieri and L Hyer (Eds). [change to 10.5 type size] *Clinical applied gerontological interventions in long-term care* (pp. 295-314). New York: Springer.

Camp, C. J. (Ed.). (1999). *Montessori-based activities for persons with dementia:Volume 1.* Beachwood, OH: Menorah Park Center for Senior Living.

Camp, C. J. (1996). The return of Sherlock Holmes: A pilgrim's progress in memory and aging research. In M. R. Merrens and G. G. Brannigan (Eds.), *The developmental psychologists* (pp. 217-232). New York: McGraw-Hill.

Camp, C. J. (1981). The use of fact retrieval versus inference in young and elderly adults.*The Journal of Gerontology, 36,* 715-721.

Camp, C. J. and Foss, J. W. (1997). Designing ecologically valid memory interventions for persons with dementia. In D. G. Payne and F. G. Conrad (Eds.), *Intersections in basic and applied memory research* (pp. 311-325). Mahwah, NJ: Lawrence Erlbaum and Assoc.

Camp, C. J., Foss, J. W., Stevens, A. B., Reichard, C. C., McKitrick, L. A., and O'Hanlon, A.M. (1993). Memory training in normal and demented populations: The E-I-E-I-O model. *Experimental Aging Research, 19,* 277-290.

Camp, C. J., Judge, K. et al. (1997). An intergenerational program for persons with dementia using Montessori methods. *The Gerontologist, 37:* 688-692.

Camp, C. J., Koss, E. and Judge, K. S. (1999). Cognitive assessment in late stage dementia. In P. A. Lichtenberg (Ed.), *Handbook of assessment in clinical gerontology* (pp. 442-467). New York: John Wiley and Sons.

Camp, C. J., Markley, R. P., and Kramer, J. J. (1983a). Naive mnemonics: What the "do-nothing" control group does. *The American Journal of Psychology, 96,* 503-511.

Camp, C. J., Markley, R. P. and Kramer, J. J. (1983b). Spontaneous use of mnemonics by elderly individuals. *Educational Gerontology, 9,* 57-71.

Camp, C. J., Orsulic-Jeras, S. et al. (2004). Effects of a Montessori-based intergenerational program on engagement and affect for adult day care clients with dementia. In M. L. Wykle, P. J. Whitehouse, and D. L. Morris (Eds.), *Successful aging through the life span: Intergenerational issues in health.* (pp. 159-176) New York: Springer.

Camp, C. J., Schneider, N., Orsulic-Jeras, S., Mattern, J., McGowan, A., Antenucci, V. M., Malone, M. L., and Gorzelle, G. J. (2006). *Montessori-based activities for persons with dementia: Volume 2.* Beachwood, OH: Menorah Park Center for Senior Living.

Camp, C. J., and Skrajner, M. J. (2004). Resident-Assisted Montessori Programming (RAMP): Training persons with dementia to serve as group activity leaders. *The Gerontologist, 44:* 426-431.

Camp, C. J., Skrajner, M. J. and Kelly, M. (2005). Early stage dementia client as group leader. *Clinical Gerontologist, 28:* 81-85.

Camp, C. J., Skrajner, M. J., Lee, M. M. and Judge, K. S. (in press). Cognitive assessment in late stage dementia. In P. A. Lichtenberg (Ed.), *Handbook of assessment in clinical gerontology (2nd edition).* New York: John Wiley and Sons.

Etxeberria, I.,Yanguas, J. J., Buiza, C., Zulaica, A., Galdona, N., and Gonzalez, M. F. (2006). Montessori-Based intervention study of patients with severe cognitive impairment and their caregivers. *The Gerontologist, 46 (special issue 1):* S260.

Foss, J. W. and Camp, C. J. (1994). "Effortless" learning in Alzheimer's disease: Evidence that spaced-retrieval training engages implicit memory. Poster presented at the fifth biennial Cognitive Aging Conference, Atlanta, GA.

Gigliotti, C., Morris, M. et al. (2005). An intergenerational summer program involving persons with dementia and preschool children. *Educational Gerontology, 31:* 425–441.

Gorzelle, G. J., Kaiser, K. and Camp, C. J. (2003). Montessori-based training makes a difference for home health workers and their clients. *CARING Magazine, 22:* 40-42.

Joltin, A., Camp, C. J., Noble, B. H. and Antenucci, V. M. (2005). *A different visit: Activities for caregivers and their loved ones with memory impairment.* Beachwood, OH: Menorah Park Center for Senior Living.

Judge, K.S., Camp, C.J. and Orsulic-Jeras, S. (2000). Use of Montessori-based activities for clients with dementia in adult day care: Effects on engagement. American Journal of Alzheimer's Disease, 15, 42-46.

Lee, M. M., Camp, C. J. and Malone, M. L. (2007). Effects of Intergenerational Montessori-based Activities Programming on Engagement of Nursing Home Residents with Dementia. *Clinical Interventions in Aging, 2(3),* 1-7.

Lillard, A. S. (2005). *Montessori: The science behind the genius.* New York: Oxford University Press.

Lin, L. et al. (2009). Using acupressure and Montessori-based activities to decrease agitation in residents with dementia: A cross-over trial. *Journal of the American Geriatrics Society, 57:* 1022-1029.

Mattern, J. M. and Kane, E. (2007). Hutington's disease client as activity leader. *Clinical Gerontologist, 30:* 93-100.

Orsulic-Jeras, S., Judge, K. S. and Camp, C. J. (2000). Montessori-based activities for long-term care residents with advanced dementia: Effects on engagement and affect. *The Gerontologist, 40,* 107-111.

Rose, M., Camp, C. J., Skrajner, M. and Gorzelle, G. (2003). Enhancing the quality of nursing home visits with Montessori-based activities. *Activities Directors' Quarterly, 3:* 4-10.

Schneider, N. M. and Camp, C. J. (2002). Use of Montessori-based activities by visitors of nursing home residents with dementia. *Clinical Gerontologist, 26*: 71-84.

Skrajner, M. J. and Camp, C. J. (2007). Resident-assisted Montessori programming (RAMP™): Use of a small group reading activity run by persons with dementia in adult day health care and long-term care settings. *The American Journal of Alzheimer's Disease and Other Dementias, 22(1):* 27-36.

Skrajner, M. J., Malone, M. L., Camp, C. J., McGowan, A. and Gorzelle, G. J. (2007). Research in practice I: Montessori-based dementia programming® (MBDP). *Alzheimer's Care Quarterly, 8(1):* 53-64.

Skinner, B. F. (1954). The science of learning and the art of teaching. *Harvard Educational Review, 24(1),* 86-97.

Vance, D., Camp, C. J., Kabacoff, M. and Greenwalt, L. (1996). Montessori methods: Innovative interventions for adults with Alzheimer's disease. *Montessori Life, 8:* 10-12.

Vance, D. E. and Porter, R. J. (2000). Montessori methods yield cognitive gains in Alzheimer's day cares. *Activities, Adaptation, and Aging, 24,* 1-22.

Van der Ploeg, E., Eppingstall, B., Griffith, J. and O'Connor, D. (2009). Design of two studies on non-pharmacological interventions to reduce agitated behaviours in persons with dementia. *Alzheimer's and Dementia, 5:* e17.

Vygotsky, L. S. (1978). *Mind in society.* Cambridge, MA: Harvard University Press.

Zeisel, J. (2009) *I'm still here: A breakthrough approach to understanding someone living with Alzheimer's.* New York: Penguin.

In: Dementia: Non-Pharmacological Therapies
Editor: Elisabetta Farina, pp. 173-188

ISBN: 978-1-61470-736-3
© 2012 Nova Science Publishers, Inc.

THE EFFICACY OF A VISUAL BARRIER TO REDUCE ROOM INTRUSIONS IN NOCTURNAL WANDERING: PILOT EVIDENCE FROM TWO SPECIAL CARE UNIT RESIDENTS

*Luc Pieter De Vreese**

Special Care Unit,
Teaching Nursing Home Facility RSA 9 Gennaio, Modena.

ABSTRACT

Introduction: Nocturnal wandering when associated with entering bedrooms uninvited is a disruptive behaviour even in Special Care Units (SCU), increasing the risk of aggressions and worsening the quality of sleep of the other residents. The study aimed at verifying the efficacy of concealing from the view of two nocturnal wanderers with advanced Alzheimer's disease, the door handles of other residents' bedrooms in terms of a reduction both of inappropriate room intrusions and challenging morning behaviour of the other SCU residents.

Methods. Masking consisted in covering the door handles of the bedrooms with small shoe boxes of the same colour as that of the bedroom doors. A single-case ABA'B' design was applied, where A and A' denote no masking and B and B', masking, each lasting 15 nights, with a one-week washout period between the experimental phases. The number of room intrusions and residents' awakenings by the two nocturnal wanderers were recorded. At the end of each morning, the presence or absence of ten kinds of agitated behaviour of the Brief Agitation Rating Scale, were recorded for the entire SCU population. Data of the two cases were analysed by means of the C test which computes at the single-case level the probability whether a behaviour observed in a temporal series is distributed at random or not. Morning behaviour of the other SCU residents were analysed by means of MANOVA for repeated measures.

Results. Case 1 reduced her nocturnal room intrusions by 97,2% (C test for combined series: 0.47; $p<0.05$) during phase B compared to baseline (phase A) and increased again her inappropriate room entering by 25% (C test for combined series: 0.38; $p<0.05$) when visual barriers were removed (phase A'). A statistically significant variation in nocturnal intrusive behaviour by case 2 was also found but only in the second part of the experiment, *i.e.*, a decrease of inappropriate entering by 77,4% (C test for combined series: 0.31; $p<0.05$) during phase B' compared to phase A'. The overall prevalence of

---

* Correspondence to: Luc P. De Vreese, PhD, MD c/o Nucleo Specialistico per le Demenze, RSA 9 Gennaio, Via Paul Harris, 165, 41100 Modena. E-mail: luc.devreese@comune.modena.it. Phone: +39592034741. Fax: +39592034790.

agitated behaviour displayed by the other 16 SCU residents was significant lower in the morning during the periods where door handles were camouflaged.

Conclusion. These preliminary findings support the contention that this user-friendly and extremely low-cost intervention may significantly reduce bedroom intrusions though with an inter-individual variability, ameliorating other SCU residents' quality of sleep with a positive effect on their morning behaviour. Further larger studies are needed to confirm the present findings.

Keywords: Alzheimer's disease, bedroom intrusion, nocturnal wandering, Special Care Unit, visual barriers.

INTRODUCTION

Persistent sleep disturbances are common in persons living with Alzheimer's disease (AD), affecting up to 44 per cent of subjects in clinic [1] and community-based samples [2-4]. These fragmented sleep/wake cycles are characterized by frequent daytime napping, prolonged night-time wakefulness, and multiple nocturnal awakenings, often resulting in increased and inappropriate levels of nocturnal activity, including wandering about in either a seemingly aimless or disorientated fashion or in pursuit of an indefinable or unobtainable goal [5]. For family caregivers, being awoken at night by a relative's wandering and other aberrant motor, vocal or verbal behaviours is one of the most disturbing aspects of care [2] and are a major risk factor for earlier institutionalisation [6-9]. It has been estimated that such behaviour occurs in around 30 per cent of subjects in nursing homes and is strongly associated with the severity of dementia and diminished visuoperceptive and navigational abilities [10].

Management of night-time wandering in traditional institutional environments comprise physical barriers, physical restraints and psychotropic medications. However, considerable ethical concerns have emerged regarding the use of barrier/restraint methods because of their potential physical consequences, such as pressure sores and infection, and psychological problems such as anxiety and distress and also physical violence [11]. Antipsychotic and other related psychotropic drugs have frequent harmful side effects including falls, excessive sedation or conversely akathisia, hasting of cognitive decline making behaviour worse, and show only modest efficacy in managing wandering in AD [12-14].

Over the last decades, the beneficial effects of restraint free care on physical and mental health of people with AD even in residential settings, have been increasingly recognised [15]. This new ethos in the management of wandering has evolved with a move towards promotion of safe ambulation, rather than its prevention, in segregated and specially designed residential settings, the so-called Special (Dementia) Care Units (SCUs) [16]. SCUs vary greatly in terms of the number, composition, and training of staff, the nature of activity programs, and patient care, but several features are generally found in all such units: they cater only for people with dementia and most often AD, there are secured entries and exits, and they have a modified physical environment, including access to a safe outdoor area [17,18].

Although there is no standardised definition of quality of care in SCUs, safety is one of the most important aspects of quality of care in this kind of dementia care settings in light of the residents' extreme vulnerability because of their cognitive and functional dependency on others [19]. Unfortunately, residents living in SCUs where a restraint free care approach is applied, in particular to wanderers, have been found to be almost three times as likely to be injured than those living in other residential services because they frequently may get themselves in trouble by 'unintentionally' provoking a physical aggression due to intrusion into other residents' personal space [20,21]. These aversive events following entering into other residents' subjective or objective personal space usually do not induce wanderers to modify their behaviour, presumably because of impaired operant conditioning. As a matter of fact, people with AD can no longer learn and act upon the association between (abnormal and/or hazardous) behaviour and the consequence because of impaired emotional nondeclarative memory such as fear conditioning [22].

Previous research on the use of visual (e.g., full-length mirror in front of the door, hiding door handles using cloth or secure cover) [23,24] or subjective barriers, defined as visual modifications that the person living with dementia may interpret as a barrier even if it is not physically so (e.g., door obscured by same colour or cotton sheet, two-dimensional grid on the floor near doors, murals on the walls above doorways) [25-29] or enhancement of the visual environment in a selected area of a residential home (e.g., "nature scene" or "home and people" environments created at purpose in nursing home corridors) [30] all focused on preventing exiting behaviour or reducing (day-time) wandering (Table 1).

Table 1. Studies of the use of objective or subjective visual barriers or enhancement of visual environment in the management of exiting behaviour

Author	Number of cases[§]	Intervention	Outcome
Hussain and Brown, 1987 [25]	8	Two-dimensional grid pattern by door of ward	Pattern of eight horizontal lines was most effective in seven out of eight male persons with dementia;
Namazi et al., 1989 [24]	9	Seven types of visual barriers (e.g., grids, door knob cover)	Cloth covering door or door handles was most effective
Chafetz, 1990 [26]	30	Grid marking on floor by exit	No reduction in exiting behaviour
Mayer and Darby, 1991 [23]	9	Full-length mirror placed in front of exit door	Significant reduction in door testing
Dickinson et al., 1995 [27]	7	Closed blind and cloth barrier used separately or in combination to obscure doors and windows	Decrease of time spent attempting to exit the ward, especially with the cloth barrier
Hewawasam, 1996 [28]	10	Two-dimensional grid pattern by door of ward	Horizontal grid pattern reduced exiting behaviour in all persons with dementia
Cohen-Mansfield and Werner, 1998 [30]	27	Enhancement of visual environment in a selected area of internal corridors in nursing home	A non significant decrease in agitation/aggression
Kincaid and Peacock, 2003 [29]	12	Murals on the walls above doorways of ward	Significant fewer exit-door contact with mural

[§] In all studies, persons living with dementia were their own comparison subjects.

The author is aware of no study to date that has examined the effects of environmental manipulation in SCU residents with nocturnal wandering who open repeatedly and randomly the doors of the other bedrooms and enter into the room often awakening and frightening the other dementia residents with the risk of resident-to-resident violence.

The aim of the present study was to replicate the findings of Namazi et al. [24], focusing on camouflaging at night-time the door handles of the bedrooms in a SCU. The primary outcome measure was a reduction in the number of intrusions by nocturnal wanderers in other residents' rooms. A secondary outcome measure was the impact of this intervention on other residents' behaviour immediately the day after in the morning.

METHODS

Participants

Two residents with a clinical diagnosis of Probable AD according to the NINCDS-ADRDA criteria [31] out of 18 SCU dementia residents, presented both persistent night-time wandering, characterised by lapping (i.e., circuitous movement revising door handles sequentially along the two corridors of the SCU) and random ambulation (i.e., haphazard movement without repeating points in sequence especially in rooms and the outdoor Alzheimer Garden).

Case 1 had lived since one year in a traditional facility from which she was transferred to the SCU of the Teaching Nursing Home Facility (henceforth called RSA 9 Gennaio) in Modena, because of clinically relevant and continuous behavioural and psychological symptoms (BPSD) [32] no longer manageable with physical restraints and resistive to numerous psychotropic drugs. Case 2 entered the SCU directly from home where an inverted sleep/wake cycle had started three months before, superimposed on violent resistance to intimate personal care. Psychotropic medications had been unsuccessful or were associated with unacceptable side effects such as sedation and iatrogenic neurological (e.g., dysphagia) and psychological (akathisia) extrapyramidal symptoms.

Table 2. Demographic and clinical characteristics of the participants in the study

	Case 1	Case 2
Gender	Female	Male
Age (expressed in years)	79	78
Schooling (expressed in years)	5	5
Presumed years of AD (expressed in years)	6	5
Mini-Mental State Examination (max 30) [§]	NA	3
Staging (Functional Assessment Staging) [¶]	7a	6d
Behavioural and psychological symptoms (Neuropsychiatric Inventory) (max. 144) [#]	45	88
Organic comorbidity index (Cumulative Illness Rating Scale) [*]	1.61	1.92

NA: not available because of non cooperativeness;
[§] Folstein et al. [33]. Reisberg et al. [34]; [#]Cummings et al. [35]. [*] Parmalee et al. [36].

Demographic and clinical characteristics of the two cases are summarised in Table 2. During the experiment, both wanderers did never present with *delirium* superimposed on dementia and there were no variations in their medications; both residents assumed an antihypertensive and an antiplatelet agent; trazodone (50mg/die) was given to case 1 for afternoon sundowning with exaggeration of obstreperous behaviour and citalopram (20mg/die) in the morning to case 2 in the attempt to treat depression, presumably exaggerating physical aggression during daily care.

Figure 1 illustrates the scores obtained by cases 1 and 2 in the twelve domains explored by NPI, filled in shortly before the beginning of the study. None of them had certified current comorbid visual impairment though case 2 underwent cataract surgery in both eyes one year before AD diagnosis.

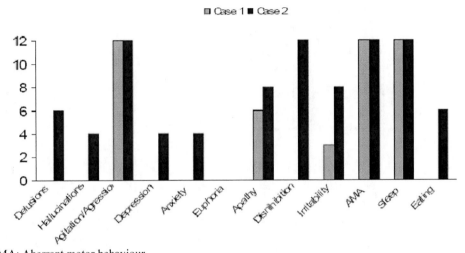

AMA: Aberrant motor behaviour.

Figure 1. Single NPI domain scores obtained by cases 1 and 2 shortly before the experiment.

Experimental Design

The SCU of the RSA 9 Gennaio admits ambulatory persons with dementia-related (i.e., primary) BPSD not responsive to psychotropic drugs, and is intended to offer temporary respite care for either family caregivers at home or staff members of traditional institutional care settings. The SCU is located at the ground floor of the RSA 9 Gennaio and has 12 bedrooms, eight with two beds, and four single bedrooms, distributed along two corridors separated by a catering room and a large community room, which communicates directly with an outdoor green space with non circular wandering paths and floor illumination allowing residents for safe walking 24 hours a day, at least in summertime (Figure 2).

At the night shift (i.e., from 8:00 p.m. to 6:00 a.m.) one nursing aid is stably present in the SCU, whereas one nurse may be called for urgencies (e.g., falls, severe agitation) who otherwise is constantly at work in the Rehabilitation Unit at the first floor. The first aid station or an ambulance may be called whenever necessary.

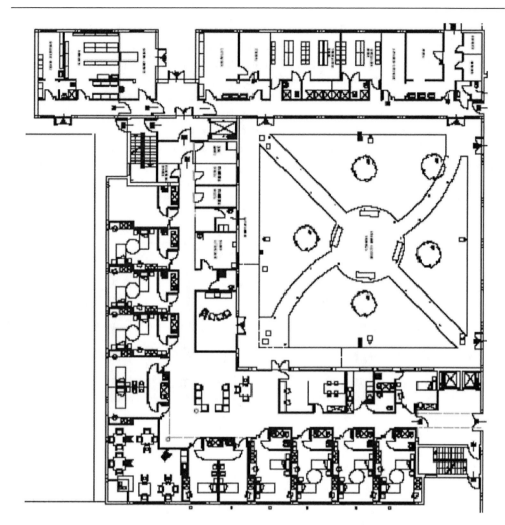

Figure 2. Planimetry of the Special Care Unit of the RSA 9 Gennaio.

At the time of the study, all but one double bedroom were occupied. This empty bedroom was always kept locked during the experiment. A single bedroom was assigned to the two wanderers because of a disturbed sleep/wake cycle. Night-time inappropriate entering of cases 1 and 2 in other resident's bedrooms was monitored in two different conditions: without *vs.* with masking of the external black coloured door handles of white coloured doors of the bedrooms. Masking consisted in covering the door handles of the nine bedrooms occupied by the other residents with small white coloured shoe boxes in such a way as to allow door opening from the inside. Shoe boxes were put with a transparent adhesive over the door handles in the evening as soon as all residents had been accompanied to bed and were removed short before the morning shift.

A single-case ABA'B' design was applied, where A and A' denote no masking and B and B', masking, each lasting 15 days, with a one-week washout period between the experimental phases in order to diminish potential carryover effects, including the sensation to be observed [37]. The nursing aid besides usual care and routine behaviour recorded at the end of the night shift, was invited to sign in a schedule created at purpose each time the wanderer opened the door of another resident's bedroom and walked into his room, specifying also whether or not the victim(s) of the intrusion was awoken. All other nocturnal behaviours such as entries and door opening of their own bedrooms as well as opening other bedroom doors and immediately closing them, and door-testing (i.e., staying in front of the door, holding and moving the door handle for a while but without opening the door) were not taken into account. During the entire experiment, this schedule could not be consulted neither by the morning shift care staff nor by the author (see below). The number of intrusions in the nine bedrooms occupied by the other 16 residents in the SCU during the four observation periods was the primary outcome measure.

In the morning, four nursing aides beside a nurse are stably present in the SCU. At the end of the morning shift, they are requested to fill in a graphic created at purpose listing items borrowed from the Cohen-Mansfield Agitation Inventory [38] to facilitate daily recording of the frequency and intensity of any disruptive behaviour displayed in the morning by each of the SCU residents [39]. This quick and reliably way of behaviour recording serves to the care staff at the afternoon shift. During the experiment, this recording by the morning care staff was done blind to the number of room intrusions and awakenings of the 16 SCU residents by the two wanderers the night before. The information contained in the graphics served as a basis for the retrospective compilation by the author, blind to the two wanderers' nocturnal behaviour the night before, of a modified *Brief Agitation Rating Scale* (BARS) [40]. The scale was applied to all the SCU residents, signing whether or not ten types of agitated behaviour (i.e., hitting, grabbing, pushing, pacing or aimless walking, repetitious mannerism, restlessness, screaming, repetitive sentences or questions, strange noises, complaining) had been observed in the morning during the entire experiment. The variation in BARS scores during the four observation periods was considered the secondary outcome measure of the study.

All nursing assistants participating in the study were female with at least five years of work experience and with at least three years of work experience in the SCU. Informed consent was obtained from the relatives of all residents directly (cases 1 and 2) or indirectly involved in the study.

Statistical Analyses

The primary outcome was measured by means of the C test [41]. This test computes at the single-case level the probability that a behaviour observed in a temporal series is distributed at random or not. The experimental hypothesis is confirmed when a series of data (i.e., behaviour) remains stable at baseline, whereas that of an intervention undergoes a significant modification.

C test was applied to the number of room intrusions by the two nocturnal wanderers, either within each of the four observation periods or between them comparing control (no masking) with experimental (with masking) periods. The secondary outcome was analysed by means of a multivariate analysis of variance (MANOVA) for repeated measures using the Statistical Program for Social Science, package version 15.01, whereas variation in morning behaviour of the two wanderers was again verified by means of the C test.

RESULTS

Primary Outcome

Figures 3-4 display the number of intrusions by cases 1 and 2 in other residents' bedrooms at night, where phases A and A' refer to the control periods and phases B and B' to the camouflage of the door handles of the nine bedrooms. C test showed a non significant trend in the variation of the number of inappropriate other residents' bedroom intrusions by cases 1 and 2 within each phase of the study experiment, suggesting a constant nocturnal wandering behaviour over each of the four 15-night periods, on the one hand, and an indirect indicator of a good inter-rater accuracy in monitoring the target behaviour by the different nurse aids at the night shifts, on the other.

By contrast, C test comparison of the variations in room intrusions by case 1 between the control and experimental phases of the study showed a significant reduction by 97.2% (C test for combined series: 0.47; $p<0.05$) during phase B in which door handles were masked compared to baseline (phase A). When visual barriers were again removed (phase A') inappropriate room entering increased by 25% (C test for combined series: 0.38; $p<0.05$). A statistically significant variation in nocturnal intrusive behaviour by case 2 was also found but only from phase A' to phase B' (C test for combined series: 0.31; $p<0.05$) with a reduction of inappropriate entering by 77,4%. All other C test comparisons did not reach the level of statistical significance.

During the study, case 2 fell accidentally twice at night: one fall during phase A, and the second one during the washout period between phases B and A', both without physical consequences.

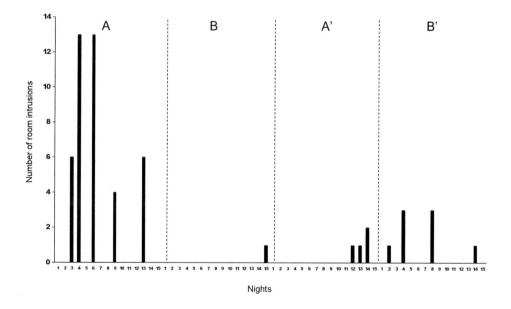

Figure 3. Trend of nocturnal room intrusions by case 1.

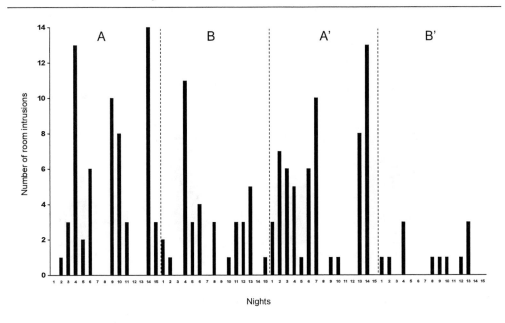

Figure 4. Trend of nocturnal room intrusions by case 2.

Two episodes of physical aggressions occurred, however, between the same nursing assistant and case 2 while trying to take him back outside another resident's bedroom, one during the washout period between phases A and B, and the other in phase B' of the study. The nurse at the night shift was called in the SCU, besides for the two aforementioned falls as indicated by the internal protocol, three other times during the experiment, once for a fall of another resident, and two times respectively for a vomit of another resident and a severe agitation episode, the latter following a room intrusion by case 2 during phase A.

Secondary Outcome

Figure 5 displays the mean (± S.D.) scores of the modified BARS [40] obtained by the 16 residents at the end of the morning shift during each observation period. A MANOVA for repeated measures showed a significant overall (Wilks' Lambda $F_{(3,13)}$ = 19.11; $p < 0.0001$) and time effect (F $_{(1,9.36)}$ = 5.06; p < 0.046). As expected, a highly significant between-subject effect was also found (F $_{(1,163.35)}$ = 99.96; p < 0.0001). By contrast, C test did not show a significant variation in the modified BARS scores obtained by cases 1 and 2 at the end of the morning shift, neither within each phase nor between phases of the experiment.

The number of residents with recorded awakenings provoked by the intruders during the study were eight, four, six, and two, respectively for phases A, B, A', and B'. Almost all of them were due to disruptive vocalisation under the form of a verbal stereotype "mamma mia, mia mamma" [my mom, my mom] in case 1 and to aberrant motor behaviour, including inappropriate voiding in case 2. Awakenings were followed by three resident-to-resident aggressions in phase A, but without clinically relevant physical consequences both for the intruder and other residents.

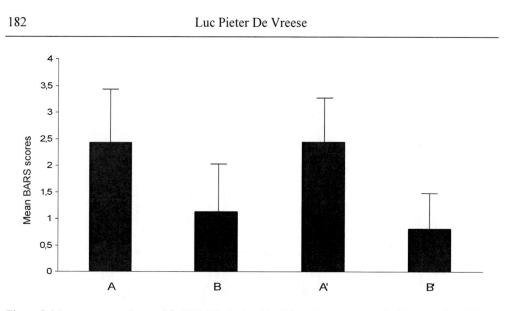

Figure 5. Mean scores on the modified BARS obtained by 16 residents at the end of the morning shift in the four observation periods.

CONCLUSION

Previous research [23-30] has examined the efficacy of environmental modifications by means of visual or subjective barriers and enhancement of visual environment in reducing wandering and exit seeking in different institutional settings (Table 1). However, none of these studies used a single case ABAB design. Staging of dementia was not always specified and where these data were available, persons with dementia' dementia severity considerably differed among the participants. The absence of comorbid visual impairment, though frequent in dementia, amplifying persons with dementia' confusion and distress [42], was not certified in these studies. These above variables may in part explain contradictory findings in efficacy [26,28], on the one hand, and an intersubject variability in responsiveness to the same type of visual barrier [25], on the other. As a matter of fact, a recent systematic review of psychological approaches to the management of neuropsychiatric symptoms of dementia [43], considered the level of consistency of evidence of these studies low (i.e., 4) with an overall grade of recommendation of C, according to the Oxford Centre for Evidenced-Based Medicine criteria.

The current study is the first to our knowledge that aimed at reducing nocturnal wanderers' intrusions in other residents' bedrooms of a SCU using through a single case ABAB design, a simple visual barrier such as shoe boxes of the same colour as that of the bedroom doors fixed over the exterior door handles, and at verifying the impact of this concealment technique on morning behaviour of the other residents.

The present study highlights the following findings. Responsiveness to the intervention differed in the two cases notwithstanding a similar degree of AD severity and a certified absence of concurrent visual impairment. In case 1 the first period of masking of door handles (phase B) was efficacious compared to baseline observation (phase A) and after a one-week washout period, removal of the shoe boxes (phase A') slightly but significantly increased again entering bedrooms uninvited at night. The application of this visual barrier for a second time (phase B') did no longer significantly modify nocturnal intrusion behaviour with respect to the second control period (phase A'). It should be noted that already during the washout period between phase B and phase A' of the study, case 1 had started to spent much more time in bed at night, reducing wandering time in the SCU corridors and consequently intrusions in other residents' bedrooms. As a matter of fact, her nocturnal wandering, that had started several months before in a traditional nursing home, disappeared completely shortly after the current study. By contrast, hiding door handles resulted efficacious in case 2 only in the second part of the experiment. There was a significant reduction in bedroom intrusions applying again shoe boxes over the door handles (phase B') after the second control phase (phase A'). The reason for this delayed benefit is not straightforward. From the comments in the recording charts created at purpose for the study, it emerged that in phase B of the experiment, case 2 had rapidly learned that is was sufficient to lift or remove the shoe boxes to grasp and to turn the door handles. By contrast, in phase B', the resident appeared to be frequently less aware of the presence of the visual barriers or in other instances wasted his time in studying the shoe boxes and in scrutinising what was concealed under them, more often than not desisting after a while without evident signs of frustration or nervousness, from opening the doors. This changed behaviour compared to the first part of the experiment, might indicate a worsening either of his visuospatial capabilities (e.g., visual agnosia, Balint's syndrome) or of his working memory, with an accelerated forgetting of the programmed intention to enter the bedrooms.

The strengths of the primary outcome of the present study include: a) the application of an ABAB design, spaced by washout periods in order to avoid placebo or carryover effects, judged as the most compelling evidence of causality in single-case interventions [37]; b) the control of text integrity i.e., medication and non-pharmacological interventions in cases 1 and 2 were kept constant throughout the experiment [44]; c) the use of a direct observation technique devoid of recall biases; d) analysis of the data by means of a valid statistical test purported at probing modification in behaviour at the single-case level [41].

At least three potential methodological limitations should be noted as well. First, According to the Emilia-Romagna regional contract stipulations in public nursing home assistance, the presence of only one nursing aid is foreseen at the night shift in SCUs. Therefore, it was not possible to obtain reliability data on the observation method by means of a contemporary second observer whose data collection should have been compared with those of the primary observer. Secondly, the presence of only one nursing aid in the SCU might have engendered errors in signing a number of inappropriate bedroom entries both in the periods with or without door handles masking, because of emergency baths, cleaning the places of inappropriate voiding, giving to eat or drink something at the awakenings of the other residents or taking them back to bed. Thirdly, at the time of the study, there were other residents with recurrent night-time insomnia regardless of the awakenings provoked by the intruders, who repeatedly got up of bed and passed several hours of the night in the community rooms, manifesting more or less obstreperous or hazardous behaviours, which might have exacerbated or on the contrary diminished wanderers' bedroom intrusions, independently of the presence or absence of the shoe boxes over the door handles. Yet, the finding that the frequency of room intrusions within each of the four observation periods did not vary significantly in neither case, proves, though indirectly, that the accuracy of nursing assistants' surveillance was maintained constant along the entire experiment, on the one hand,

and that wandering behaviour and bedrooms' intrusions by cases 1 and 2 were independent of other residents' nocturnal behaviour, on the other.

The other relevant finding of the study was a statistically significant reduction in the frequency of morning agitated behaviour of the other residents taken as a whole, as indexed by a modified BARS [40], in the phases B and B' (with masking). However several limitations are apparent and therefore the secondary outcome measure of the study should be interpreted with caution. First, although nurse aids' routine recordings of morning behaviour exhibited by the SCU residents and the compilation of BARS by the author were done blind to what had happened the night before during the study experiment, both the care staff and the author were not so as to the phases of the study. Second, the modified BARS has not yet been validated in Italy, ignoring therefore its validity and reliability. Third, BARS scores were exclusively derived from the information in the graphics which in turn were filled in by the care staff at the end of the morning shift. Therefore, BARS scores might not have been exempt from methodological biases such as recall bias or simplification of the complex A(ntecedent) B(ehaviour) C(onsequences) mechanisms underlying agitated behaviour. Last but not least, it was not possible to keep constant medication of the other SCU residents because of intervening organic or psychiatric co-morbidities during the four study periods. Notwithstanding these short-comings, a significant tendency to more adequate morning behaviour of the other residents taken as a whole, emerged twice during the phases B and B' with door handles masking. Reduction in nocturnal room intrusions and hence an amelioration of sleep quality, is in line with previous research which demonstrated that disrupted sleep in persons living with dementia negatively interferes with subsequent day-time behaviour [45,46].

Finally, the present study did not establish directly the views of cases 1 and 2 on the acceptability of the use of visual barriers, considered a necessary but quite often neglected secondary outcome in non-pharmacological interventions to reduce wandering in dementia [47]. Yet, the finding that morning behaviour of the two wanderers as indexed by their individual BARS scores did not change significantly neither within each phase nor between phases of the experiment, and that anecdotally recorded nocturnal behaviour remained constant throughout the different conditions of the study, indirectly suggests a good acceptability by the experimental cases of this kind of visual barrier used in the current study.

In conclusion, nocturnal wandering is one of the most disruptive behaviours of AD usually persistent over time and more often than not refractory to psychotropic medications. In residential settings, nocturnal wandering when associated with entering repeatedly in other residents' bedrooms uninvited, is difficult to treat and increases the risk of resident-to-resident or wanderer-to-staff member violence. The current study showed that the camouflage of door handles significantly decreases the number of room intrusions though with a considerable inter-individual variability. Consequent less disturbed sleep also improved morning agitation of the residents taken as a whole.

These findings obtained by means of a simple device such as shoe boxes, preserving freedom and autonomy of the nocturnal wanderers and ameliorating the other residents' quality of sleep, minimising the risk of violent resident-to-resident incidents, should stimulate clinicians to replicate this user-friendly and extremely low cost intervention in other residential settings.

CONFLICT OF INTEREST

None

ACKNOWLEDGMENTS

The author is grateful to the nursing assistants and the SCU residents who took part in the study.

REFERENCES

[1]   Ritchie, K. (1996). Behavioral disturbances of dementia in ambulatory care settings. *International Psychogeriatrics*, 8, 439–442.

[2]   McCurry, S.M., Logsdon, R.G., Teri, L. et al. (1999). Characteristics of sleep disturbance in community-dwelling Alzheimer's disease patients. *Journal of Geriatric and Psychiatry Neurology*, 12, 53–59.

[3]   Carpenter, B.D., Strauss, M.E., Patterson, M.B. (1995). Sleep disturbances in community dwelling patients with Alzheimer's disease. *Clinical Gerontology*, 16, 35–49.

[4]   Lyketsos , C.G., Lopez, O., Jones, B. et al. (2002). Prevalence of neuropsychiatric symptoms in dementia and mild cognitive impairment: results from the cardiovascular health study. *Journal of the American Medical Association*, 288, 1475-1483.

[5]   Bliwise, D.L. (2004). Sleep disorders in Alzheimer's disease and other dementias. *Clinical Cornerstone*, 6(suppl 1A), S16-S28.

[6]   Pollak, C.P., Perlick, D. (1991). Sleep problems and institutionalization of the elderly. *Journal of Geriatric Psychiatry and Neurology*, 4, 204–210.

[7]   Hope, T., Keene, J., Gedling, K. et al. (1998). Predictors of institutionalization for people with dementia living at home with a carer. *International Journal of Geriatric Psychiatry,* 13:682–690.

[8]   Gaugler, J.E., Edwards, A.B., Femia, E.E. et al. (2000). Predictors of institutionalization of cognitively impaired elders: Family help and the timing of placement. Journal of Gerontology. *Psychological Sciences and Social Sciences*, 55B, P247–P255.

[9]   Phillips, V.L. and Diwan, S. (2003). The incremental effect of dementia-related problem behaviours on the time to nursing home placement in poor, frail, demented older people. *Journal of the American Geriatric Society*, 52, 188-193.

[10] Algase, D.L. (1999). Wandering in dementia. *Annual Review of Nursing Research*,17, 185-217.

[11] Cotter, V.T. (2005). Restraint free care in older adults with dementia. *Keio Journal of Medecine*, 54, 80-84.

[12] Howard, R., Ballard, C.G., O'Brien, J., Burns, A., on behalf of the UK and Ireland Group for Optimization of Management in Dementia. (2001). Guidelines for the management of agitation in dementia. *International Journal of Geriatric Psychiatry*, 16, 714-717.

[13] Omelan, C. (2006). Approach to managing behavioural disturbances in dementia. *Canadian Family Physician*, 52, 191-199.

[14] Hermann, N and Gauthier, S. (2008). Diagnosis and treatment of dementia: 6. Management of severe Alzheimer disease. *Canadian Medical Association Journal*, 179, 1279-1287.

[15] Coltharp, W.J., Richie, M.F., Kaas, M.J. (1996) Wandering. *Journal of Gerontological Nursing*, 22, 5-10.

[16] Leon, J. (1994). The 1990/1991 national survey of special care units in nursing homes. *Alzheimer Disease and Associated Disorders*, 3, 24-29.

[17] Lai, C.K.Y., Yeung, J.H.M., Mok, V., Chi, I. (2007). Special care units for dementia individuals with behavioural problems (Protocol). *The Cochrane Library*, Issue 4.

[18] Grumeir, A., Lapane, K.L., Miller, S.C., Mor, V. (2008). Is dementia special care really special? A new look at an old question. *Journal of the American Geriatric Association*, 56, 199-205.

[19] Albert, S.M. (2004). The special care unit as a quality-of-life intervention for people with dementia. *Journal of the American Geriatric Society*, 52, 1214-1215.

[20] Shinoda-Tagawa, T., Leonard, R., Pontikas, J., McDonough, J.E., Allen, D., Dreyer, P.I. (2004). Resident-to-resident violence in Nursing Homes. *Journal of the American Medical Association*, 291, 591-598.

[21] Bridges-Parlet, S., Knopman,D, Thompson, T. (1994). A descriptive study of physically aggressive behavior in dementia by direct observation. *Journal of the American Geriatric Society*, 42, 192-197.

[22] Hamann, S., Monarch, E.S., Goldstein, F.C. (2002). Impaired fear conditioning in Alzheimer's disease. *Neuropsychologia*, 40, 1187-1195.

[23] Mayer, R and Darby, S. (1991). Does a mirror deter wandering in demented older people? *International Journal of Geriatric Psychiatry*, 6, 607-609.

[24] Namazi, K., Rosner, T., Calkins, M. (1989). Visual barriers to prevent ambulatory Alzheimer's patients from exiting through an emergency door. *Gerontologist*, 29, 699-702.

[25] Hussain, R.A. and Brown, D.C. (1987). Use of two-dimensional grid patterns to limit hazardous ambulation in demented patients. *Journal of Gerontology*, 42, 558–560.

[26] Chafetz, P. (1990). Two-dimensional grid is ineffective against demented patients' exiting through glass doors. *Psychology and Aging*, 5, 146-147.

[27] Dickinson, J., McLain-Kark, J., Marshall-Baker, A. (1995). The effects of visual barriers on exiting behavior in a dementia care unit. *Gerontologist*, 35, 127-130.

[28] Hewawasam. L. (1996). Floor patterns limit wandering of people with Alzheimer's. *Nursing Times*, 92, 41–44.

[29] Kincaid, C. and Peacock, JR. (2003). The effect of a wall mural on decreasing four types of door-testing behaviors. *Journal of Applied Gerontology*, 22, 76–88.

[30] Cohen-Mansfield, J. and Werner, P. (1998). The effects of an enhanced environment on nursing home residents who pace. *Gerontologist*, 38, 199-208.

[31] McKhann, G., Drachman, D., Folstein, M. et al. (1984). Clinical diagnosis of Alzheimer's disease: report of the NINCDS/ADRDA Work Group under the auspices of Department of Health and Human Services Task Force on Alzheimer's disease. *Neurology*, 34, 939-944.

[32] Finkel, S.I. and Burns, A. (eds.) (2000). Behavioral and Psychological Signs and Symptoms of Dementia (BPSD): A clinical and research update. *International Psychogeriatrics*, 12 (suppl 1), S9-S18.

[33] Folstein, M.F., Folstein, S.E., McHugh, P.R. (1975). Mini-mental state. A practical method for grading the cognitive state of patients for the clinician. *Journal of Psychiatric Research*, 12, 189-198.

[34] Reisberg, B., Ferris, S.H., Anand, R. et al. (1984). Functional staging of dementia of the Alzheimer's type. *Annals of the New York Academy of Sciences*, 435, 481-483.

[35] Cummings, J.L. (1997). The Neuropsychiatric Inventory: assessing psychopathology in dementia patients. *Neurology*, 49 (suppl), S10-S17.

[36] Parmalee, P.A., Thuras, P.D., Katz, IR, Lawton, M.P. (1995). Validation of the Cumulative Rating Scale in a geriatric residential population. *Journal of the American Geriatric Society*, 43, 130-137.

[37] Barlow, D.H., Hersen, M. *Single-Case Experimental Designs: Strategies for Studying Behavior Change*. 2nd ed. Eimsford, NY: Pergamon, 1984.

[38] Cohen-Mansfield, J. and Billig, N. (1986). Agitated behaviours in the elderly I: A conceptual review. *Journal of the American Geriatric Society*, 34, 711-721.

[39] De Vreese, L.P. and Belloi, L. (2002.) L'esperienza del Nucleo Specialistico per le Demenze:da un approccio di stile di vita (*Life Style Approach*) a una qualità di vita migliore del malato di demenza.[The experience of a Dementia Special Care Unit: from a Life Style Approach to a better quality of life of people with dementia]. Pro Terza Età, 8, 4-11.

[40] Finkel, S.I. et al. (1993). A Brief Agitation Rating Scale (BARS) for nursing home elderly. *Journal of the American Geriatric Society*, 41, 50-52.

[41] Di Nuovo, S. La sperimentazione in psicologia applicata. Problemi di metodologia e analisi dei dati. [*Experiments in applied psychology. Methodological problems and data analysis*] Milano: Franco Angeli, 1992.

[42] Lawrence, V., Murray, J., Ffytche, D., Banerjee S. (2009). "Out of sight, out of mind": a qualitative study of visual impairment and dementia from three perspectives. *International Psychogeriatrics*, 21, 511-518.

[43] Livingston, G., Johnston, K., Katona, C. et al. (2005). Systematic review of psychological approaches to the management of neuropsychiatric symptoms of dementia. *American Journal of Psychiatry*, 162, 1996-2021.

[44] Landreville P., Bédard, A., Verreault, R. et al. (2006). Non-pharmacological interventions for aggressive behaviour in older adults living in long-term care facilities. *International Psychogeriatrics*, 18, 47-73.

[45] Alessi, C.A., Yoon E.J., Schnelle, J.F., Al-Samarrai, N.R., Cruise, P.A. (1999). A randomized trial of a combined physical activity and environmental intervention in nursing home residents: do sleep and agitation improve? *Journal of the American Geriatric Society*, 47, 784-791.

[46] McCurry, S.M., Gibbons, L.E., Logsdon, R.G., Vitiello M.V., Teri, L. (2005). Nighttime insomnia treatment and education for Alzheimer's disease: a randomised, controlled study. *Journal of the American Geriatric Society*, 53, 793-802.

[47] Robinson, L., Hutchings, D., Dickinson, H.O. et al. (2007). Effectiveness and acceptability of non-pharmacological interventions to reduce wandering in dementia : a systematic review. *International Journal of Geriatric Psychiatry*, 22, 9-22.

In: Dementia: Non-Pharmacological Therapies
Editor: Elisabetta Farina, pp. 189-208

DEVELOPMENT OF AN EVIDENCE-BASED EXTENDED PROGRAMME OF MAINTENANCE COGNITIVE STIMULATION THERAPY (CST) FOR PEOPLE WITH DEMENTIA

Elisa Aguirre[1]*, Aimee Spector[2], Juanita Hoe[1], Amy Streater[1], Ian T. Russell[3], Robert T. Woods[4] and Martin Orrell[1]

[1] Department of Mental Health Sciences, University College London,
Charles Bell House, 67-73 Riding House Street, London, UK.
[2] Department of Clinical, Educational and Health Psychology,
University College London, 1- 19 Torrington Place, London, UK.
[3] North Wales Organisation for Randomised Trials in Health and Social Care,
Institute of Medical and Social Care Research, Bangor University,
Ardudwy Hall, Normal Site, Holyhead Road, Bangor, UK.
[4] Dementia Services Development Centre Wales,
Institute of Medical and Social Care Research,
Bangor University, Ardudwy Hall, Normal Site,
Holyhead Road, Bangor, UK.

ABSTRACT

Psychosocial interventions for dementia have often been developed without a sound theoretical, empirical and clinical basis, and most evaluations of these interventions have had serious methodological limitations. This highlights the need to link intervention development with evaluation and design issues during the early stages of phase 1 or development of an intervention. Best practice is to develop interventions systematically, using the best available evidence and appropriate theory. This study focuses on the developmental stage of the Medical Research Council (MRC) guidelines (2008) to develop an evidence-based Maintenance Cognitive Stimulation Therapy (MCST) programme for dementia.

The intervention was developed based on a mixed methods approach, using evidence obtained from the Cochrane review of Cognitive Stimulation for dementia followed by a Delphi consultation process with key stake-holders. Four techniques were used: (1) Cochrane review of cognitive stimulation for dementia, (2) a consultation with key stake holders using a Delphi Consensus Process (including an expert consensus conference),

* Corresponding author: Email: e.aguirre@ucl.ac.uk

(3) focus groups with the target population and (4) a Delphi survey. These techniques were used to complete the theoretical preclinical and phase I modelling of the MRC framework for developing the MCST intervention for dementia.

It was feasible and effective to use a systematic development process to produce successive modifications of the draft manual for an evidence based maintenance CST programme for dementia. Close involvement of users and carers ensured that the manual was well targeted on the preferences and abilities of people with dementia.

The final Maintenance CST programme and manual is currently being tested as part of a large multicentre, randomised controlled trial.

Keywords: Cognitive Stimulation Therapy (CST), Complex intervention, Medical Research Council (MRC) guidelines, psychosocial intervention, dementia.

INTRODUCTION

Psychosocial interventions for dementia have often been developed without a sound theoretical, empirical and clinical basis, and most evaluations of these interventions have had serious methodological limitations (Woods et al., 2005). In our earlier work, the Cochrane Review on Reality Orientation (RO) was used to develop an evidence based Cognitive Stimulation Therapy (CST) programme for dementia (Spector et al., 2000; 2001; 2003). The results of a randomised controlled trial (RCT) of CST compared favourably with trials of cholinesterase inhibitors for Alzheimer's disease, in terms of the size of the effects on cognition (Spector et al, 2003) and the economic analysis showed that CST was likely to be cost-effective (Knapp et al, 2006). The NICE guidelines (NICE-SCIE, 2006) recommended that people with mild/moderate dementia should be 'given the opportunity to participate in a structured group cognitive stimulation programme'. Cognitive stimulation approaches may have long-term effects (Zanetti et al., 1995; Metitieri et al., 2001) and a 16 week pilot study of maintenance CST (Orrell et al., 2005) following the initial 7 weeks of CST, found a significant improvement in cognitive function (MMSE) and identified the need for a large-scale, multi-centre RCT. Best practice is to develop interventions systematically, using the best available evidence and appropriate theory (Craig at al., 2008). This highlights the need to link intervention development with evaluation and design issues during the early stages of phase 1 or development of an intervention. This study focuses on the developmental stage of the Medical Research Council guidelines (2008) for the development and evaluation of complex interventions (Figure 1). Modelling a complex intervention prior to a full-scale evaluation can provide important information about the design of both the intervention and the evaluation (Clancy et al., 2002; Wortman, 1995; Nazaret et al., 2002). The aim was to develop a programme of Maintenance CST for dementia, as a complex long-term intervention in preparation for its evaluation in a large RCT. The three main steps for the development of the programme (MRC, 2008) were: identifying the evidence; identifying and developing theory and modelling process and outcomes.

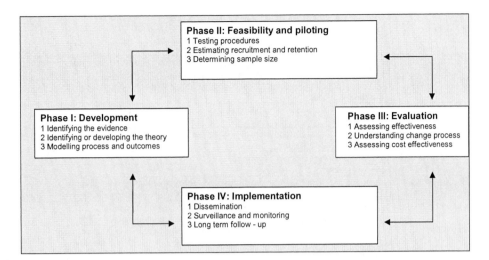

Figure 1. Key elements of the development and evaluation process (MRC framework 2008).

METHODS

Identifying the Evidence Base

An updated Cochrane Systematic Review on the effectiveness of cognitive stimulation programmes for people with dementia was conducted. Searches were based on the Cochrane Dementia and Cognitive Improvement Group (CDCIG) methods guidelines. The therapeutic content of each study and subsequent outcomes were tabulated (Table 1). Priority was given to studies with stronger methodology, such as RCTs. Studies, which did not match the inclusion criteria for the Cochrane Review, but were classified as high quality studies were also included in our analyses (Table 1). The criteria for classification as high quality studies were: 1) extensive description of the intervention classified as being cognitive stimulation, 2) positive outcome and 3) strong methodological design (although not a RCT). Studies with positive outcomes were drawn out from the tables, and the contents of the intervention examined. Through this process, potentially beneficial elements of each type of therapy were identified, and were incorporated into the design of the new maintenance CST programme on the basis of consensus agreement amongst the expert group (EA, BW, AS, MO). In Table 1, the studies and elements, which contributed to the design of this programme, are highlighted in italic type.

Table 1. Included studies for the development of the draft Version 1 of the manual

Authors	Description	Outcome
Studies in the Cochrane Review Woods et al., 2010 (Also included in Spector et al., 2000) C /B*		
Baines 1987	RO Board, old and current newspapers, personal and local photos, materials to stimulate all senses (e.g. cinnamon, silk, honey)	+ B*
Baldelli, 1993	No info given	
Breuil 1994	Copying pictures, associated words, naming and categorising objects.	+C
Ferrario, 1991	No info given	

Table 1. (Continued).

Authors	Description	Outcome
Gerber 1991	Simple exercises, self-care, food preparation, orientation room with RO board, large clock, coloured illustrations.	+C
Hanley 1981	RO Board, clocks, calendars, maps, posters, and room overlooked garden area to enable discussion.	+C
Wallis 1983	Repetition of orientation information (e.g., time, place, weather), charts, pictures, touching objects and material.	-C
Woods 1979	Daily personal diary, group activities (dominoes, spelling, bingo) naming objects, reading RO board.	+C
New studies included in the Cochrane Review Woods et al., 2010		
Baldelli 2002	No info given	+C
Bottino 2005	Temporal and spatial orientation, discussion of interesting themes, reminiscence activities, naming people, daily activities, *planning use of calendars and clocks*	+C
Chapman, 2004	Current events; discussion of hobbies and activities; education regarding Alzheimer's disease; life story work; links with daily life encouraged.	+C
Onder 2005	Current information, topics of general interest, historical events and famous people, attention, memory and visuo-spatial exercises; *use of clocks, calendars and notes*	+C
Requena 2007	Orientation, Body awareness, family and society, *caring for oneself*, reminiscing, *household tips*, animals, people and objects	+C
High quality studies used in the development of the manual but not included in the Cochrane Review		
Olazaran 2004	Reminiscing parents home, significant event, sounds, favourite sports, word game, visual clues to make a trajectory, similarities, *what to do in case of fire*, verbal calculations, serial additions, current affairs, write a letter, orientation, make a cake, make budget from shopping.	+C
Farina, 2002	Searching for words in a text, naming pictures, ranging words in alphabetical order, identifying specific visuospatial stimuli, matching figures, drawing figures, puzzles.	+C
Farina 2006	Conversation, singing, comments on pictures, collage, and poster creation.	+C, +B
Zanetti 2001	Procedural memory training stimulation. Basic and instrumental activities of daily living train, washing face, closing door, writing a letter, locking door.	+C

*C: Cognition.
B: Behaviour.

Identifying and Developing Appropriate Theory: The Theoretical Basis for CST in Dementia

A theoretical understanding of the likely process of change in the primary outcomes (cognition and quality of life) was developed by drawing on existing evidence and theory.

Global Stimulation of Cognitive Abilities: Changes in Cognition

Dementia is characterised by declining cognition but nevertheless, people with dementia often have reserve capacity for cognitive information processing (Katzman et al., 1988, 1993). Implicit memory in people with Alzheimer's is preserved for a longer period than episodic memory, and also responds to regular stimulation (Fleischman et al., 2005) and beneficial effects on cognition may not only be based on implicit memory, but may enhance facilitation of residual explicit memory (Hunkin et al., 1998; Tailby and Haslam, 2003). Offering people with dementia a set of mental activities that takes this remaining reserve capacity into account, allows them to maintain, for a certain period, a relatively enhanced level of cognitive performance. CST provides global stimulation of cognition: memory, concentration, language, executive functioning, spatio-temporal orientation and visuo-constructive abilities. Strategies such as including multi-sensory stimulation, mental imagery, categorical classification, and semantic association, have the aim of maximising episodic and semantic memory functions as well as consolidating implicit memory. The CST activities are adapted to the interests and activities of the participants. Each theme contains exercises of different types including categorical classifications, old /new comparisons of objects, numerical and musical exercises designed to enrich the general cognitive stock as well as the use of implicit strategies for recalling words or concepts. The latter is particularly important in that lack of confidence due to cognitive problems and the consequent anxiety of forgetting words in the middle of a conversation constitutes a risk factor for social withdrawal (Rubin, 1982; Rubin, LeMare, & Lollis, 1990).An important element is stimulation of orientation and each session includes an orientation board with information about the day, time, place and current news so participants can discuss current information and news. CST uses reminiscence as an aid to orientation; this may contribute to the psychological health of people with dementia given that the progressive deteriorating nature of the disease erodes the ability to succeed at a range of previous activities and makes individuals increasingly dependent on past accomplishments for a sense of competency (Kiernat, 1979). People with dementia may retain the capacity to recall and integrate the past because remote memory is spared through most of the disease process (Woods, 1992). Another element of the programme is the use of physical activity in the sessions, including 10 minutes of warm up activity at the beginning of each session, and a session theme called 'physical games'. This constitutes an important element of the intervention as some studies have shown that physical activity delays the onset of dementia in healthy older adults and slows down cognitive decline to prevent the onset of cognitive disability (Forbes et al., 2008). Studies using animal models suggest that physical activity has the potential to attenuate the pathophysiology of dementia. (Cotman et al., 2007).

Stimulation of Social Abilities and Person Centred Care: Changes in Quality of Life

Cognitive and affective functions influence the social roles of people with dementia, such as family activities, maintenance of social relationships and participation in social activities. CST also targets the effects of the intervention on the person's well-being and quality of life (QoL). Cognitive based approaches in dementia care have been criticised suggesting that cognitive gains after the intervention may be achieved at the expense of reduced wellbeing and adverse effects (American Psychiatric Association, 1997). In view of these concerns, person centred care has been included as the basis of the development of the CST programme (Spector et al., 2001) and it has been suggested that improvements in QoL have not arisen simply from non-specific factors, such as the enjoyment of a group activity and social interaction except insofar as these factors also contributed to cognitive change (Woods et al., 2006). CST appeared to have a single mechanism for its effects, with improvements in cognition and QoL going hand in hand. Participants in CST groups reported improved quality of life specifically in relation to memory, as well as energy, relationships and managing chores (Woods et al., 2006).

The structural framework of the CST sessions (groups of 5 to 8 people) permits the participant to meet others in similar situations, which in turn serves to reduce anxiety with respect to one's individual situation. The basis for delivering CST in groups as a psychosocial intervention is the assumption that when individuals gather together to share their concerns, they can cope with the stress better than on their own. The group supplies: (a) emotional bonding that creates closeness and reduces feelings of isolation; (b) enhanced self-esteem in having information to share about current coping strategies; and (c) information exchange that creates a sense of hope and efficacy (Toseland, 1997). Offering CST in a group might increase the performance of the cognitive tasks presented in sessions (such as problem-solving, decision-making, inference and idea generation), as it has been argued that groups can be conceptualized as information processors (Hinsz, Tindale, & Vollrath, 1997). Information processing in groups involves activities that occur at the individual as well as the group level which involves the sharing of solutions, preferences and ideas during discussion (Tindale & Kameda, 2003).

A possible mechanism for QoL change is that the CST approach is grounded in a strong value base of respecting individuality and personhood (Woods, 2001). Kitwood (1997) conceptualised person-centred dementia care in response to a reductionist biomedical view of dementia that downgraded the person to a carrier of an incurable disease ignoring personal experiences of well-being, dignity, and worth (Kitwood, 1997). Kitwood, described the characteristics that define the concept of person-centred care in his seminal work on the subject: the acknowledgment that the individual is a person that can experience life and relationships, despite the progressive disease; offering and respecting choices; the inclusion of the person's past life and history in their care; and the focus on what the person can do, rather than the abilities that have been lost owing to the disease (Kitwood 1997). Person-centred care has been defined as supporting the rights, values, and beliefs of the individual; involving them and providing unconditional positive regard; entering their world and assuming that there is meaning in all behaviour, even if it is difficult to interpret; maximising each person's potential; and sharing decision making.

The different CST principles serve as strategies to meet and fulfil the psychological needs expressed by Kitwood (1997): Identity, attachment, comfort, inclusion, occupation and love. The CST approach to deliver person-centred care incorporates:

(a) Biographical knowledge of the person that helps facilitators to adapt the different sessions according to the individual's needs and interest. Accounts of a person's previous life, routines, and occupation providing interpretative cues for their present behaviour, needs, and wishes.

(b) Reminiscence is used to promote person-centredness as an aid to the here and now. It is thought to affirm the experiences and views of the world of people with dementia and foster social interaction through sharing of autobiographical memories using multisensory stimuli such as pictures, music, and scrapbooks.

(c) Focusing on opinion rather than facts promotes the use of validation to acknowledge the person's interpretation of reality through validation of their individual experiences. This unconditional positive regard may promote confidence and well being (Overshott & Burns 2006; Neal & Wright 2003). CST sessions offer freedom of expression and a release from previous constraints and concerns to present new sources of pleasure and satisfaction for the person with dementia.

(d) Giving consistency between sessions using the same place and session structure providing home-like surroundings. This has been associated with positive effects on the behaviour and mood of people with dementia (Cohen-Mansfield & Werner 1998), and smaller-sized groups show increased social interaction and community formation (McAllister & Silverman 1999; Moore, 1999).

(e) Valuing every person in the group and helping them feel content; offering dignity and striving to preserve a sense of self; accepting everyone's ways of being and opinions; sharing everyday life with a sense of togetherness (15 minutes included before the session with refreshments for extra social interaction); encouraging a sense of belonging to the group (selecting their group name and song in the first session of the programme); offering a secure environment; providing opportunities for occupation through the different proposed activities; and promoting a sense of power and control (including encouraging different roles within the group).

Using Consensus Methods Drawing on Evidence and Theory to Develop the Programme

In the absence of a large body of good quality evidence regarding the effectiveness of long-term CST programmes for dementia and theory behind this, a consensus conference was convened. This brought together the knowledge and expertise of local and external professionals, researchers and family caregivers involved in cognitive programmes in the dementia care field. Maintenance CST programme Version 1 was presented at an international consensus conference in London compromising key academics, research staff, clinical staff and family caregivers. A consensus method provides a means of synthesising the available information (Jones and Hunter, 1995). The aim of the consensus conference was to develop indicators for the successfulness of CST activities by considering the research evidence for the effectiveness of this therapy, and to use the feedback from participants to validate and review the draft Version 1. Participants reviewed the different presented themes in the programme and considered which activities they felt would be successful or unsuccessful for a long term intervention. The conference began with a presentation of the evidence from the Cochrane review (Woods et al., 2010), a presentation about the evidence from the CST trial (Spector et al., 2003) and a presentation about the development of the Maintenance CST programme Version 1. The participants worked in small multidisciplinary groups that facilitated the discussion about the presented themes (old and new) in the maintenance programme. Each group included clinical and research professionals plus family caregivers. Each group was asked to appoint a chairman whose role was to ensure that the group worked to the brief and to report back to the other groups. The groups worked on their brief for one and a half hours and drew up a list of the themes that they were reviewing. The groups were asked to split the themes into pros and cons for each of the activities. Subsequently, the groups came together and presented their opinions about the themes to the whole group. After the consensus conference, the different discussed points were typed and circulated to the Maintenance CST panel and consensus attendees, in the first phase Delphi survey, to encourage comments on the points. The changes from the consensus conference were included and integrated into the programme, leading to the maintenance CST programme draft Version 2. A list of the key principles of CST underlying the relevant theory behind the success of this therapy was also established among the CST panel (AS, BW, MO, JH, EA).

MODELLING PROCESS

To improve the therapy programme in terms of clarity, appropriateness and effectiveness asoutlined in Phase I (modelling) of the MRC guidelines (2008), we included qualitative testing of the intervention through focus groups. Focus groups were undertaken separately with the three main groups of users who constituted key stakeholders in the project; people with dementia, family carers and staff, in order to identify strengths and weaknesses in the programme and refinement of the therapy. Focus groups were the natural choice since the aim was to gain as comprehensive a picture as possible of the views of the key stakeholders with regards to the Maintenance CST programme. Two members of the research team conducted nine (one-hour each) focus groups (3 with people with dementia, 3 with family caregivers and 3 with care staff). The groups focused on the 19 themes developed for the Maintenance CST programme and cognitive stimulation as defined by Clare et al (2003). Clare & Woods (2003) has made headway in categorising cognitive interventions by attempting to draw together the different ideas into three main types: 'Cognitive Stimulation', 'Cognitive Training' and 'Cognitive Rehabilitation'. Accordingly 'Cognitive Stimulation' is applied to interventions which involve the engagement in a range of activities and discussions aimed at general enhancement of cognitive and social.

The focus group interviews were tape-recorded and subsequently transcribed. The authors used an inductive thematic analysis approach (Boyatzis, 1998) to code and analyze the data. Using the final codebook, all transcripts were coded independently by both raters and then compared to reach 100% consensus (Aguirre et al, 2010).

ESTABLISHING CONSENSUS

In order to establish the extent of agreement and consensus among the consensus conference participants with regards to the therapy programme Version 3, a final step was taken. A Delphi survey was sent to the consensus conference attendees that consisted of a covering letter introducing and explaining the steps followed for the development of the manual Version 3, plus a survey questionnaire that aimed to clarify points of the development of the programme and reach consensus about its development and key features.

RESULTS

The different stages that were undertaken for the development of the intervention resulted in different therapy programme manual versions (Figure 2). These are detailed below:

Draft Manual Version 1

The systematic review found 5 new studies published from 2002 to 2007 meeting the inclusion criteria since the last Cochrane review (Spector et al., 2000). Combining the results from 15 RCTs (8 included in the previous review, 5 new and 2 from our team; Spector et al., 2001; Spector et al., 2003) (Table 1), the meta-analyses showed that people receiving cognitive stimulation improved significantly more than controls in cognition and quality of life (Woods et al., 2010). In addition to Spector et al., 2003 two other studies were the most influential studies in the design of this Maintenance programme: Requena et al., 2004 and Onder et al., 2005. Requena et al., 2004 was a single blind RCT demonstrating improvements in cognition and memory over a two-year period. They included a new technique using 'visual clips' that was included in the draft Version 1 of our programme. Onder et al, 2005 was a single blind RCT that demonstrated improvements in cognition over 25 weeks of therapy, delivered individually by family care-givers for 30 minutes three times a week. They included a session about the use of calendars, notes and clocks that was adapted and included in the draft Version 1 of the manual as a new theme called "useful tips - caring for oneself".

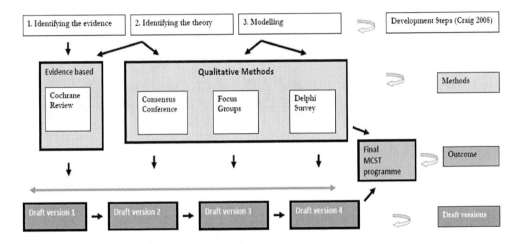

Figure 2. Development of the Maintenance CST programme manual.

As a result of the process of identifying and developing appropriate theory for the programme, a table identifying themes and properties of the manuals was developed. A database was also created including the different elements, guiding principles and session themes that were found in the Cochrane review included studies. The key themes from the initial CST manual (Spector et al., 2006) guiding principles and sessions were organised in the database including the 16 sessions developed for the Maintenance CST pilot project (Orrell et al., 2005). From the analysed interventions of the Cochrane review studies, a 24 weekly session of Maintenance CST programme Version 1 was developed (Table 2). The MCST programme was based on the structural model of CST (Spector et al., 2003) and had similar criteria set out for it before development was started, as its aim was to complement it. This criterion was that the programme sessions had to be flexible, with stimulating exercises grouped by theme (e.g. food, childhood, sounds, physical exercises, famous faces, word game, and number games). Each theme had to contain exercises of different types, focusing on memory, concentration, linguistic, and executive abilities and each session had to follow the following structure: beginning with introductions and a warm-up activity (such as ball game), followed by a main activity and finishing with a closing to the session.

Draft Manual Version 2

The maintenance programme themes in the draft Manual Version 1 were validated and reviewed through the application of a Delphi consensus process. The consensus conference took place at University College London (UCL) over one afternoon and was attended by 34 participants comprising key academics, research staff, clinical staff and family caregivers. As a result the activities included in the different presented themes were extended and adapted to be more suitable for the target population. Some theme titles were also modified, 'using objects' was replaced by 'household treasures', 'golden expression cards' was replaced by 'thinking cards' and 'childhood' by 'my life'. 'My life' theme was incorporated twice in the programme, about the first one focussing on childhood and the second one focusing on occupations. The overall format of the programme Version 1 was preserved, although it was suggested that the programme should incorporate activities that could be drawn on by different cultural communities. At the consensus conference, it was fed back that the way that CST was defined and how this differed to other cognitive therapies or other occupational activities normally run in day centres and care homes was not entirely clear. In the response to this, '18 key principles' were developed. These were subsequently included in the manual and used as an additional measure of adherence and continuous training for group facilitators and co-facilitators.

Draft Manual Version 3

The programme Version 2 was presented in nine focus groups. In total 17 people with dementia, 13 staff and 18 family carers participated (Aguirre et al., 2010). Thematic analysis revealed themes relating to perceptions and opinions of 'mental stimulation/use it or lose it'; 'examples of mental stimulating activities of daily life '; 'factors influencing successfulness and unsuccessfulness of a mental stimulation activity' and 'opinions and perceptions of specific themes of the presented Maintenance CST programme'. Patterns of themes were found among the different groups (people with dementia, family caregivers, staff). Positive agreement was found among the presented 14 CST session themes and suggestions were made for the 5 remaining new session themes. The feedback from the analyses of the focus groups involved the organisation of the different session themes in a different order and reclassification of the session themes that were planned to run twice during the 24 weeks of intervention. Two session themes (current affairs and thinking cards) that were originally planned to run twice on the Version 2 of the programme were reduced to once, and replaced by two session themes that were rated very highly in the focus groups with people with dementia: word games and household treasures. Detailed information about the modification of the programme themes from Version 1 to Version 3 is shown in Table 2. These results were used to produce the manual for the Maintenance CST programme Version 3 of the programme.

Table 2. CST and Maintenance CST programme themes

Programme	Pilot MCST	Version 1	Version 2	Version 3	Final Version
1	Childhood	Childhood	My life / Childhood	My life / Childhood	My life / Childhood
2	Current affairs	Current affairs	Current affairs	Current affairs	Current affairs
3	Current affairs	Food	Food	Food	Food
4	Using objects	Being creative	Being creative	Being creative	Being creative
5	Number Games	Number Games	Number Games	Number Games	Number Games
6	Team Games, Quiz	Team Games, Quiz	Team Games, Quiz	Team Games, Quiz	Team Games, Quiz
7	Sound	Sound	Sound	Sound	Sound
8	Physical Games	Physical Games	Physical Games	Physical Games	Physical Games
9	Categorising objects	Categorising Objects	Categorising Objects	Categorising Objects	Categorising Objects
10	Using objects	Using objects *P	Household treasures	Household treasures	Household treasures
11	Useful tips	Useful tips (Household) *P	Useful tips (Household)	Useful tips (Household)	Useful tips (Household)
12	Golden Expression cards	Golden Expression cards *P	Thinking cards	Thinking cards	Thinking cards
13	Golden Expression cards	Visual Clips *C	Visual Clips	Visual Clips	Visual Clips
14	Art Discussion	Art Discussion *P	Art Discussion	Art Discussion	Art Discussion
15	Famous faces/Scenes	Famous faces/Scenes	Famous faces/Scenes	Famous faces/Scenes	Famous faces/Scenes
16	Word Games	Word Games	Word Games	Word Games	Word Games
17		Food	Food	Food	Food
18		Associated words	Associated words	Associated words	Associated words
19		Orientation	Orientation	Orientation	Orientation
20		Using money	Using money	Using money	Using money
21		Current affairs	Current affairs	Word Games	Word Games

Table 2. (Continued).

Programme	Pilot MCST	Version 1	Version 2	Version 3	Final Version
22		Golden Expression cards *P	Thinking cards	Household treasures	Household treasures
23		Childhood	My life / Occupations	My life / Occupations	My life / Occupations
24		Useful tips (Health/Memory) *C	Useful tips (Health/Memory)	Useful tips (Health/Memory)	Useful tips (Health/Memory)

*C: Themes developed from the systematic review.

*P: Themes from the pilot maintenance CST.

Themes included from the original CST programme

FINAL MAINTENANCE CST PROGRAMME

As the final round of the Delphi process, 23 questionnaires were sent to the consensus conference participants. Six were returned and considering the multiple feedback processes inherent in the Delphi process, the potential exists for low response rates. Striving to maintain robust feedback can be a challenge as poor response rate is magnified fourfold as a maximum of four surveys may be sent to the same panellists (Witkin & Altschuld, 1995). All participants who replied to the survey felt that the draft Version 3 included all the elements discussed at the consensus conference and felt that would be a beneficial programme for people with dementia, as well as a useful tool for professionals working in the field. Although a low response rate was achieved in this survey, consensus in the long-term maintenance programme was expressed by the number of professionals that replied.

The feedback from the surveys resulted in some minor editorial changes and survey participants expressed their concerns about preparation time in order to run the sessions. They suggested that in order to make the manual more user friendly for staff, the appendixes of the manual could be extended. Appendixes were added with: resources for each session, and guidance for co-facilitators of CST, recommending steps to help prepare for the sessions, and procedures to follow when co facilitating a group. Following the feedback from these questionnaires the final Version of the Maintenance programme was prepared. Table 2 shows how each theme within the programme has evolved through the different developmental stages from Version 1 to final version.

DISCUSSION

This study shows that it is feasible to develop a psychological therapy as a complex intervention following the Medical Research Council (2008) guidelines using the three stages of: identifying the evidence, developing the theory and modelling. The original MRC framework 2000 identified designing, describing, and implementing a well defined intervention as: "the most challenging part of evaluating a complex intervention and the most frequent weakness in such trials." By developing a programme following the framework we have ensured that the intervention has been developed to the point where it can reasonably be expected to have a worthwhile effect. Although several studies have described using the MRC framework for the development of their intervention, the interpretation of the content and purpose of phases seems to differ between the studies (Rowlands et al., 2005; Robinson et al., 2005; Haw et al., 2007). It appears that carefully developing complex interventions is regarded as a good thing, but details of how to achieve phase 1 (review of theory and evidence) and modelling of the framework are lacking.

The specific model (Figure 2) shows the use of mixed methods along phase I: the use of a systematic review; qualitative methods including the involvement of service users through consensus conference and focus groups; and a final Delphi survey. The involvement of service users as well as being ethically preferable represents practical advantages for the future phases of the evaluation of the intervention. Recruitment and retention are likely to be better if the intervention is valued by potential participants, concerns about fairness are addressed and the knowledge that community leaders support the evaluation in the case of community-based interventions (MRC framework 2008). The use of focus groups as a modelling exercise to prepare for the trial, also allowed us to think about implementation at an early stage (before embarking on a lengthy and expensive evaluation process) as recommended by some studies (Glasgow et al., 2003; Tunis et al., 2002). Although there is growing awareness of the role that qualitative research can play in the design and evaluation of interventions, a recent methodological study about the use of qualitative methods alongside randomized controlled trials of complex interventions (Lewin et al., 2009) identified that less than one third of recently completed trials of complex interventions in the Cochrane Effective Practice and Organisation of Care register included some form of qualitative research. Of these, only about two thirds were published studies. This may contribute to the view that earlier phases of research, such as efficacy trials, do not need to incorporate qualitative studies to explore the effects of contextual and other moderating factors. Such methods are seen as important only in the later phases of evaluation (Glasgow et al., 2003).

Some limitations included in the development of this programme included the number of questions we sought to answer in relation to developing the theory step from our literature review and the limited resources we found from the included studies, meant relying predominantly on expert knowledge. The generalisability of our qualitative results may also have been limited as our consensus conference steering group relied on individuals participating, and the small number of participants in the focus groups. Definitive evidence of effectiveness of our intervention requires an evaluation in a randomized trial. We now have an intervention worthy of further evaluation although comprehensive development of intervention is not synonymous with efficacy. Harderman et al., (2005) developed an intervention to encourage people at risk of diabetes to be more physically active and followed the MRC framework but the intervention was subsequently shown to be ineffective in the RCT. Therefore, the results of the maintenance CST RCT (Phase III) are needed before drawing conclusions about its effectiveness.

In order to better understand the effectiveness of the developed intervention and as recommended by the MRC guidelines (2008) that suggests a more circular approach to their understanding, a process evaluation, phase IV study will be carry out following the evaluation through the RCT (Aguirre et al., 2010). The purpose of the final phase will be to examine the implementation of the intervention into practice, paying particular attention to the rate of uptake, the stability of the intervention, any broadening of subject groups, and the possible existence of adverse effects. Furthermore, this phase study will provide valuable insight into why the intervention fails or has unexpected consequences, or why the intervention results successful and works and how it can be optimised.

CONCLUSIONS

This study demonstrates that an evidence-based approach, tempered with the input of experienced professionals and input from service users, is feasible and productive. The involvement of people with dementia ensured that the maintenance CST sessions included in the programme were appropriate to their preferences and abilities. The detailed manual to accompany the Maintenance programme is also being prepared (available from the authors). A large, multi-centre RCT is now under way, representing phase III of the development of a complex intervention (Aguirre et al., 2010), which uses the final version of the Maintenance CST programme.

Competing Interests

AS runs the CST training course on a commercial basis.

AS, BW and MO have co-authored a CST manual, the royalties from which are received by the Dementia Services Development Centre Wales.

Authors' Contributions

Contributions: MO, RTW, ITR developed the original concept of the trial, and EA and MO drafted the original protocol; AS, ASt and JH co authored the treatment manual; all authors reviewed and commented on drafts of the protocol and paper.

ACKNOWLEDGEMENTS

Maintenance Cognitive Stimulation Programme (ISRCTN26286067) is part of the Support at Home - Interventions to Enhance Life in Dementia (SHIELD) project (Application No RP-PG-0606-1083) which is funded by the NIHR Programme Grants for Applied research funding scheme. The grant holders are Professors Orrell (UCL), Woods (Bangor), Challis (Manchester), Moniz-Cook (Hull), Russell (Swansea), Knapp (LSE) and Dr Charlesworth (UCL).

The views and opinions expressed in this paper are those of the authors and do not necessarily reflect those of the Department of Health/NIHR.

REFERENCES

[1]   Aguirre, E; Spector, A; Streater, A; Burnell, K; Orrell, M. Service users' involvement in the development of a maintenance Cognitive Stimulation Therapy (CST) programme: A comparison of the views of people with dementia, staff and family carers. *Dementia Journal*, 2010, in press.

[2]   Aguirre, E; Spector, A; Hoe, J; Russell, TI; Knapp, M; Woods, TR; Orrell M. Maintenance Cognitive Stimulation Therapy (CST) for dementia: A single-blind, multi-centre, randomized controlled trial of Maintenance CST vs. CST for dementia. *Trials*, 2010, 11:46.

[3]   American Psychiatric Association. Practice guideline for the treatment of patients with Alzheimer's disease and other dementias of late life. *American Journal of Psychiatry*, 1997, 154 (5): 1–39.

[4]   Baines, S; Saxby, P; Ehlert, K. Reality orientation and reminiscence therapy A controlled cross-over study of elderly confused people. *British Journal of Psychiatry* ,1987;151:222-31.

[5]   Baldelli, MV; Pirani, A; Motta, M; Abati, E; Mariani, E; Manzi, V. Effects of reality orientation therapy on elderly patients in the community. *Archives of Gerontology and Geriatrics,* 1993a;1 7(3):21 1-8.

[6]   Baldelli, MV; Boiardi, R; Fabbo, A; Pradelli, JM; Neri, M. The role of reality orientation therapy in restorative care of elderly patients with dementia plus stroke in the subacute nursing home setting. Archives of Gerontology and Geriatrics, 2002; 35(8):1 5-22.

[7]   Bottino,CM; Carvalho, IA; Alvarez, AM; Avila, R; Zukauskas, PR; Bustamante, SE; Andrade, FC; Hototian, SR; Saffi, F; Câmargo, CH. Cognitive rehabilitation combined with drug treatment in Alzheimer's disease patients: a pilot study. *Clinical Rehabilitation,* 2005, 19(8):861-9.

[8]   Boyatzis RE. *Transforming qualitative information: thematic analysis and code development.* London: Sage; 1998.

[9]   Breuil, V; De Rotrou, J; Forette, F. Cognitive stimulation of patients with dementia: preliminary results. *International Journal of Geriatric Psychiatry,* 1994, 9, 211–217.

[10] Chapman, SB; Weiner, MF; Rackley, A; Hynan, LS; Zientz, J. Effects of cognitive-communication stimulation for Alzheimer's disease patients treated with donepezil. *Journal of Speech, Language, and Hearing Research,* 2004;47(5):1 149-63.

[11] Clancy, L; Goodman, P; Sinclair, H; Dockery, DW. Effect of air pollution control on death rates in Dublin, Ireland: an intervention study. *Lancet,* 2002, 360:1210-4.

[12] Clare, L; Woods, RT. Cognitive training and rehabilitation for people with early-stage Alzheimer's disease: a review, *Neuropsychological Rehabilitation,* 2003, 14, 385-401

[13] Craig, P; Dieppe, P; Macintyre, S; Michie, S; Nazareth, I; Petticrew, M. Developing and evaluating complex interventions: the new Medical Research Council guidance. *British Medical Journal,* 2008, 337: a1655.

[14] Cohen-Mansfield, J; Werner, P. The effects of an enhanced environment on nursing home residents who pace. *Gerontologist,* 1998, 38: 199–208.

[15] Cotman, CW; Berchtold, NC. Physical activity and the maintenance of cognition: Learning from animal models. *Alzheimer's & Dementia Journal,* 2007, 3:S30-S37.

[16] Farina, E; Fioravanti R; Chiavari, L; Imbornone, E;Alberoni, M;Pomati, S; Pinardi, G; Pignatti, R; Mariani, C. Comparing two programs of cognitive training in Alzheimer's disease: a pilot study. *Acta Neurologica Scandinavica,* 2002, 105 (5), 365-3

[17] Farina, E; Mantovani, F; Fioravanti, R; Pignatti, R; Chiavari, L; Imbornone, E; Olivotto' F; Alberoni' M; Mariani, C; Nemni, R.Evaluating two group programmes of cognitive training in mild-to-moderate AD: is there any difference between a 'global' stimulation and a 'cognitive-specific' one? *Aging & Mental Health,* 2006, 10(3): 211-8.

[18] Ferrario, E; Cappa, G; Molaschi, M; Rocco, M; Fabris, F. Reality orientation therapy in institutionalized elderly patients: Preliminary results. *Archives of Gerontology and Geriatrics,*1991 ;12(2):1 39-42.

[19] Fleischman, DA; Wilson, RS; Gabrieli, JD. Implicit memory and Alzheimer's disease neuropathology. *Brain,* 2005, 128: 2006-2015.

[20] Forbes, D; Forbes, S; Morgan, DG; Markle-Reid, M; Wood, J; Culum, I. Physical activity programs for persons with dementia. *Cochrane Database of Systematic Reviews* 2008, Issue 3. Art. No.: CD006489. DOI: 10.1002/14651858. CD006489.pub2.

[21] Gerber, GJ; Prince, PN; Snider, HG; Atchison, K; Dubois, L; Kilgour, JA. Group activity and cognitive improvement among patients with Alzheimer's disease. *Hospital and Community Psychiatry*, 1991 ;42(8):843-5.

[22] Glasgow, RE; Lichtenstein, E; Marcus, AC. Why don't we see more translation of health promotion research into practice? Rethinking the efficacy-to-effectiveness transition. *American Journal of Public Health*, 2003, 93(8): 1261-7.

[23] Hanley, IG; McGuire, RJ; Boyd, WD. Reality orientation and dementia: A controlled trial of two approaches. *British Journal of Psychiatry*, 1981, 138:10-4.

[24] Hardeman, W; Sutton, S; Griffin, S; Johnston, M; White, A; Wareham, NJ. A causal modelling approach to the development of theory-based behaviour change programmes for trial evaluation. *Health Education Research*, 2005, 20: 676-87.

[25] Haw, SJ; Gruer, L. Changes in exposure of adult non-smokers to 26 secondhand smoke after implementation of smoke-free legislation in Scotland: national cross sectional survey. *British Medical Journal*, 2007, 335:549-52.

[26] Hinsz, VB, Tindale, RS; Vollrath, DA. The emerging conceptualization of groups as information processors. *Psychological Bulletin*, 1997, 121,43–64.

[27] Hunkin, NM; Squires, EJ; Parkin, AJ; Tidy, JA. Are the benefits of errorless learning dependent on implicit memory?. *Neuropsychologia*, 1998, 36, 25- 36.

[28] Jones, J; Hunter, D. Qualitative research: Consensus methods for medical and health services research. *British Medical Journal*, 1995, 311: 376-380

[29] Katzman, R; Terry, R; DeTeresa, R; Brown, T; Davies, P; Fuld, P; Renbing, X; Peck, A. Clinical, pathological, and neurochemical changes in dementia: A subgroup with preserved mental status and numerous neocortical plaques. *Annals of Neurology*, 1988, 23, 138–144.

[30] Katzman, R. Education and the prevalence of dementia and Alzheimer's disease. *Neurology*, 1993, 43, 13 - 20.

[31] Kiernat, JM. The use of life review activity with confused nursing home residents. *American Journal of Occupational Therapy*, 1979, 33, 306-310

[32] Kitwood, T. Dementia reconsidered: The person comes first. Buckingham: Open University Press; 1997

[33] Kitwood, T. The concept of personhood and its relevance for a new culture of dementia care. In: Miesen, BML, Jones, GMM. *Care giving in dementia: research and applications, vol. 2*. London, Routledge; 1997; 3-13.

[34] Knapp, M; Thorgrimsen, L; Patel, A; Spector, A; Hallam, A; Woods, B; Orrell, M. Cognitive Stimulation Therapy for people with dementia: Cost Effectiveness Analysis . *British Journal of Psychiatry*, 2006, 188: 574-580.

[35] Lewin, S; Glenton, C; Oxman, A. Use of qualitative methods alongside RCTs of complex healthcare interventions: methodological study. *British Medical Journal*, 2009, 339:b3496 doi:10.1136.

[36] Medical Research Council. *A framework for development and evaluation of RCTs for complex interventions to improve health*. London, MRC guidelines; 2000.

[37] Medical Research Council. A framework for development and evaluation of RCTs for complex interventions to improve health. London, MRC guidelines; 2008.

[38] Metitieri, T; Zanetti ,O; Geroldi, C. Reality Orientation Therapy to delay outcomes of progression in patients with dementia: A retrospective study. *Clinical Rehabilitation*, 2001, 15: 471-478.

[39] McAllister, CL; Silverman, MA. Community formation and community roles among persons with Alzheimer's disease: a comparative study of experiences in a residential Alzheimer's facility and a traditional nursing home. *Quality Health Research*, 1999, 9: 65 – 85.

[40] Moore, K. Dissonance in the dining room: a study of social interaction in a special care unit, *Quality Health Research*, 1999, 9:133–155

[41] National Institute of Clinical Excellence. *Clinical Guideline number 42. In Supporting people with dementia and their carers in health and social care*. Department of Health, London; 2006.

[42] Nazareth, I; Freemantle, N; Duggan, C; Mason, J; Haines, A. Evaluation of a complex intervention for changing professional behaviour: the evidence based outreach (EBOR) trial. *Journal of Health Services Research Policy*, 2002, 7: 230-8.

[43] Neal, M; Wright, PB. Validation therapy for dementia, *Cochrane Database of Systematic Reviews,* 2003, Issue 3. Art. No.: CD001394. DOI: 10.1002/14651858. CD00139

[44] Olazaran, J; Muniz, R; Reisberg, B; Pena-Casanova, J; del Ser, T; Cruz-Jentoft, AJ. Benefits of cognitive-motor intervention in MCI and mild to moderate Alzheimer disease. *Neurology,* 2004, 63:2348-53.

[45] Onder, G; Zanetti, O; Giacobini, E. Reality orientation therapy combined with cholinesterase inhibitors in Alzheimer's disease: randomised controlled trial. *British Journal of Psychiatry*, 2005, 187: 450-455.

[46] Orrell, M; Spector, A; Thorgrimsen, L; Woods, B. A pilot study examining the effectiveness of maintenance Cognitive Stimulation Therapy (MCST) for people with dementia. *International Journal of Geriatric Psychiatry*, 2005, 20:446-451

[47] Overshott, R; Burns, A. Non-pharmacological treatment of severe dementia: an overview. In: A Burns and B Winblad, Editors, *Severe dementia*, Wiley, Chichester. 2006, 164–175.

[48] Requena, C; Ibor, MI; Maestu, F; Campo, P; Ibor, JJ; Ortiz, T. Effects of cholinergic drugs and cognitive training on dementia. *Dementia Geriatric Cognitive Disorders*, 2004, 18: 50–54.

[49] Robinson, L; Francis, J; James, P; Tindle, N; Greenwell, K; Rodgers, H. Caring for carers of people with stroke: developing a complex intervention following the Medical Research Council framework. *Clinical Rehabilitation*, 2005, 19:560–571

[50] Rowlands, G; Sims, J; Kerry, S. A lesson learnt: the importance of modelling in randomized controlled trials for complex interventions in primary care. *Family Practice*, 2005, 22:132–139

[51] Rubin, KH. Social and social-cognitive developmental characteristics of young isolate, normal, and sociable children". In Peer Relationships and Social Skills in Childhood, ed. K. H. Rubin, H. S. Ross, New York: Springer-Verlag; 1982, 353-74

[52] Rubin, KH; LeMare, LJ; Lollis, S. Social withdrawal in childhood: developmental pathways to rejection. In S. R. Asher, SR; Coie JD. *Peer Rejection in Childhood*. New York: Cambridge Univeristy Press; 1990; 217-49.

[53] Spector, A; Davies, S; Woods, B; Orrell, M. Reality orientation for dementia: a systematic review of the evidence of effectiveness from randomised controlled trials. *Gerontologist*, 2000, 40, 206–212.

[54] Spector, A; Davies, S; Woods, B; Orrell, M. Can reality orientation be rehabilitated? Development and piloting of an evidence-based programme of cognition-based therapies for people with dementia. *Neuropsychological Rehabilitation*, 2001, 11, 377–397.

[55] Spector, A; Thorgrimsen, L; Woods, B; Royan, L; Davies, S; Butterworth, M; Orrell, M. (Efficacy of an evidence-based cognitive stimulation therapy programme for people with dementia: Randomised Controlled Trial. *British Journal of Psychiatry*, 2003, 183: 248-254

[56] Spector, A; Thorgrimsen, L; Woods, B; Orrell, M. *Making a difference: An evidence-based group programme to offer cognitive stimulation therapy (CST) to people with dementia: Manual for group leaders*. United Kingdom: Hawker Publications; 2006.

[57] Tailby, R; Haslam ,C. An investigation of errorless learning in memory-impaired patients: Improving the technique and clarifying theory. *Neuropsychologia*, 2003, 4 (9), 1230-1240.

[58] Tindale, RS; Kameda, T. Social sharedness as a unifying theme for information processing in groups. *Group Processes Intergroup Relations*, 2003, 3 (20) 123-140.

[59] Toseland, RW; Diehl, M; Freeman, K; Manzanares, T; McCallion, P. The impact of validation group therapy on nursing home residents with dementia. *Journal of Applied Gerontology*, 1997, 16, (1), 31–50

[60] Tunis, SR; Stryer ,DB; Clancy, CM. Practical clinical trials: increasing the value of research for *decision-making in clinical and health policy. Journal of the American Medical Association*, 2002, 290(12): 1624-32.

[61] Wallis, GG; Baldwin, M; Higginbotham, P. Reality orientation therapy-a controlled trial. *British Journal of Medical Psychology*, 1983, 56(3): 271 -7.

[62] Witkin, BR; Altschuld, JW. *Planning and conducting needs assessment: A practical guide*. Thousand Oaks, CA: Sage Publications, Inc.; 1995.

[63] Woods, RT. Reality Orientation and Staff attention: A Controlled Study. *British Journal of Psychiatry*, 1979, 134:502- 7.

[64] Woods, B. What can be learned from studies on reality orientation? In Jones GMM. & Miesen BL. *Care-giving in dementia: Research and applications*. New York: Tavistock/Routledge; 1992, 21-136.

[65] Woods, RT. Discovering the person with Alzheimer's disease: Cognitive, emotional and behavioural aspects. *Aging & Mental Health*, 2001, 5 (1), S7–S16.

[66] Woods, B; Spector, A; Jones, C; Orrell, M; Davies, S. Reminiscence therapy for dementia. *Cochrane Database Systematic Reviews*: 2005, Issue 2. Art. No.: CD001120. DOI: 10.1002/14651858.CD001120.pub2.

[67] Woods, B; Thorgrimsen, L; Spector, A; Royan, L; Orrell, M. Improved quality of life and cognitive stimulation therapy in dementia. *Aging and Mental Health*, 2006, 10(3):219–226.

[68] Woods, RT; Aguirre, E; Spector, A; Orrell, M. Cognitive Stimulation Therapy for dementia: a review of the evidence of effectiveness. *Cochrane Database Systematic Reviews*: 2010, in press

[69] Wortman, PM. An exemplary evaluation of a program that worked: the High/Scope Perry preschool project". *American Journal of Evaluation*, 1995, 16:257-65.

[70] Zanetti, O; Frisoni, GB; De Leo, D; Buono, MD; Bianchetti, A; Trabucci ,M. Reality Orientation Therapy in Alzheimer's disease: Useful or not? A controlled study. *Alzheimer's disease and Associated Disorders*, 1995, 9: 132-13

In: Dementia: Non-Pharmacological Therapies
Editor: Elisabetta Farina, pp. 209-228

ISBN: 978-1-61470-736-3
© 2012 Nova Science Publishers, Inc.

COMPUTER-ASSISTED SPACED RETRIEVAL TRAINING OF FACES AND NAMES FOR PERSONS WITH DEMENTIA

Nidhi Mahendra[*]

Department of Communicative Sciences &
Disorders California State University East Bay.

ABSTRACT

This study was designed to investigate the feasibility and document the outcomes of computer-assisted spaced retrieval training (SRT) for persons with dementia. Twenty three participants with mild to moderate dementia participated in computer-assisted SRT for learning novel and familiar face-name associations. Study results reveal that computer-assisted SRT is feasible for persons with dementia and yielded positive treatment outcomes for a majority of participants. Specifically, twenty participants were successful in recalling face-name associations and related factual information over a 32-minute, within-session time interval. Nineteen of these twenty participants maintained this new learning for 6 weeks after the intervention ceased. These data add to the growing empirical evidence on the benefits of spaced retrieval for persons with dementia. Further, study findings extend the existing research on the outcomes of SRT by demonstrating feasibility and robust outcomes with use of a laptop computer as a medium for training.

Keywords: computer-assisted spaced retrieval training (SRT), face-name associations, dementia.

INTRODUCTION

Dementia is characterized by acquired and persistent impairment of multiple cognitive domains that is severe enough to interfere with activities of daily living, occupation, and social interaction (Grabowski & Damasio, 2004). Affected cognitive domains include memory, attention, executive function, language and communicative function, and visuospatial abilities. Alzheimer's disease (AD) is the most common cause of dementia in older adults over the age of 65 years, accounting for approximately 50% of clinical diagnoses of dementia (Alzheimer's Association, 2010). There is substantial evidence that cognitive

---

[*] Corresponding author: Phone: 510-396-1098, Fax: (510) 885-2186, Email: mahendranidhi@gmail.com

interventions for persons with dementia (PWD) are efficacious and can facilitate maintenance or improvement of performance on discrete cognitive tasks and on functional activities of daily living (Bayles & Kim, 2003; Bourgeois et al., 2003; Camp, 1989; Mahendra, 2001; Mahendra & Arkin, 2003; McKitrick, Camp, & Black, 1992). Given the rapidly rising incidence of dementia and the limited benefit from existing pharmacological treatments using acetylcholinesterase (ACE) inhibitors and N-methyl-D-aspartate (NMDA) antagonists, it is imperative that researchers continue to aggressively develop and study outcomes of innovative, non-pharmacological interventions. Further, it is noteworthy that there is emerging empirical evidence supporting better outcomes for PWD following a synergistic combination of pharmacological and nonpharmacalogical interventions, as compared to drug treatments alone (Chapman et al., 2004; Requena et al., 2004; Requena et al., 2006). In this paper, we report the outcomes of computer-assisted spaced retrieval training (SRT) for teaching face-name associations to persons with dementia. Spaced retrieval training is described in the next section, followed by a brief review of existing research on its application for designing interventions for persons with dementia.

SPACED RETRIEVAL TRAINING

Spaced retrieval training (SRT) was first described by Landauer and Bjork (1978) as a technique for facilitating memory in healthy young adults. Subsequently, Schacter, Rich, and Stampp (1985) demonstrated its efficacy for teaching face-name associations to persons with memory disorders followed by Camp (1989) adapting this technique for PWD. Spaced retrieval training is best understood as a shaping paradigm for memory training (Brush & Camp, 1998a) and has been shown to facilitate new learning in PWD. In SRT, new facts are presented (Brush & Camp, 2000; Lee et al., 2009) or a new motor procedure is demonstrated (Lin et al., 2010; Mahendra & Tomoeda, 2009) followed by PWD recalling or demonstrating newly learned information immediately after it has been presented. Subsequently, facts are recalled or procedures demonstrated repeatedly over gradually increasing time intervals. Time intervals following successful recall attempts are doubled whereas intervals following failed recall attempts are maintained or reduced in their duration (see Figure 1 for a visual display of recall trials in SRT). In this way, PWD learn to recall functionally relevant information over longer periods of time and this improved recall, in turn, supports independent functioning for specific activities. Findings of multiple researchers have revealed the success of SRT for persons with dementia (Bourgeois et al., 2003; Cherry, Walvoord, & Hawley, 2010; Hopper et al., 2005; Lee et al., 2009; Ozgis, Rendell, & Henry, 2009), traumatic brain injury (Bourgeois, Lenius, Turkstra, & Camp, 2007), and amnesia (Schacter, Rich, & Stampp, 1985). SRT has been used to teach dementia patients word lists (Lee et al., 2009), names of people (Cherry, Walvoord, & Hawley, 2010; Hopper, Drefs, Bayles, Tomoeda, & Dinu, 2010), prospective memory tasks (Ozgis, Rendell, & Henry, 2009), and compensatory techniques to promote safe swallowing (Brush & Camp, 1998b), safe mobility and transfers (Brush & Camp, 1998c) and to facilitate positive communicative behaviors (Brush & Camp, 1998c). See Hopper et al (2005) for an evidence-based systematic review on the outcomes of SRT for persons with AD.Much attention has been focused on detailing the precise mechanism by which SRT facilitates recall and retention in PWD, despite their significant episodic memory deficits. This mechanism is not fully understood. However, current research points to some important factors that underlie the success of SRT. It is likely that SRT works because of repeated opportunities to retrieve target information (Mahendra, 2001), gradual building up of duration over which recall is maintained (Bourgeois et al., 2003), and emphasis on retrieval success (Brush & Camp, 2000). Further, some have suggested that SRT capitalizes on relatively spared implicit memory processes (Hopper, 2003) and requires little cognitive effort from dementia patients (Lee et al., 2009). Hopper (2003) also discusses that SRT may work especially well because of the incidental use of errorless learning in its implementation. For persons with intact episodic memory, trial and error learning works well because individuals remember the erroneous response and subsequent corrective feedback as a learning episode. This retention of the learning episode reduces the likelihood of future occurrences of the same error. However, for PWD, the very act of making an error is undesirable early on during learning new information. This is because the severe episodic memory deficits in PWD render them unable to remember errors or corrective feedback. This leads directly to the same errors being repeated (Baddeley & Wilson, 1994) and being reinforced. Therefore, using errorless learning principles (Baddeley, 1992; Clare & Jones, 2008) to constrain stimulus presentation, task instructions, and permitted responses may further facilitate new learning when using SRT. Successful implementation of SRT requires that persons always end a recall trial or a therapeutic session with a correct desired response. Two noteworthy components of SRT deserve mention. The first concerns whether treatment outcomes differ by fixed interval or spaced interval retrieval schedules. Although most researchers reporting successful outcomes with SRT have used gradually lengthening intervals, two groups of researchers have recently documented comparable success with spaced and fixed length of recall intervals. Hochhalter, Overmier, Gasper, Bakke, and Holub (2005) compared expanding intervals to other rehearsal schedules (random intervals, uniformly distributed intervals) with a small group of persons with AD. They found no significant advantage for expanded retrieval over equally spaced practice schedules. Similarly, Balota, Duchek, Sergent-Marshall, and Roediger (2006) found no advantage of expanded retrieval over an equal interval schedule, in improving the memory performance of persons with AD and healthy older adults. Based on the results of these two studies, it appears that spaced intervals are not critical to the success of SRT. Thus, it may be that the repeated presentation of information and frequent generation of a correct response are more compelling reasons for the success of SRT. A second aspect of SRT that merits attention is whether intervals between recall attempts are best spent doing task-related activities or unrelated activities. It is reasonable to assume that task-related activities during the intervals may further enhance learning whereas unrelated activities might interfere with new learning and adversely impact subsequent recall performance. However, this assumption is not supported by empirical evidence. Indeed, Hopper and colleagues (2010) demonstrated that tasks unrelated to a target face-name association, completed during intervals, did not negatively impact learning by PWD. This important finding has practical applications during SRT implementation because activities such as conversation, a snack, or brief recreational or therapeutic activity can be nested within these recall intervals.

Spaced Retrieval Training and Computers: A Powerful Combination

Given the widespread use, low cost, and versatility of laptop computers, improving levels of computer literacy among older adults, and emerging evidence about the benefits of computer-assisted cognitive interventions for PWD (Galante, Venturini, & Fiaccadori, 2007; Hofmann et al., 2003; Mahendra et al., 2005), we wanted to assess the feasibility and document the outcomes of computer-assisted SRT for PWD. Specifically, we employed computer-assisted SRT for teaching face-name associations to persons with mild and moderate dementia. Our interest in using a laptop computer to facilitate SRT implementation was motivated by wanting to deliver SRT with more control of stimulus presentation, better tracking of interval duration, and greater consistency of activities completed during intervals. Our set-up included a laptop PC with a high-resolution monitor and a wireless computer mouse. Using a laptop computer allowed us to present high-resolution, digital, color photos of persons with accompanying text about the person appearing sequentially. This was done by creating animated slide shows in which the person's photo appeared first, followed by their first and last name, their occupation, place of residence, and one other biographical detail. During the intervals between recall attempts, participants played commercially available computer games or games from therapy software packages. The first broad goal of this study was to assess the feasibility of computer-assisted cognitive interventions for PWD. We wanted to know if PWD could be taught basic computer operations using a wireless mouse or a Magic Touch™ Screen. The second goal of this study was to document the outcomes of computer-assisted SRT for teaching novel (unfamiliar, never known) and familiar face-name associations to PWD. To our knowledge, this is the first investigation of computer-assisted SRT for individuals with dementia. It was also of interest to document the number of treatment sessions needed for PWD to learn someone's name according to apriori established learning criteria. Finally, once faces and names were learned to a specific criterion, we stopped SRT and assessed maintenance of learned face-name associations for six to eight weeks after training ceased.

METHOD

Participants

Participants were recruited via flyers placed in newsletters of the Northern California Alzheimer's Association and the Family Caregiver Alliance as well as at local senior centers and assisted living and skilled nursing facilities in the San Francisco Bay area of Northern California. All participants were literate, fluent speakers of English, with no history of alcohol or drug dependency, psychiatric disease, seizures, acute cerebrovascular accident, or traumatic brain injury. Informed consent was obtained from participants and their caregivers as appropriate. When a caregiver provided proxy consent, participants were approached and the study activities explained, followed by obtaining verbal assent. Fifty participants with dementia were initially recruited into the study. Each potential participant was diagnosed with dementia (probable Alzheimer's disease or probable vascular dementia) based on combined findings from a neurological examination and a 2-3 hour long neuropsychological evaluation.

Forty of these fifty participants also had detailed brain imaging studies (e.g. structural/functional MRI or PET scan) that corroborated a dementia diagnosis. Of these fifty recruited PWD, three persons withdrew after completing initial assessments and another seven were unable to complete the study due to illness (n=2), injury (n=3), or death (n = 2). The remaining forty participants were enrolled in the study. This paper details the outcomes of computer-assisted SRT for twenty three participants (6 men, 17 women) with mild to moderate dementia who have completed all phases of this ongoing study. Another 17 participants are receiving computer-assisted SRT to learn face-name associations and novel motor procedures. Of the 23 participants, 20 had a medical diagnosis of probable AD, based on clinical criteria established by the National Institute of Neurologic and Communicative Disorders and Stroke and Alzheimer's Disease and Related Disorders Association (NINCDS-ADRDA; McKhann et al., 1984). Three individuals had a diagnosis of probable vascular dementia, based on the standardized, consensus diagnostic criteria established by the National Institute of Neurological Disorders and Stroke and the Association Internationale pour la Recherche et l'Enseignement en Neurosciences (NINDS-AIREN; Roman et al., 2003). Thirteen of the 23 participants were not on any drug treatment for dementia at the time of enrolment into this study. Of the ten remaining participants, six were taking an acetylcholinesterase inhibitor (Aricept), and four were taking an N-methyl D-aspartate (NMDA) receptor antagonist (Namenda). Three of these 23 participants lived in a dementia unit; 13 lived in assisted living settings, and 7 participants lived independently in the community. Regarding ethnicity, twenty participants were Caucasian, 2 were Asian, and 1 person was Latino.

Screening and Assessment

Prior to beginning intervention, each participant completed a comprehensive screening and evaluation to document medical history, sensory status (hearing, vision), affective state, severity of cognitive impairment, and a profile of areas of greatest impairment and relative strengths. The screening consisted of the *Mini Mental State Exam* (Folstein, Folstein, & McHugh, 1975), the *Geriatric Depression Scale-Short Form* (Sheikh & Yesavage, 1986), vision screening tests from the *Arizona Battery for Communication Disorders of Dementia* (ABCD; Bayles & Tomoeda, 1993), and a hearing screening consisting of otoscopy, audiometric screening, and assessment of word recognition ability. The MMSE, GDS-SF, and the ABCD are described in the following section. Participants' medical records also were reviewed and a health history obtained directly from participants or professional/personal caregivers. Finally, because this study involved using computers, participants and their caregivers answered questions about prior and current computer usage, and about specific activities for which they used computers (e.g., sending email, paying bills, etc). Based on their responses, participants were characterized as having no familiarity with computers, limited familiarity, or high familiarity (see Table 1).

Mini Mental State Exam (MMSE)
Participants were administered the MMSE (Folstein, Folstein, & McHugh, 1975), which is a widely used and well known, 11-item test that yields a maximum score of 30 points. An MMSE score below 24 is a strong indicator of cognitive impairment (Tombaugh & McIntyre,

1992), although scores of 25 and 26 typically also indicate some degree of cognitive impairment (Azuma et al., 1997). We interpreted participants' MMSE scores using population-based, age- and education-stratified norms for the MMSE (Crum, Anthony, Bassett, and Folstein, 1993). Study participants had a mean MMSE score of 23.3, with scores ranging from 13 to 30. Only one participant with mild dementia had a score of 30 (Table 1), which was determined to be an artifact from having completed the MMSE multiple times, at the facility where he lived. Despite this spuriously high MMSE score, this individual had a clinical diagnosis of probable AD, based on findings from neurological, neuropsychological, and brain imaging investigations.

Geriatric Depression Scale-Short Form (GDS-SF)

The GDS-Short Form (Sheikh & Yesavage, 1986) consists of fifteen questions presented to an older adult that require a yes or no response (e.g., "Do you have more problems with memory than most people?", "Is it wonderful to be alive now?"). Depending on participants' responses, a score out of 15 is generated with scores of 5 or greater requiring referral to a physician to address the possibility of clinical depression. Study participants had a mean GDS-SF score of 1.59, with scores ranging from 0 to 5. Two participants had scores of 5 on the GDS-SF; both were receiving counseling services and one was on anti-depressant medication.

Hearing and Vision Screening

Participants were administered a brief vision screening to rule out gross visual defects and to ensure that participants could see text and pictures presented via computer. This screening comprised tasks of letter cancellation, picture identification (of 4 common objects), and sentence reading (of 2 short sentences) from the ABCD (Bayles & Tomoeda, 1993). Based on recommendations of the American Speech Language Hearing Association (1997), PWD were administered a hearing screening comprising otoscopy, pure tone audiometric screening, and assessment of word recognition ability. Word recognition ability was assessed by asking PWD to repeat two, 10-word, isophonemic word lists (Boothroyd, 1968), each containing the same 30 phonemes (10 vowels, 20 consonants). Two participants did not have hearing aids but demonstrated difficulty hearing examiners during the screening. These persons were provided assistive listening devices for use during SRT sessions. Table 1 provides information on participant demographic data and performance on all screening measures.

Following this screening, we used the *Global Deterioration Scale* (GDS; Reisberg, Ferris, deLeon, & Crook, 1982) to stage dementia. The GDS is a seven stage rating scale used to determine the stage of dementia, based on presenting clinical features. Stages 1 to 3 are considered pre-dementia stages whereas Stages 4 to 7 are mild to severe stages of dementia. Based on results of the MMSE and GDS, we classified our participants into 19 persons with mild dementia (GDS Stage 4 and MMSE scores $\geq$ 17) and 4 persons with moderate dementia (GDS Stage 5 and MMSE scores between 10 and 16). Next, we administered the *Dementia Rating Scale* (DRS-2; Mattis, Jurica, & Leitten, 1982) to assess performance across cognitive domains, and the *Rivermead Behavioral Memory Test* (RBMT-2; Wilson, Cockburn, & Baddeley, 1985) to quantify the severity of memory impairment. The DRS-2 is a widely used, neuropsychological measure of cognitive status for adults over the age of 55 years. It consists of thirty six tasks that provide raw and age- and education-corrected scaled scores on five domains – attention, initiation/preservation, construction, conceptualization, and memory. We used a total DRS-2 raw score of less than or equal to 132 (out of a maximum possible score of 144 points), as a cut-off for dementia because this score corresponds to 1.5 standard deviations below an age- and education- matched control group (Rajji et al., 2009). The RBMT-2 (Wilson et al., 1985) is a standardized test designed to quantify spared and impaired aspects of memory. It consists of nine subtests that assess episodic memory (verbal, visual, and spatial) in immediate and delayed contexts, face-name recognition, orientation, and prospective memory. Whereas the DRS-2 and the RBMT-2 could have been re-administered after completing SRT, we intentionally did not use these tests as outcome measures. This was because we did not expect our stimulus-specific, computer-assisted SRT to impact performance on standardized tests or result in fundamental changes in overall cognitive functioning. Rather, we expected task- and stimulus-specific learning with maintenance of learned faces and names over time. Finally, a brief dynamic assessment was conducted to determine participants' candidacy for participating in SRT. Dynamic assessment techniques are designed to determine if specific manipulations facilitate patient performance on a task. Such manipulations may include use of teach-test-retest methods, interactive coaching, or trial therapy (Bourgeois & Hickey, 2009) to identify a dementia patient's restorative potential. We adapted a published screening protocol for SRT (Brush & Camp, 2000), in which we had participants recall the examiner's place of work (e.g. California State University) over 1-and 2-minute short delays and a longer delay of 5 minutes. If participants were successful in recalling this information over 5 minutes, we considered this a "pass", indicating that participants were candidates for computer-assisted SRT. Table 2 provides data on participant performance on the GDS, DRS-2, RBMT-2, and on the assessment of candidacy for SRT.

Table 1. Participant demographics and screening data

Participant Demographics	n = 23 participants (6 men, 17 women)
Age (in years)	Mean = 84.17 (Range: 75-93)
Years of Education	Mean = 13.2 (Range: 8-19)
Language History	Monolingual: 21/23 Bilingual: 2/23
Computer Use/Exposure	No familiarity/use: 12/23, Limited familiarity/use: 10/23, High familiarity/use: 1/23
Screening data	
MMSE Scores	Mean = 23.13 (Range: 13-30[1])
GDS-SF Scores	Mean = 1.59 (Range: 0-5)
Vision Screening	Letter Cancellation: Mean = 18/20 (Range: 11-20; 3 PWD scored < 16/20)
	Picture identification: Mean = 4/4 (Range: 0; all scored 4/4)
	Sentence reading: Mean = 1.8/2 (Range: 0-2; two PWD scored 1/2)
	Number passed in both ears: 5/23
Hearing Screening	Number passed in one ear: 6/23
	Number failed in both ears: 12/23[2]
	Word Recognition Score: Mean = 85% (Range: 50-100%)[3]

1-Only one participant had an MMSE score of 30. This participant had been given the MMSE multiple times likely resulting in a spurious score. Scores on a neuropsychological examination, the DRS-2, and results of brain imaging confirmed a clinical diagnosis of probable AD disease.

2-All participants who failed hearing screening wore their hearing aids or an assisted listening device for treatment sessions.

3- All but one participant had scores of 60% or better at comprehending spoken words in the absence of visual cues.

Table 2. Participant data on evaluation measures

Evaluation Data	n = 23 participants
Dementia Diagnosis	Probable Alzheimer's disease: 20/23 participants Probable Vascular dementia: 3/23 participants
Global Deterioration Scale (GDS)	Stage 4 (Mild dementia): 19/23 participants Stage 5 (Moderate dementia): 4/23 participants
Dementia Rating Scale (DRS-2) Rivermead Behavioral Memory Test (RBMT-2)	Mean Total Raw Score = 117.7/144 Range: 91-132 out of 144 Mean Standardized Profile Score = 10.25/24 Range: 1-19 out of 24
Dynamic Assessment of Candidacy for SRT	% participants who passed (i.e., had correct recall at a 5-minute delay): 100%

Study Hypotheses

First, we hypothesized that computer-assisted SRT would be feasible for the majority of our dementia participants. Next, we expected computer-assisted SRT to yield positive outcomes for teaching face-name associations to PWD, based on the extensive, published evidence on treatment outcomes of traditional SRT (see Hopper et al., 2005 for a review). Third, we anticipated that it would take longer to train a novel face-name association than it would take to train a familiar face-name association. This hypothesis was based on unpublished pilot data (Mahendra, Bayles, & Tomoeda, 2000) in which PWD demonstrated some resistance to learning a novel face-name association and greater motivation to learn names of familiar persons. Further, PWD also learned familiar names faster than names of novel persons. Finally, we expected that after training was stopped, familiar names would be better retained over time than novel names.

Intervention

Clinician Training

Computer-assisted SRT was administered by the author and her trained research assistants. A comprehensive procedure manual was developed that provided detailed instructions for conducting computer-assisted SRT. This manual included step-by-step instructions on baseline testing, presentation of photos via laptop computer, to-be-trained responses, clinician reinforcement, inter-interval activities, and data sheets for tracking and recording participant performance. Research assistants met with the author/investigator after completing the pre-intervention training and the first two SRT sessions. Session notes, activities, and data sheets were reviewed for accuracy. Further, actual sessions and videotapes of ten, randomly selected, participants were viewed by the author to assess compliance with the research protocol. No procedural errors were noted in implementing computer-assisted SRT or in completing activities during intervals. However, some initial errors were identified in clinician scoring of participant performance on SRT trials, using the data sheets provided. This was addressed by revising the procedure manual and including samples of completed data sheets for review.

Pre-intervention Training

Each participant began with three or four, 45-minute sessions of pre-intervention training to facilitate familiarity with the laptop computer set-up and to allow researchers to assess participant ability to interact with a laptop computer. Specifically, research assistants assessed participants' ability to use a mouse to click on objects or to use a touch screen (MagicTouch™ screen), to read text and identify images on the screen, and respond to voice prompts from the computer. These initial sessions also were used to introduce computer games and to obtain baseline data on participants' ability to identify names of people familiar to them. We incorporated this pre-intervention training into this study based on pilot work preceding this research (Mahendra, Bayles, & Tomoeda, 2000). In our pilot work, older adults with limited prior exposure to a personal computer sometimes became anxious about using technology and this interfered with the intervention. We also found that in fewer than five, short sessions of using a computer and playing games, PWD began to begin to respond with more confidence and enthusiasm about computer-assisted interventions. In this study, we used card games (e.g. Solitaire, Pinochle), word games (e.g. Scrabble, Lexicon, Wheel of Fortune), therapy software (e.g. Twenty Questions, Memory from Laureate Learning Systems), hand-held games, or other computer applications (e.g. ArtPad™ digital canvas).

Training Stimuli

The novel and familiar face stimuli were high-resolution, digital, color photographs. To prepare these stimuli, a 10.1 megapixel, Canon digital camera was used to take head shots of persons. These photographs were edited using Adobe Photoshop software so that they were all of the same size, orientation, and pixel resolution. For each person whose name and face were presented, three additional facts also were presented to provide semantic context. These facts were the person's occupation (e.g., Maria is a social worker), place of residence (e.g. Maria lives in San Francisco), and another biographical detail (e.g. Maria has two children). All faces, names, and related facts were assembled into an animated slide show, prepared using Microsoft Powerpoint software.

Prior to initiating the study, we established a learning criterion for successful recall of a face-name association, over what we considered to be a clinically significant time interval for PWD. This criterion was that participants had to correctly recall the trained name over a 32-minute time delay, and achieve this delayed recall on four consecutive sessions, over 2 weeks. This strict learning criterion was chosen to ensure that PWD demonstrated stable retention of a face-name association over a reasonable, functional length of time before the intervention was stopped and post-training retention assessed. See Figure 1 for an illustration of the recall trials in a typical SRT session.

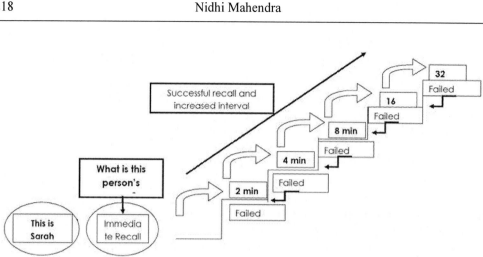

Figure 1. Visual illustration of an SRT session.

Novel Face-Name Association

Following pre-intervention training, participants were taught one novel face-name association. A color photograph of a research collaborator was used. This individual was a middle-aged, Caucasian, woman who lived in a different state and geographic region. Thus, there was no possibility of participants' prior exposure to her face. This allowed us to have complete experimental control and to avoid any confound with differential exposure among participants. The pictured person was assigned a fictitious first and last name, *Sarah Johnson*, an occupation, a place of residence, and one personal detail (e.g., she has three cats). Participants were presented this novel face-name association via an animated slideshow that revealed the name first, followed by sequential presentation of the other facts. Participants had to recall this first and last name correctly over gradually increasing time intervals until they could retain it over a 32-minute interval, within a single treatment session. Participants began by retaining the first and last name over a 1-minute interval (Figure 1). If the first and last name were successfully recalled after one minute, the next recall interval was doubled to 2 minutes. If the first and last name were again recalled accurately, the next recall interval was doubled to 4 minutes. However, if a participant could not recall the first and last name after 4 minutes, the correct name was re-presented and its immediate recall assessed after presentation. Following this correct immediate recall, the next interval was reset to 2 minutes to establish correct delayed recall. Thus, a shaping paradigm was used to allow PWD to build up to correct recall of the first and last name over a 32-minute time interval. Two unique aspects of our computer-assisted SRT intervention merit discussion. First, an explicit errorless instruction (Figure 1) was embedded into the SRT. At each recall trial, when participants were asked to name a target person, they also simultaneously were instructed 'not to guess' (Figure 1) and to respond only with information that they were sure was accurate. It was hoped that this instruction might reduce error frequency and subsequent error persistence that could significantly interfere with learning. Another interesting aspect was that activities during the intervals were unrelated to the face-name association being trained. During the intervals between recall attempts, PWD engaged in casual conversation during the short intervals (e.g., 1 to 4 minutes in length) and played computer games during longer intervals (e.g. 8 minutes or more). Researchers offered PWD choices of computer games and provided cueing and prompting to facilitate performance, as needed. For computer games attempted at each interval, simple log sheets were filled out indicating the games played, the level (e.g. Beginner, Intermediate) and noted objective aspects (game score, number of prompts needed, number of errors committed, etc). On occasion, a participant's preferred game was purchased and set up on the laptop computer to provide motivation and to expand the types of computer games offered to study participants. Figure 2 is a photograph of a study participant independently using a laptop computer and wireless mouse to play a card game.

Familiar Face-Name Association

After training the novel face-name association and tracking post-SRT maintenance, one familiar face-name association was individually chosen for each participant. Familiar persons whose names were trained were persons who were relevant in the daily lives and living environments of PWD, had regular interactions with them, and were recognized by participants as being familiar but could not be named. For each study participant, a digital camera was used to take pictures of multiple people (e.g. family members, friends, nurses, activities personnel, social worker, therapists, personal aide, clergy members, etc). At baseline, PWD were tested for their ability to name several persons identified as familiar. Multiple baselines were obtained during three sessions preceding SRT. If a participant correctly named a person even once on any of three baseline sessions, that name was discarded as a training target. This was done to ensure that PWD were consistently unable to name a targeted familiar person, prior to initiating SRT. Establishing this stable, pre-intervention baseline was necessary for an unbiased evaluation of the benefit of computer-assisted SRT for teaching names to PWD. For 21 out of 23 PWD, names of professional caregivers were trained with two remaining participants being taught names of a grandchild. It is important to mention some differences in training learning and retention of familiar face-name associations. First, familiar faces and names were variable for each participant and differed in their length (number of syllables), phonetic complexity, and ethnic familiarity. This occasionally resulted in the novel name, *Sarah Johnson*, perhaps being easier to learn than a familiar name (e.g. *Maria DeCaprio*, or *Teresa Gallegos*). Second, as mentioned, most familiar face-name associations were of professional caregivers with at least weekly interactions with participating PWD. Some caregivers interacted with participants daily (e.g., a certified nurse's aide) whereas others interacted once or twice a week (e.g., a granddaughter or a clergy member). Next, for the familiar name, we were interested in documenting any transfer of the learned name from the context of the training sessions to actually addressing caregivers by name in subsequent interactions. Following PWD learning familiar names to criterion, we collected data twice weekly for 3 weeks to assess participants' incidental use of a caregiver's name during routine interactions. This was done by a regular phone call or email to caregivers asking whether participants had addressed them by name. A simple frequency count was maintained of the number of times a caregiver reported that a study participant had addressed them by name.

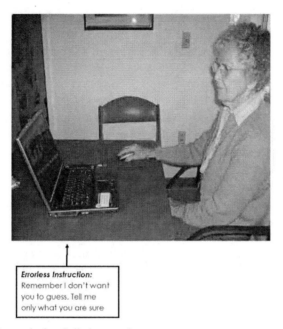

Figure 2. Participant playing Solitaire on a laptop computer.

RESULTS

Feasibility of Computer-Assisted Interventions

All 23 participants completed pre-intervention training and fully participated in computer-assisted SRT, for anywhere between 3 to 6 months from initial screening, SRT, and post-treatment maintenance probes. Each of these participants was able to learn some aspects of computer use and to play computer games as demonstrated by improving accuracy and improving scores on games, and need for less clinician assistance over time. Eleven of these 23 participants (47.8%) learned to independently locate a game icon on the laptop screen, click on it, and initiate playing a computer game. Four of these 23 participants (17.3%) also began to play the same computer games on desktop or laptop computers at their facilities or in their homes. Another noteworthy fact was that four out of 23 participants (17.3%) purchased a personal laptop computer, for the first time, while participating in this study.

Qualitative data on participant and caregiver reactions to computer-assisted interventions

We did not formally and systematically assess participant and caregiver reactions to computer-assisted SRT. However, we noted any spontaneous comments and reactions from participants and their caregivers. Fifteen out of 23 participants (65.2%) overtly mentioned enjoying the computer games (e.g. *'I'm on a roll with this'*, *'This is a lot of fun'*) and verbally stated feeling positive about the interventions (e.g. *'This is good for my mind'*, *'I need this because my memory sure is getting bad'*, *'My grandson thinks it's cool I am learning to use the computer'* etc). Eleven participants (47.8%) expressed disappointment to researchers when the SRT training ended, either directly or indirectly through their caregivers. These qualitative data endorse the perceived value of cognitively stimulating activities and computer-assisted interventions by PWD.

Outcomes of Computer-Assisted SRT: Learning of Face-Name Associations

Twenty out of 23 participants (86.9%) successfully learned novel face-name associations in 5 to 19 SRT sessions (mean number of sessions = 8.4), each lasting 45 to 50 minutes. Only one outlier participant required 19 sessions to learn a novel name to criterion with the remaining 19 (out of 20) participants learning a novel name in 5 to 13 sessions. This outlier participant had been diagnosed with AD longer than any other study participant (approximately 7 years post-diagnosis) and was among only four study participants with moderate dementia. Next, 20 out of 23 participants (86.9%) learned familiar names to criterion in 5 to 13 sessions (mean number of sessions = 8.6), each lasting 45 to 50 minutes. Because we presented the first and last name along with three facts about each person, we were able to differentially assess recall of the name versus recall of related biographical information. We broke down the facts presented about each person into 7 distinct information units (including the first name, last name, occupation, city and state of residence, and personal detail). Impressively, PWD recalled a mean 6.1 out of 7 information units for the novel person and 5.4 out of 7 information units for a familiar person. Three participants did not learn novel or familiar names to meet learning criterion, after a reasonable attempt lasting over 6 weeks. We hypothesized that previously familiar names would be easier to learn to criterion, than novel names. Contrary to our expectations, our data (Table 3) did not support this hypothesis. Compared to the number of sessions required to learn a novel face-name association to criterion (mean number of sessions=8.4), on average, most participants needed the same number of sessions or slightly more to achieve learning criterion for familiar names (mean number of sessions = 8.6). This difference in mean number of sessions to learn names of novel versus familiar persons was not statistically significant [t (22) = 0.011, p < 0.5].

Table 3. Data on learning of novel and familiar face-name associations

Number of participants who achieved learning criterion	Number of Sessions	Mean Information Units Recalled (out of 7)
Novel Face-Name		
20/23 86.9%	Mean = 8.4 Range: 5-19*	Mean = 6.1/7 Range: 2-7
Familiar Face-Name 20/23 86.9%	Mean=8.6 Range: 5-13	Mean = 5.6 Range: 2-7

*Only 1 person with moderate AD needed 19 sessions to learn the novel face-name to criterion. Remaining PWD took between 5 to 13 sessions.

Transfer of Familiar Names from Training Sessions to Real-Life Interactions

Of the 20 participants who learned familiar names to criterion in SRT sessions, 17 participants (85%) were reported by caregivers to address them by their correct name in at least one interaction per week. Sixteen participants (80% of those who met criterion) addressed caregivers by their correct name in two weekly interactions. Ten of these 20 PWD (50%) were reported to explicitly acknowledge working on caregiver names in their conversations with caregivers.

Table 4. Post-SRT retention of novel face-name association

n = 23	Week 1	Week 2	Week 3	Week 4	Week 6
Number or participants who met criterion = 20/23 86.9%					
Number who recalled first and last name	20 86.9%	19 82.6%	18 78.2%	19 82.6%	19 82.6%
Mean number of information units recalled (out of 7)	6.2	6.2	5.7	6	5.5
Range of information units recalled, across participants	2-7	4-7	3-7	2-7	2-7

Post-SRT Retention of Novel and Familiar Names

After face-name associations were learned to criterion, maintenance of learned names was assessed at one week, two weeks, three weeks, four weeks, and six weeks post-SRT. These data are presented in Table 4 (novel face-name associations) and Table 5 (familiar face-name associations). Our data reveal that out of twenty participants that met learning criterion for both novel and familiar name acquisition, 19 (95%) retained the novel name and 18 (90%) retained the familiar name six weeks post-SRT. The mean number of information units recalled by participants at each post-SRT time point was comparable for novel and familiar face-name associations, with a trend for slightly better recall of information about the novel person.

Table 5. Post-SRT retention of familiar face-name association

n = 23	Week 1	Week 2	Week 3	Week 4	Week 6
Number of participants who met learning criterion = 20/23 86.9%					
Number who recalled first and last name	19 82.6%	19 82.6%	18 78.2%	19 82.6%	18 78.2%
Mean number of information units recalled (out of 7)	5.89	5.94	5.5	5.69	5.8
Range of information units recalled, across participants	4-7	4-7	3-7	4-7	4-7

DISCUSSION

This study was designed to assess the feasibility of computer-assisted cognitive interventions for PWD and to document the outcomes of computer-assisted SRT for face-name association training. Our findings support the customized application of computer-assisted cognitive interventions and specifically, computer-assisted SRT, for teaching face-name associations to persons with mild and moderate dementia. It is noted that the relatively high educational level of this participant sample likely influenced motivation for study participation and the feasibility of conducting and completing a study on computer-assisted interventions. Data from the pre-training phase confirmed findings of our pilot work (Mahendra, Bayles, & Tomoeda, 2000) in that several PWD became less anxious, more receptive and enthusiastic about using a laptop computer after completing pre-intervention training. This was designed to ease PWD into interacting with a computer and to experience some initial success at using a mouse and playing computer games. Such pre-training may be crucial for facilitating optimal responsiveness to technology-assisted interventions among PWD. Regarding face-name learning, twenty out of 23 participants (86.9%) succeeded in learning novel and familiar names and related biographical information to criterion. Nineteen of these participants (82.6%) retained the learned name at 6 weeks post-intervention and eighteen (78.2%) retained the familiar name at 6 weeks post-SRT. These findings support published literature (Cherry et al., 2010; Hopper et al., 2005; Hopper et al., 2010) in which the efficacy of SRT has been demonstrated, for teaching new information to persons with dementia. Three participants (13%) did not benefit from computer-assisted SRT for learning novel or familiar names to criterion. Upon closely examining these participants' performance, four interesting observations emerged. First, two of these three participants had vascular dementia with fluctuating cognitive impairments and variable performance during intervention and while playing computer games. A third participant who failed to meet learning criterion had been diagnosed with probable AD for 9 years, the longest time post-diagnosis among our study participants. Next, all three participants had moderate dementia severity; one also had depressive disorder. Finally, all three individuals had no prior exposure to or experience with using a laptop computer. It is likely that these factors together influenced these participants' limited response to computer-assisted SRT. Despite being unable to achieve or maintain delayed recall of a trained name over a 32-minute interval, all three participants learned and recalled 2-3 out of 7 information units (e.g., occupation, place of residence, etc) besides the person's name. This suggests that new learning is possible for persons with moderate dementia, and that SRT is successful for teaching new information. This finding also suggests that the efficacy of SRT for moderate dementia patients may vary by the type of information taught. For instance, failure to learn names to criterion (but not other related facts) supports the notion that face-name associations are arbitrary, uniquely complex, and learning them may rely more on episodic memory abilities (Werheid & Clare, 2007). Finally, all study participants (with mild and moderate dementia) received twice weekly SRT sessions. Therefore, it is possible that persons with moderate dementia severity may need increased weekly frequency of SRT to achieve the same learning criterion as persons with mild dementia. Contrary to our prediction, dementia participants, as a group, did not differ in the mean number of sessions required to learn a novel name versus a familiar name. We expected participants to take longer (i.e., more sessions) to learn the novel name to criterion. However, we underestimated the variability in length (number of syllables), phonetic complexity, and ethnic origin (e.g. Anglo Saxon vs. non Anglo Saxon names) of names of familiar persons. Undoubtedly, some of these names were inherently harder to retain than others (e.g. *Maria DeCaprio* or *Teresa Gallegos* were more complex names than *Katie Smith*) and some PWD acknowledged this when making repeated errors (e.g. *Teresa Gallagher* for *Teresa Gallegos*). Once learning criterion for recalling novel or familiar names had been achieved, PWD, as a group, had comparable retention of both types of learned names over time. From our results, it appears that the number of sessions needed to learn a face-name association may have less to do with name familiarity and more to do with the delay over which recall had to be maintained (learning criterion), particularly when familiar names being learned belong to professional caregivers. With the exception of two PWD who learned names of grandchildren, the remaining 21 were taught a familiar name of a professional caregiver. Perhaps this implicitly affected participant motivation and resulted in PWD taking more time than expected to learn familiar face-name associations. However, this finding deserves further investigation.In an effort to inform future research endeavors, some discussion of this study's limitations is warranted. The first obvious limitation is the modest sample size, and variable type and severity of dementia among study participants. Next, we acknowledge that our clinically-motivated, strict learning criterion may have been too stringent for persons with moderate dementia severity to achieve with just two weekly treatment sessions. Indeed we offered SRT treatment sessions twice a week to all PWD, regardless of the severity of their everyday memory deficits or overall cognitive status. It is plausible that persons with greater dementia severity or those experiencing difficulty learning the face-name associations to criterion might have had better treatment outcomes, with more frequent weekly SRT sessions. Also, we did not employ a control condition in which participants' naming performance was documented on an untrained, familiar face-name association. Further, this study would be enhanced by including a small control group of dementia participants who are taught face-name associations, not by SRT, but by ordinary repetition, to examine the difference in learning outcomes by teaching technique. Finally, it is important that learning outcomes of computer-assisted SRT be documented beyond 6 weeks post-SRT. In conclusion, results from this study support the robust success of computer-assisted SRT for facilitating recall and retention of face-name associations and related facts for persons with dementia. Additional research is needed to replicate these findings with a larger sample of persons with mild and moderate dementia, with participants who have vascular dementia, and who have more varied educational levels. Follow-up investigations are required to document the effects of varying weekly SRT treatment frequency on learning outcomes, and the efficacy of computer-assisted SRT for teaching procedural skills (e.g., using an appliance, a safety strategy, etc) to persons with dementia.

DISCLOSURE

Some of the data reported in this paper have been presented at annual conventions of the International Neuropsychological Society (Mahendra, Apple, & Reed, 2008) and the 2009 Everyday Technology for Alzheimer Care Research Symposium (Mahendra & Tomoeda, 2009).

ACKNOWLEDGMENTS

This research was funded by an Everyday Technology for Alzheimer Care (ETAC) research grant awarded to the author by the Alzheimer's Association and Intel Corporation. The author thanks Dr. Kathryn Bayles, Cheryl Tomoeda, and Dr. Mitchell Watnik for their significant input during this project.

REFERENCES

[1]   Alzheimer's Association (2010). 2010 Alzheimer's disease facts and figures. *Alzheimer's and Dementia, 6,* 4-65.

[2]   American Speech Language Hearing Association (1997). Guidelines for audiology service delivery in nursing homes. Retrieved July 14, 2007 from: http://www.asha.org/docs/html/GL1997-00004.html

[3]   Azuma, T., Bayles, K., Cruz, R., Tomoeda, C. K., Wood, J. A., McGeagh, A. et al. (1997). Comparing the difficulty of letter, semantic, and name fluency tasks for normal elderly and patients with Parkinson's disease. *Neuropsychology, 11*(4), 1-10.

[4]   Baddeley, A. D. (1992). Implicit memory and errorless learning: A link between cognitive theory and neuropsychological rehabilitation? In L. R. Squire & N. Butters (Eds.). *Neuropsychology of Memory (2ⁿᵈ Edition,* pp. 309-314). New York: Guilford Press.

[5]   Baddeley, A. and Wilson, B. A. (1994). When implicit memory fails: Amnesia and the problem of error elimination. *Neuropsychologia, 32*(1), 53-68.

[6]   Balota, D. A., Duchek, J. M., Sergent-Marshall, S. and Roediger, H. L. III. (2006). Does expanded retrieval produce benefits over equal-interval spacing? Explorations of spacing effects in healthy aging and early stage Alzheimer's disease. *Psychology and Aging,21*(1),19–31.

[7]   Bayles, K. A. and Kim, E. S. (2003). Improving the functioning of individuals with Alzheimer's disease: Emergence of behavioral interventions. *Journal of Communication Disorders, 36,* 327-343.

[8]   Bayles, K. A. and Tomoeda, C. K. (1993). *The Arizona Battery for Communication Disorders of Dementia.* Tucson, AZ: Canyonlands Publishing.

[9]   Boothroyd, A. (1968). Statistical theory of the speech discrimination score. *Journal of the Acoustical Society of America,* 43(2), 362-367.

[10]   Bourgeois, M. S., Camp, C. J., Rose, M., White, B., Malone, M., Carr, J., Rovine, M. (2003). A comparison of training strategies to enhance use of external aids by persons with dementia. *Journal of Communication Disorders, 36,* 361-378.

[11]   Bourgeois, M. S. and key, E. (2009). *Dementia from diagnosis to management: A functional approach.* Psychology Press.

[12]   Bourgeois, M. S., Lenius, K., Turkstra, L. and Camp, C. (2007). The effects of cognitive teletherapy on reported everyday memory behaviours of persons with chronic traumatic brain injury. *Brain Injury, 21* (12), 1245-1257.

[13]   Brush, J. A. and Camp, C. J. (1998a). Using spaced-retrieval training as an intervention during speech-language therapy. *Clinical Gerontologist, 19*(1), 51-64.

[14] Brush, J., A. and Camp, C. J. (1998b). Spaced retrieval during dysphagia therapy. *Clinical Gerontologist, 19(2)*, 96-99.

[15] Brush, J. A. and Camp, C. J. (1998c). Using spaced retrieval as a therapeutic intervention during the rehabilitative process (J. Chitwood, Director). In C. K. Tomoeda (Producer), *Telerounds*. Tucson, AZ: The University of Arizona.

[16] Brush, J. A. and Camp, C. J. (2000). *Spaced retrieval: A therapy technique for improving memory.* Available at http://www.nss-nrs.com (Northern Speech Services, Inc. and National Rehabilitation Services)

[17] Camp, C. J. (1989). Facilitation in learning of Alzheimer's disease. In G. Gilmore, P. Whitehouse, & M. Wykle (Eds.). *Memory and aging: Theory, research, and practice.* New York: Springer.

[18] Chapman, S. B., Weiner, M. F., Rackley, A., Hynan, L., S. and Zientz, J. (2004). Effects of cognitive-communicative stimulation for Alzheimer's disease patients treated with donepezil. *Journal of Speech Language and Hearing Research, 47*, 1149-1163.

[19] Cherry, K. E., Walvoord, A. G. and Hawley, K. S. (2010). Spaced retrieval enhances memory for a name-face-occupation association in older adults with probable Alzheimer's disease. *The Journal of Genetic Psychology, 171* (2), 168-181.

[20] Clare, L. and Jones, R. S. P. (2008). Errorless learning in the rehabilitation of memory impairment: A critical review. *Neuropsychology Review, 18*, 1-23.

[21] Crum, R. M., Anthony, J. C., Bassett, S. S. and Folstein, M. F. (1993). Population-based norms for the Mini-Mental State Examination by age and education level. *Journal of the American Medical Association, 269* (18), 2386-2391.

[22] Folstein, M. F., Folstein, S. E. & McHugh, P. R. (1975). Mini-Mental State: A practical method for grading the cognitive state of patients for the clinician. *Journal of PsychiatricResearch, 12*, 189-98.

[23] Galante, E., Venturini, G. and Fiaccadori, C. (2007). Computer-based cognitive intervention for dementia: preliminary results of a randomized clinical trial. *Giornale Italiano di Medicina del Lavoro ed Ergonomia, Supplemento B, Psicologia, 29*(3), B26-B32.

[24] Grabowski, T. J. and Damasio, A. R. (2004). Definition, clinical features, and neuroanatomical basis of dementia. In M. Esiri, V. Lee, and J. Trojanowski (Eds). *Neuropathology of dementia* (2nd edition, pp. 1-10). UK: Cambridge University Press.

[25] Hochhalter, A. K., Overmier, J. B., Gasper, S. M., Bakke, B. L. and Holub, R. J. (2005). A comparison of spaced retrieval to other schedules of practice for people with dementia. *Experimental Aging Research, 31*, 101–118.

[26] Hofmann, M., Rösler, A., Schwarz, W., Müller-Spahn, F., Kräuchi, K., Hock, C. and Seifritz, E. (2003). Interactive computer-training as a therapeutic tool in Alzheimer's disease. *Comprehensive Psychiatry, 44*(3), 213-219.

[27] Hopper, T. (2003). "They're just going to get worse anyway": Perspectives on rehabilitation for nursing home residents with dementia. *Journal of Communication Disorders, 36*, 345-359.

[28] Hopper, T., Drefs, S., Bayles, K. A. Tomoeda, C. K and Dinu. I. (2010). The effects of modified spaced-retrieval training on learning and retention of face-name associations by individuals with dementia. *Neuropsychological Rehabilitation, 20*(1):81-102.

[29] Hopper, T., Mahendra, N., Kim, E., Azuma, T., Bayles, K., Cleary, S. and Tomoeda, C. K. (2005). Evidence-based practice recommendations for working with individuals with dementia: Spaced retrieval training. *Journal of Medical Speech Language Pathology*, 13(4), xxvii-xxxiv.

[30] Lee, S. B., Park, C. S., Jeong, J. W., Choe, J. Y., Hwang, Y. J., Park and C-A. ... Kim, K. W. (2009). Effects of spaced retrieval training on cognitive function in Alzheimer's disease patients. *Archives of Gerontology and Geriatrics, 49*, 289-293.

[31] Lin, L-C., Huang, Y-J., Su, S-G, Watson, R., Tsai, B. W. and Wu, S-C. (2010). Using spaced retrieval and Montessori-based activities in improving eating ability for residents with dementia. *International Journal of Geriatric Psychiatry*, DOI: 10.1002/gps.2433.

[32] Landauer, T. K. and Bjork, R. A. (1978). Optimum rehearsal patterns and name learning. In M.M. Grunenberg, P. S. Morris, & R. N. Sykes (Eds.). Practice aspects of memory (pp. 625-632). New York: Academic Press.

[33] Mahendra, N. (2001). Direct interventions for improving the performance of individuals with Alzheimer's disease. *Seminars in Speech & Language, 22*(4), 289-302.

[34] Mahendra, N. and Tomoeda, C. K. (September, 2009). *Computerized cognitive interventions for persons with Alzheimer's disease: Facts, surprises, and challenges.* Technical paper presented at the Everyday Technology for Alzheimer Care (ETAC) Consortium Conference, Hillsboro, Oregon.

[35] Mahendra, N., Apple, A. and Reed, D. (February, 2008). *Computer-assisted training of face-name associations in persons with dementia.* Poster presented at the annual meeting of the International Neuropsychological Society Meeting, Waikoloa, Hawaii.

[36] Mahendra, N. and Arkin, S. M. (2003). Effect of four years of exercise, language, and social interventions on Alzheimer discourse. *Journal of Communication Disorders*, 36(5), 395-422.

[37] Mahendra, N., Bayles, K. A. and Tomoeda, C. K. (2000). *Computer assisted cognitive stimulation.* Paper presented at the annual convention of the Arizona Speech and Hearing Association, Tucson, Arizona.

[38] Mahendra, N., Kim, E., Bayles, K., Hopper, T., Cleary, S. and Azuma, T. (2005). Evidence-based practice recommendations for working with individuals with dementia: Computer-assisted cognitive interventions. *Journal of Medical Speech Language Pathology,*13(4), xxxv-xliv.

[39] Mattis, S., Jurica, P. and Leitten, C. (1982) *Dementia Rating Scale (DRS-2)*. Lutz, FL: Psychological Assessment Resources, Inc.

[40] McKhann, G., Drachman, D., Folstein, M., Katzman, R., Price, D. and Stadlan, E. M. (1984). Clinical diagnosis of Alzheimer's disease: Report of the NINCDS-ADRDA work group under the auspices of the Department of Health and Human Services task force on Alzheimer's disease. *Neurology*, 34, 939-44.

[41] McKitrick, L. A., Camp, C. J. and Black, F. W. (1992). Prospective memory intervention in Alzheimer's disease. *Journal of Gerontology: Psychological Sciences*, 47(5), 337-343.

[42] Ozgis, S., Rendell, P. G. and Henry, J. D. (2009). Spaced retrieval significantly improves prospective memory performance of cognitively impaired older adults. *Gerontology, 55*, 229-232.

[43] Rajji, T.K., Miranda, D., Mulsant, B., Lotz, M., Houck, P., Zmouda, M.D. and Butters, M. A. (2009). The MMSE is not an adequate screening cognitive instrument in studies of late-life depression. *Journal of Psychiatric Research*, 43(4), 464-470.

[44] Reisberg, B., Ferris, S., deLeon, M. and Crook, T. (1982). The global deterioration scale: An instrument for the assessment of primary degenerative dementia. *American Journal of Psychiatry, 139*, 1136-1139.

[45] Requena, C., Ibor, M. I., Maestu, F., Campo, P., Ibor, J. J. and Ortiz, T. (2004). Effects of cholinergic drugs and cognitive training on dementia. *Dementia and Geriatric Cognitive Disorders, 18*, 50-54.

[46] Requena, C., Maestu, F., Campo, P., Fernandez, A. and Ortiz, T. (2006). Effects of cholinergic drugs and cognitive training on dementia: Two year follow-up. *Dementia and Geriatric Cognitive Disorders, 22*, 339-345.

[47] Román G .C., Tatemichi T. K., Erkinjuntti T., Cummings J. L., Masdeu J. C., Garcia J. H., Amaducci L., Orgogozo J. M., Brun A., Hofman A., et al. (1993). Vascular dementia: diagnostic criteria for research studies. Report of the NINDS-AIREN International Workshop. *Neurology, 43*(2), 250-260.

[48] Schacter, D. L., Rich, S. A. and Stampp, M. S. (1985). Remediation of memory disorders: experimental evaluation of the spaced retrieval technique. *Journal of Clinical and Experimental Neuropsychology, 7*(1), 79-96.

[49] Sheikh, J. I. and Yesavage, J. A. (1986). Geriatric Depression Scale (GDS): Recent evidence and development of a shorter version. *Clinical Gerontologist, 5*(1-2), 165-173.

[50] Tombaugh, T. and McIntyre, N. (1992). The Mini-Mental State Examination: A comprehensive review. *Journal of American Geriatrics Society*, 40, 922-35.

[51] Werheid, K. and Clare, L. (2007). Are faces special in Alzheimer's disease? Cognitive conceptualization, neural correlates, and diagnostic relevance of impaired memory for faces and names. *Cortex, 43* (7), 898-906.

[52] Wilson, B. A., Cockburn, J. and Baddeley, A. (1985). *The Rivermead Behavioral Memory Test*. San Antonio, TX: Psychological Corporation.

In: Dementia: Non-Pharmacological Therapies
Editor: Elisabetta Farina, pp. 229-238

ISBN: 978-1-61470-736-3
© 2012 Nova Science Publishers, Inc.

NPT-ES: A MEASURE OF THE EXPERIENCE OF PEOPLE WITH DEMENTIA DURING NON-PHARMACOLOGICAL INTERVENTIONS

R. Muñiz[1]*, J. Olazarán[1], S. Poveda[1], P. Lago[2] and J. Peña-Casanova[3]

[1] Maria Wolff Foundation. Madrid. Spain.
[2] National University of Distance
Education (UNED). Madrid. Spain.
[3] Department of Behavioral Neurology.

ABSTRACT

Introduction. The non-pharmacological therapy (NPT) field lacks an easy-to-use instrument that measures the experience of people with dementia (PWD) while undergoing non-pharmacological interventions. The NPT Experience Scale (NPT-ES) was designed and validated to cover this need.

Methods. A multi-disciplinary team developed 15 candidate items of which five items were selected on the basis of objectivity, emotional valence, complementarity and inter-rater reliability. The properties of NPT-ES were studied in people with Alzheimer's disease (AD) receiving several NPTs at two day-care centers. Scale validation was conducted via administration of NPT-ES by independent raters in four successive steps: I. Rating by two external observers. II. Rating by one external observer and one therapist. III. Rating by two internal observers and one therapist. IV. Rating by one internal observer and one therapist that alternated roles.

Results. NPT-ES internal consistency was good or excellent (Cronbach α ranged from 0.68 to 0.88). Good inter-rater agreement was attained by internal observers (intra-class correlation coefficient [ICC] 0.83) and by external observers (ICC 0.79). Fair-moderate agreement was obtained between observers and therapists (ICC 0.49-0.69), but almost excellent agreement was achieved when therapist and internal observer alternated roles (ICC 0.90). Properties of the scale improved with frequent use and with increased evaluator's acquaintance of the assessed PWD.

Conclusion. NPT-ES is an adequate and easy-to-use instrument to measure the affective and social experience of people with dementia while receiving non-pharmacological interventions. The scale displayed good properties under varied testing conditions. Best results were obtained when therapists were trained as internal observers.

* Corresponding author: Ruben Muñiz, Fundación Maria Wolff, C/Río Sil 15 Bis, 28669 Boadilla del Monte, Madrid, Spain Fax: +34-91-2663178 E-mail: ruben@mariawolff.es

INTRODUCTION

The increase in prevalence of Alzheimer's disease and related dementias (ADRD) and the lack of curative therapies is fuelling the development of non-pharmacological therapies (NPT) to improve quality of life of both people with dementia (PWD) and their caregivers (Woods 2003). Offering NPTs to PWD has two main objectives: a) convey as many positive experiences as possible while minimizing the negative ones whilst the PWD is in a session.and b) provide clinically relevant carryover effects in domains like cognition, function, behaviour or mood, amongst other.

A positive affective and social experience is possibly the main objective in dementia care, particularly for those persons in advanced stages of the disease (Kitwood 1997a). However, people from moderate dementia onwards have increasing difficulties expressing their likes and dislikes about NPTs or the care they receive. For this reason, the immediate experience of PWD has to be induced from careful observation of patients. Although several instruments have been utilized, some were too narrowly focused (Lee and Kieckhefer 1989; Hurley et al., 1992; Kovach and Henschel 1996; Lawton et al., 1996; Holliman et al., 2001), other required high expertise (Kitwood 1997b), or were time-consuming (Baker and Dowling, 1995). Moreover, some of the scales were not designed for the evaluation of discrete interventions (Lee and Kieckhefer 1989; Hurley et al., 1992; Kitwood 1997b).

The Philadelphia Geriatric Center Affect Rating Scale was designed to measure the affect of PWD in an Alzheimer special care unit. It contains six items, three of them measuring positive affect and the other three measuring negative affect (Lawton et al., 1996). This simple and easy to use instrument would appear to be adequate to evaluate PWD experience during non-pharmacological interventions, but it was not designed for that purpose, and relevant items related to participation and relation with others are not included. The Copper Ridge Activities Index was specifically designed to measure the success of activity therapy sessions. It included participation (1–6 points), cueing (1–3 points), and enjoyment (1-5 points). Interater reliability of these subscales, when administered independently after session by two 'therapists' was, respectively, 0.69, 0.78 and 0.92, but details about the roles of these two 'therapists' were not given. The properties of the scale under other testing conditions (e.g. evaluation by external observer) were also not investigated (Politis et al., 2004).

We developed a brief scale to measure the immediate affective and social effect of any kind of discrete non-pharmacological intervention delivered to people with ADRD. The feasibility and validity of this NPT Experience Scale (NPT-ES) was tested under different rating conditions. We analysed the properties of the scale when administered by out-of-session observers (i.e., external video observers), in-session observers (i.e., internal observers) and therapists at the end of sessions. The hypothesis was that the NPT-ES would work well in those three key settings. By doing so, the scale could help to improve the design of NPTs and monitor therapist skills in both daily-care and research settings.

METHOD

1) Development of the NPT-ES

A) Selection of Items by Multi-Disciplinary Team

Candidate items were elaborated from observations and in-depth interviews (Ibáñez 1985) run by the first author (RM) with PWD and Maria Wolff staff of two day care centres (four occupational therapists, two psychomotor-therapists, one music-therapist [PL], one social worker, one geriatrician and one general physician). After discussion of the multi-disciplinary team, 15 items were pre-selected (Table 1). Pre-selected items should help inferring affective experience and social interaction of PWD during sessions of NPTs.

Pre-selected items were piloted by two independent observers using video-recorded sessions of different kinds of NPT sessions. Raters were instructed to take notes and score every item at the end of the observation period. Items were initially scored on a five-point basis, according to the percentage of time that PWD manifested those items.

After piloting, five items were selected on the basis of objectiveness of the measure, emotional valence, lack of redundancy and inter-rater reliability. For instance, items like "smiles", "frowns", "relaxed face muscles", etc., were difficult to observe and interpret, and their inter-rater reliability was low. Other items ("time patient participates" and "time patient does not participate") were too concordant and therefore redundant. Inadequate items were dropped or reformulated to yield the final 5 item scale presented here. In addition, a simpler four-level grading of items was chosen to facilitate a potential use of the scale by therapists after group interventions. Therefore, the total score of the final NPT-ES ranged from zero to 15, higher scores indicating more positive experience.

B) Translation and Back-Translation

The Spanish scale was translated to English and then back-translated to Spanish by two independent translators. Only minor discrepancies emerged between the original and final Spanish versions, which were analyzed and resolved with the help of a third translator (Appendix 1 and 2).

2) Validation of NPT-ES

The validation of NPT-ES was performed in four steps that are described in Table 2. Steps I and II were planned to assess NPT-ES' properties in the most differing testing conditions: external observers that did not know the participants and watched the sessions on video versus therapists that were familiar with participants. Stages III and IV were designed *post-hoc* to investigate the reasons of discrepancy between external observers and therapists found at stage II. The evaluators received 10-minute training of NPT-ES rationale, objectives and use. The study design, however, was not disclosed. They were just requested to complete the NPT-ES for each participating PWD at the end of session. Taking notes during sessions was not permitted. When several raters had to be together in the same sessions (Stages III and IV) they were instructed to use the NPT-ES independently of each other.

Therapy sessions were conducted at two Maria Wolff day-care centers. Sessions of cognitive stimulation, use of music, psychomotor exercises, training of activities of daily living and massage were conducted following a pseudo-random sequence. Session duration was 45 minutes. Patients were people with moderate or moderately severe Alzheimer's disease (AD) that attended Maria Wolff day-care centers regularly. Both patients and their caregivers were informed about the study and asked consent to participate.

Internal consistency of NPT-ES was analysed using Cronbach α coefficient. This indicator gives an estimate of global correlation among the different items of the scale. Since all scale items are targeted at the same concept, a high α (desirably ranging between 0.70 and 0.95) would support face validity. Inter-rater reliability was assessed using intra-class correlation coefficient (ICC). This is the most appropriate indicator of agreement when dealing with quantitative variables. An ICC between 0.7 and 1 is desirable (Argimón & Jiménez, 1998).

Table. Process of validation of NPT-ES

Stage (rater characteristics)*	Sample description	Number of sessions, number of observations	Internal consistency (α)	Inter-rater reliability (ICC)
I. Two psychologists (A,B) after watching videos of sessions	45 AD, 60% Female Mean age 78, SD 7 FAST 5-6a	45, 385	0.81 (A) 0.77 (B)	0.79 (A-B)
II. Therapist (C) after conducting sessions and psychologist (A) after watching videos of those sessions	11 AD, 82% female Mean age 78, SD 5 FAST 5-6a	5, 55	0.82 (C) 0.63 (A)	0.49 (A-C)
III. Therapist (D) and two raters (C,E) that were present but not involved in sessions	10 AD, 70% female Mean age 79, SD 5 FAST 5-6a	5, 50	0.88 (E) 0.86 (C) 0.73 (D)	0.83 (C-E) 0.69 (C-D) 0.61 (D-E)
IV. Two raters (C,E) that alternated roles of therapist and internal observer every session	Same as above	8, 80	0.86 (E) 0.84 (C)	0.88 (C-E)

*Raters completed NPT-ES for each PWD at the end of intervention session.

A and B were psychologists with neither knowledge of PWDs nor experience as therapist. C,D and E were therapists that knew PWDs and had similar working experience.

α: Cronbach coefficient (> 0'70, good; > 0'80, excellent); ICC: intra-class correlation coefficient (< 0'30, bad; 0'31-0'50, fair; 0'51-0'70, moderate; 0'71-0'90, good; >0'91, excellent).

AD: Alzheimer's disease; FAST: Functional Assessment Staging (Reisberg 1988); NPT-ES: non-pharmacological therapies experience scale; PWD: person with dementia.

RESULTS

Internal consistency of NPT-ES was good or excellent in virtually all testing conditions (α 0.73-0.88). Internal consistency was slightly inferior in one instance that involved relatively few observations of new patients by external observer (stage II, α 0.63) (Table 2). In the majority of instances, the elimination of the different items of the scale reduced α coefficient (data of α coefficients if the individual items are eliminated are not shown).

Inter-rater agreement between raters that watched videos of sessions was good (ICC 0.79, step I) but agreement between video assessment and assessment by therapist was fair (ICC 0.49, step II). After these results, validation stage III was designed to assess a hypothetical effect of being out of sessions in NPT-ES reliability. Agreement between observers present during sessions and therapist reached the moderate range (ICC 0.61 and 0.69, step III) but agreement between those two internal observers was still superior (ICC 0.83, step III). After these results, it was hypothesized that acting as an evaluator would train and improve the therapist's rating capacity. This hypothesis was confirmed at step IV, where the highest inter-rater agreement was attained by internal observers and therapists that changed their roles on every session (ICC 0.88) (Table 2).

DISCUSSION

Several instruments have been used to measure the effects of non-pharmacological interventions in PWD. In most instances these instruments were not specifically designed to measure the effect of interventions. Typically, existing scales were adapted to evaluate specific intervention targets, particularly agitation (Gerdner 2000; Sloane et al., 2004) or affect (Sloane et al., 2004). When reported, psychometric characteristics of these scales were usually good (Lawton et al., 1996; Mitchell and Maercklein 1996; Vogelpohl and Beck, 1997; Politis et al., 2004; Sloane et al., 2004).

In contrast, our NPT-ES was specifically designed to measure the immediate affective and social effect of discrete non-pharmacological interventions in PWD. The NPT-ES was well accepted and easily used by different kind of professionals in various settings, evaluating a variety of non-pharmacological interventions. The high internal consistency of NPT-ES indirectly supports content validity of the selected five items.

In addition, to the authors' knowledge, this is the first time that properties of a scale of this kind were measured and compared under different rating conditions. Consistency and reliability of NPT-ES when used by observers that watched videos of sessions were good (Table, step I). Moreover, these external observers were neither therapists nor familiar with non-pharmacological interventions for dementia. However, agreement between intervening therapist and external observer was fair (Table, step II). This result, possibly due to missing information of PWD characteristics and responses by external observer, do not permit to conclude on the adequacy of NPT-ES in research contexts where intervention sessions should ideally be evaluated at minimal costs by raters that are neither present in the sessions nor aware of study design.

Results obtained when NPT-ES was rated by an internal observer (i.e., a therapist present, but not involved in the sessions) were better than those obtained by external observers. However, agreement between intervening therapist and internal observers were just moderate (Table, step III). This could be due to lack of rater experience or missing information of PWD responses by therapist. This explanation was confirmed in our validation step IV, when agreement between internal observers and therapists clearly improved after therapists also acted as internal observers. In other words, step IV results suggest that acting as an internal observer for several sessions train and improve the therapist's observational skills. This training, later qualifies the therapist to rate his or her own sessions.

This study bears some limitations. Only group sessions of AD PWDs at moderate or moderately severe stages of dementia were analysed. Our data do not allow us to extrapolate the performance of the scale with severe stages, where patients' behavioural or psychological signs might be less apparent. We also have not measured the scale in individual settings where expressivity might be different than in a group.

In conclusion, the NPT-ES emerges as a feasible and reliable tool to measure the experiences of PWD during NPT. It is particularly adequate to be used by therapists trained also as internal observers. This instrument has several immediate applications. It allows therapists to evaluate their own sessions, it may facilitate the adjustment of interventions to improve patient's experience (satisfaction) with NPTs, and it may be used to compare patient response to different NPTs (e.g., Music Therapy vs. Cognitive Stimulation). More research is needed to further ascertain the use of NPT-ES in research settings, either in its present, or modified form, (e.g.: some added items). An instrument like the NPT-ES for research use is needed, since poor response to NPTs might be associated to poor clinical prognosis.

APPENDIX 1. NON-PHARMACOLOGICAL THERAPY EXPERIENCE SCALE (NPT-ES): ENGLISH VERSION

Instructions

The NPT-ES seeks to measure aspects of patients' experience at the time of intervention. Experience is awareness of the present moment, conditioned by the possibilities of each patient. Some of the observable consequences of a this experience are expressed through behaviour and social relationships.

The scale consists of five items, which must be scored as per the guidelines included below. In the case of ambiguous or dubious answers, the evaluator has to make a judgement call according to his/her knowledge of the patient, without losing sight of the aim of the scale outlined above.

The time used for evaluation must be the entire period required for the target intervention. In other words, the evaluation period may be a complete session, from the first to the last therapeutic element (e.g., from greeting to closure, both inclusive), or only a part of the session (e.g., psychomotor activity).

Item scores will be allocated at the end of the intervention. The use of watches or other aids (notes, etc.) is not permitted. One item may possibly determine the scoring of another: for instance, if a patient has abandoned the session, any time that he/she spends out of the room will be counted as "rejection" as well as "non-participation", though not necessarily as "displeasure". 'Not assessable' will be endorsed when information is not available for more than half of the evaluation period.

A. Participation

The patient shows signs of paying attention and responding to the therapists' indications, through his/her posture, looks, gestures, words or actions. Should the patient not understand or be unable to perform the task, his/her efforts to collaborate will be viewed positively for scoring purposes. Spontaneous responses as well as responses to the therapist's indications are all scored.

3. Always
2. Frequently
1. Sometimes
0. Never   Not assessable

B. Pleasure
The patient shows signs of wellbeing and pleasure, through smiles, other gestures and expressions, posture, words or actions. Please note that participation does not necessarily mean pleasure.

3. Always
2. Frequently
1. Sometimes
0. Never   Not assessable

C. Relationship with others
The patient communicates positively (respectfully, in a friendly manner, etc.) or neutrally with other patients in the session or with the therapist, through looks, gestures, words or actions, whether spontaneously or at the therapist's indication.
3. Always
2. Frequently
1. Sometimes
0. Never   Not assessable

D. Displeasure
The patient displays negative feelings, such as uneasiness, anxiety, sadness, discomfort, shame, boredom, through posture, gestures and expressions, or words. Motor and other more complex actions will only be scored as displeasure if accompanied by some other indication of negative mood (e.g., leg tremble accompanied by tense posture or facial expression of anxiety, or drumming of the fingers accompanied by facial expression of boredom). Likewise, actions of rejection (question E) will only be included here if accompanied by signs of displeasure.

0. Always
1. Frequently
2. Sometimes
3. Never   Not assessable

E. Rejection
The patient actively rejects the therapist's indications. This includes gestures (e.g., shaking his/her head), postures (e.g., folding arms and staring at the floor), words, motor actions (e.g., pushing away or throwing objects), and more complex actions (e.g., pacing

about, retreating, leaving). Should the patient leave, the length of time he/she is out of the room is also counted as rejection. To qualify as rejection, there is no need for displeasure to be present.

0. Always
1. Frequently
2. Sometimes
3. Never   .Not assessable

APPENDIX 2. NON-PHARMACOLOGICAL THERAPY EXPERIENCE SCALE (NPT-ES): SPANISH VERSION

Instrucciones

La NPT-ES pretende medir aspectos de la experiencia del paciente en el momento de la intervención. La experiencia es la vivencia del momento presente, condicionada por las posibilidades de cada paciente. Algunas de las consecuencias observables de esta experiencia se expresan en la conducta y en las relaciones sociales.

El tiempo de evaluación ha de ser todo el que abarque la intervención que se quiera puntuar. Por tanto, el tiempo de evaluación puede ser una sesión completa, desde el primer elemento terapéutico hasta el último (p.e., desde la acogida hasta la despedida, incluyendo ambas), o bien sólo una parte de la sesión (p.e., la psicomotricidad).

Las puntuaciones en cada ítem se realizarán al finalizar la intervención. No se permite el uso de reloj ni de otras ayudas (notas, etc.). Es posible que un ítem condicione la puntuación en otros. Por ejemplo, si un paciente ha abandonado la sesión, el tiempo que permanece fuera de la sala se contabilizará como "rechazo" además de "no participación", aunque no necesariamente como "displacer". La respuesta 'no valorable' se aplicará cuando no se disponga de información para más de la mitad del tiempo de evaluación.

A. Participación

El paciente da muestras de atender y de responder a las indicaciones del terapeuta, a través de la postura, la mirada, los gestos, las palabras o las acciones. En caso de que el paciente no comprenda o no sea capaz de realizar la tarea, se valoran positivamente sus intentos de colaborar. Se puntúa tanto la respuesta espontánea como la respuesta a indicación del terapeuta.

3. Siempre
2. A menudo
1. Alguna vez
0. Nunca   No valorable

B. Disfrute

El paciente expresa bienestar y placer, a través de la sonrisa, de otros gestos, de la postura, de las palabras o de las acciones. Debe advertirse que la participación no necesariamente conlleva disfrute.

3. Siempre
2. A menudo
1. Alguna vez
0. Nunca   No valorable

C. Relación con otros

El paciente se comunica de forma positiva (respetuosa, amigable, etc.) o neutra con otros pacientes presentes en la sesión o con el terapeuta, mediante miradas, gestos, palabras o acciones, ya sea de forma espontánea o a indicación del terapeuta.

3. Siempre
2. A menudo
1. Alguna vez
0. Nunca   No valorable

D. Displacer

El paciente da muestras de sentimientos negativos tales como malestar, ansiedad, tristeza, incomodidad, vergüenza, aburrimiento, a través de la postura, los gestos o las palabras. Los actos motores y las acciones más complejas sólo se puntuarán como displacer si se acompañan de algún otro dato que indique un humor negativo (p.e. un temblor en una pierna que se acompañe de una postura tensa o de un aspecto facial de ansiedad, o un tamborilear con los dedos con cara de aburrimiento). De igual modo, las acciones de rechazo (pregunta E) sólo se incluirán aquí si se acompañan de signos de displacer.

0. Siempre
1. A menudo
2. Alguna vez
3. Nunca   No valorable

E. Rechazo

El paciente rechaza de forma activa las indicaciones del terapeuta. Se incluyen gestos (p.e., negación con la cabeza), posturas (p.e., cruzar los brazos y mirar hacia el suelo), palabras, actos motores (p.e. apartar o tirar objetos), y acciones más complejas (p.e. deambulación, alejarse, irse). En caso de irse, el tiempo que el paciente permanece fuera de la sala se contabiliza también como rechazo. Para puntuar como rechazo, no es necesario que exista displacer.

0. Siempre
1. A menudo
2. Alguna vez
3. Nunca   No valorable

REFERENCES

[1]   Argimón, JM; Jiménez, J. Diseño de estudios descriptivos (III): estudios sobre fiabilidad de una medida. Diseño y validación de cuestionarios. In: Argimón JM, Jiménez J. Diseño de investigaciones en ciencias de la salud. Barcelona: Signo, 1998.

[2]   Baker, R; Dowling, Z. INTERACT: a new measure of response to multi-sensory environments. Research Publication. Research and Development Support Unit, Poole Hospital, Dorset; 1995.

[3]   Gerdner, LA. Effects of individualized versus classical "relaxation" music on the frequency of agitation in elderly persons with Alzheimer's disease and related disorders. *Int Psychogeriatr* 2000; 12: 49-65.

[4]   Holliman, DC; Orgassa, UC; Forney, JP. Developing an interactive physical activity group in a Geriatric Psychiatry facility. Activities, Adaptation and Aging 2001; 26: 57-69.

[5]   Hurley, AC; Volicer, BJ; Hanrahan, PA; Houde, S; Volicer, L. Assessment of discomfort in advanced Alzheimer patients. *Res Nurs Health* 1992; 15:369-77.

[6]   Ibáñez, J; (1985). Del algoritmo al sujeto. Madrid: Siglo XXI.1985

[7]   Kitwood T. Dementia reconsidered: the person comes first. Buckingham: Open University Press; 1997a.

[8]   Kitwood, T. Dementia Care Mapping: the DCM method (7th ed.). Bradford: 1997b; Bradford Dementia Group, University of Bradford.

[9]   Kovach, CR; Henschel, H. Planning activities for patients with dementia: a descriptive study of therapeutic activities on special care units. *J Gerontolog Nurs* 1996; 22: 33-8.

[10]   Lawton, MP; Van Haitsma, K; Klapper, J. Observed affect in nursing home residents with Alzheimer's disease. *J Gerontol Psychol Sci* 1996; 51B: P3-P14.

[11]   Lee KA, Kieckhefer GM. Measuring human responses using visual analogue scales. *West J Nurs Res* 1989; 11:128-32.

[12]   Mitchell, LA; Maercklein, G. The effect of individualized special instruction on the behaviors of nursing home residents diagnosed with dementia. *Am J Alzheimer Dis* 1996; January/February: 23-31.

[13]   Politis, AM; Vozzella, S; Mayer, LS; Onyike, CU; Baker, AS; Lyketsos, CG. A randomized, controlled, clinical trial of activity therapy for apathy in patients with dementia residing in long-term care. *Int J Geriatr Psychiatry* 2004; 19: 1087-94.

[14]   Reisberg, B. Functional Assessment Staging (FAST). *Psychopharmacol Bull* 1988; 24: 653-9.

[15]   Sloane, PD; Hoeffer, B; Mitchell, CM; McKenzie, DA; Barrick, AL; Rader, J; et al., Effect of person-centered showering and the towel bath on bathing-associated aggression, agitation, and discomfort in nursing home residents with dementia: a randomized, controlled trial. *J Am Geriatr Soc* 2004; 52: 1795-804.

[16]   Vogelpohl, TS; Beck, CK. Affective responses to behavioral interventions. *Sem Clin Neuropsychiatry* 1997; 2: 102-112.

[17]   Woods, RT. Non-pharmacological techniques. In: Qizilbash N, Schneider LS, Chui H, Tariot P, Broday H, Kaye J, Erkinjuntti T, editors. Evidence-based dementia practice. Oxford: Blackwell; 2003: 428-446.

In: Dementia: Non-Pharmacological Therapies
Editor: Elisabetta Farina, pp. 239-257

ISBN: 978-1-61470-736-3
© 2012 Nova Science Publishers, Inc.

PREDICTORS OF EFFECTIVE SUPPORT FOR CARERS OF PERSONS WITH DEMENTIA

Franka J.M. Meiland[*][1], Cees Jonker[2] and Rose-Marie Dröes[1]

[1] Department of Psychiatry/Nursing Home Medicine,
VU University medical center.
[2] LASA, VU University medical center.

ABSTRACT

Objective: To investigate how informal carers of community dwelling persons with dementia value the Meeting Centers Support Programme (MCSP) for people with dementia and their carers, including the carer support activities, such as informative meetings, discussion groups and individual consultation, and to explore if characteristics of the carers are related to their satisfaction with and effectiveness of the support programme.

Methods: Participants were 71 informal carers of persons with mild to severe dementia who participated in the MSCP. Beside background characteristics, after 7 months of participation, a questionnaire was administered to the carers to investigate their satisfaction with the entire support programme and the different support activities offered to the carers. To measure the effectiveness of the MCSP in carers, before and after 7 months of participation in the MCSP interviews were held with regard to different outcome measures, i.e.: psychological and psychosomatic complaints, feeling of competence, experienced burden, and institutionalisation of the person with dementia.

Results: The large majority of carers were satisfied with the entire support programme (91,6%) as well as with each of the support activities offered to the carers. Several carer characteristics, such as lower age, longer duration of caregiving and higher degree of social support, were related to a more positive evaluation of the support programme. Characteristics that were related to the effect measures were loneliness, duration of caregiving, financial expenditure and formal support before starting the programme.

Conclusion: This exploratory study demonstrated that the satisfaction of carers with the MCSP, including the carer support activities, and the effectiveness of the support offered were related to characteristics of the carers. Thus it seems relevant to continue the evaluation of different types of support for carers on a larger scale and in different settings, to get insight into the relation between carer characteristics, the satisfaction with

[*] Corresponding author: Department of Psychiatry, VU University medical center Valeriusplein 9 1075 BG Amsterdam, The Netherlands Tel: +31-20-7885623 / Fax: +31-20-6737458 E-mail: fj.meiland@vumc.nl

support activities and the effectiveness of the support offered. Insight into these relations may contribute to more effective and efficient support of carers of persons with dementia.

Keywords: dementia; informal carers; support programme; predictors; evaluation.

INTRODUCTION

People are becoming increasingly aware that providing informal care to persons with chronic diseases is a heavy task [1]. This is particularly true when caring for people with dementia, because dementia deeply affects both the person concerned with the illness and his or her social environment [2]. Caring for a person with dementia frequently has negative physical, mental and social consequences for the informal carer [3-9]. These negative consequences turn out to be related with earlier institutionalization of the person with dementia [10-16].

Support should therefore focus on the persons with dementia, as well as on their informal carers. Empirical as well as academic literature [17,18] show that persons with dementia exhibit fewer behaviour and mood disorders if they are assisted in coping with the consequences of their illness, and that informal carers feel less burdened by changes in behaviour and mood of the person with dementia if they are adequately supported and assisted in dealing with them [19-23]. Effective support of the informal carers also increases the chance that people with dementia can maintain in their own home for a longer period of time [19,21,24]. Unfortunately, persons with dementia and their informal carers often still lack adequate information regarding the disease and the available care and support offers that could meet their needs [25]. Research shows that GPs and other professional carers do not always provide the informal carers and the person with dementia with adequate, tailored, and sufficient information on the available support for people with dementia and their carers [26]. One of the reasons for this could be a lack of knowledge about the effectiveness of support activities or programmes for subgroups of patients and carers. For example, it is not clear whether different types of informal carers (e.g. partners vs. children), would benefit more from particular types of support, like respite care or information, than from other types of support, such as discussion groups or an individual consultation hour. Knowledge on this could help to increase the effectiveness and efficiency of the support delivered to informal carers. Research to gain this knowledge is therefore recommended [27-31].

The goal of the exploratory study described in this paper was to investigate whether subgroups of informal carers value different types of support activities (i.e. discussion groups, informative meetings, a social club and an individual consultation hour) differently, and whether particular subgroups of informal carers benefit more from the support they receive.

The study was conducted within the framework of a multicenter study into the effect of a comprehensive support programme for people with dementia and their carers, the Meeting Centres Support Programme [18], which includes the mentioned types of support.

Meeting Centres Support Programme

In the Netherlands, since 1993 community dwelling persons with dementia and their informal carers can participate in the Meeting Centres Support Programme (MCSP)[32]. The meeting centres, which are mostly integrated into general community centres or centres for the elderly offer a variety of support activities on a small-scale base: 12 to 15 couples of persons with dementia and their informal carers. These support activities are, among other things, a *social club* where people with mild to moderately severe dementia can benefit of recreational, creative, and therapeutic activities, three days a week, and a series of eight to ten *informative, educational meetings* and a long-term (bi-weekly) *discussion group* for the carers. Both the informative meetings and discussion groups last one and a half hours and are highly interactive. While in the public informative meetings different professionals (GP, welfare worker, neurologist from the memory clinic, psychologist) present information on specific themes relevant for dealing with dementia (e.g. diagnostic screening, coping with behaviour and mood problems, psychopharmacotherapy, ethical aspects), with the main aim of (psycho)education, the discussion group is meant to emotionally and socially support the participants of the MCSP by allowing them to discuss their own problems, and is lead by the programme coordinator and a fixed co-leader (e.g. a social psychiatric nurse). A weekly *consultation hour* can be used for individual counselling. For more information about the content of the programme and the applied support strategies see Dröes, Meiland et al.[32]. At present there are 60 meeting centres across the Netherlands.

Various studies have shown that in comparison to regular psychogeriatric day treatment offered in nursing homes, the combined support programme offered in the community based meeting centres has more positive effect on the persons with dementia and the carers: persons with dementia exhibit less behaviour and mood disorders, and the carers feel less burdened, more competent and are able to provide care at home for a longer period of time. In addition, lonely carers have fewer psychological and psychosomatic complaints [18,21].

METHODS

Design

For this exploratory study into predictors of effective support a one group pretest-posttest design was used. Carers of persons with dementia were interviewed twice: at the start of participation in the MCSP, and after 7 months.

Data collection focused on a) characteristics of the informal carer, such as gender, relationship with the person with dementia, having/not having a paid job, and the emotional burden prior to participation, b) satisfaction regarding the support activities offered in the MCSP, and c) different measures in order to evaluate the effect of participation to the support programme on the carer: psychological and psychosomatic complaints, the feeling of competence, experienced burden, and quitting the support programme within seven months after the beginning of participation in the support programme.

Participants and Setting

The participants were drawn from a large multi-centre study on the conditions of successful implementation of meeting centres for people with dementia and their informal carers (IMO-project; 33). This project was approved by the Medical Ethical Committee of the VU University Medical Centre. In this project we performed a controlled impact study in eight meeting centres, spread across the Netherlands. By means of a pretest-posttest control group design people with dementia and carers who participated in the MCSP were compared with participants in regular psychogeriatric day treatment in nursing homes [18,21].

Out of the 111 dyads of persons with dementia and their carers that were approached for the exploratory study on the basis of an informed consent procedure (all of whom were new participants in the MCSP), 11 (10%) refused to participate, 8 (7%) dropped out before the baseline measurement, and 21 (19%) dropped out during the research period (figure 1). Data were collected on 71 (64%) informal carers at the start of the support and after 7 months of participation.

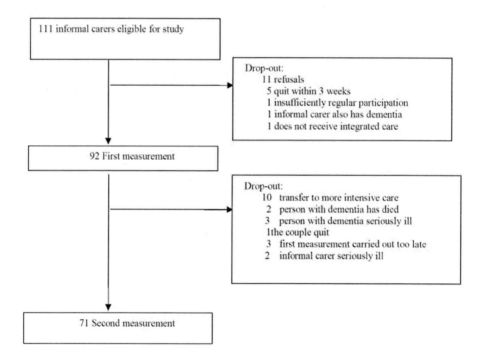

Figure 1. Flow-chart participants in the predictors-study.

Procedure and Measuring Instruments

Before participation in the MCSP all persons with dementia and carers received verbal and written information on the support programmes and procedures of the research project. This was followed by an informed consent procedure, in which people with dementia and carers were invited to participate in the study and to sign a consent form to express their consent with the data collection. Written consent was obtained from all the persons with dementia and their caregivers.

The data were collected in various ways: by means of interviewing carers and administering questionnaires, information was recorded by the programme coordinators in meeting centres, and diagnostic information was retrieved from general practitioners and/or specialists. The interviews were conducted by independent and trained interviewers. As a particular order in tests and questionnaires could result in a systematic group effect, the questionnaires were administered on the basis of a so-called balanced incomplete block design [34]. Data collection took place between 2000 and 2003.

The *satisfaction* of the carer with the entire support programme and each of the support activities was assessed seven months after the start of participation in the MCSP by means of a questionnaire.

During interviews with carers various *background characteristics* were registered for both the informal carer (age, gender, being gainfully employed, relationship to person with dementia, etc.), and the person with dementia (age, gender, education, etc.) on the basis of a checklist. Behaviour and psychological disorders of the persons with dementia and the *emotional impact* of these disorders on the carer were investigated using the Neuropsychiatric Inventory (NPI, $\alpha= 0.88$; 35,36) and the NPI-Distress scale [13]. This questionnaire is used to find out whether neuropsychiatric symptoms are present, how severe they are, and what emotional impact they have on the informal carer. Carers can indicate on a scale of 0 (no emotional burden) to 5 (very severe or extreme emotional burden) how distressing the neuropsychiatric symptom is for them. The total emotional impact score is calculated by adding up the emotional impact of the neuropsychiatric disorders that are present.

The *coping behaviour* and *loneliness* of informal carers were determined using the Jalowiec Coping Scale (JCS; α varies from 0.64 to 0.97); 37) and the Loneliness Scale (KR20=0.90; 38); *objective* support was determined by the modified Use of Services checklist [39] and the *experienced social support* from the person's own environment by the Social Support List (SSL, $\alpha=.87$; 40).

The *burden* of the informal carer was measured by means of reported *psychological and psychosomatic* complaints, as determined by the General Health Questionnaire (GHQ-28, $\alpha= 0.91$; 41); *feeling of competence*, determined by the modified version of the Sense of Competence Scale ($\alpha= 0.79$; 19, 42); *experienced burden* as compared to the burden experienced before participation in the support programme, determined by means of one question in the written survey on satisfaction with the MCSP ('Do you feel less burdened since you participate in the programme?' Answer options: Much less, somewhat less, no); and *institutionalization* within 7 months after start of the support, determined by recording the support programme starting date and the date of admission of the person with dementia into a nursing home. In order to find out the date of admission, all participants who had participated in the first interview of the impact study (n=92) were followed for a period of 7 months after the start of participation in the support programme.

Data on *diagnosis and type and severity of dementia* of the participants were retrieved from GPs and/or specialists. Diagnosis and type of dementia were assessed on the basis of the DSM-IV criteria [43] and the Standard of the Dutch Society of General Practitioners [44]. The Global Deterioration Scale [45,46] was used to assess the severity of dementia.

Analysis

SPSS-Windows version 11 was used to carry out the analyses. In order to determine whether the participants of the 8 meeting centres could be treated as one homogeneous group in the analyses, we conducted a Kruskal Wallis test: At the beginning of participation in the support programme, we investigated if the selected informal carers in these meeting centres differed in regard of sense of competence, and if the persons with dementia differed in regard of the severity of dementia and the neuropsychiatric symptoms. These variables were selected because they are frequently mentioned in the literature as relevant aspects related to the feeling of burden of informal carers. Descriptive statistics were used to describe the research sample and satisfaction with the support programme. To describe changes in the effect measures (psychological and psychosomatic complaints; feeling of competence), difference scores between baseline and follow-up measurements were calculated. As difference scores may also be based on random differences and errors of measurement, reliable changes after 7 months participation in the support programme were calculated. Based on Jacobson et al.'s research [47] we used the following criterion: the rough difference score must be at least 1.96 times larger than the standard measuring error of measurement of the variable in question. We applied the following formula:

$$X_1 - X_2 > 1.96 \, S_x \, \sqrt{1 - r_{xx}}$$

X_1	=	value found at measurement 1
X_2	=	value found at measurement 2
S_x	=	standard deviation measurement 2
r_{xx}	=	homogeneity coefficient of the dependent variable

As the data did not meet the assumption of normal distribution that applies to regression analyses, we conducted non-parametric tests. To find out whether the carers who were very satisfied with the support programme and carers whose relatives were not admitted into nursing homes differed with respect to background characteristics from the carers who were not satisfied, or those whose relatives were admitted into a nursing home, difference tests were conducted: Chi-square tests were conducted for the nominal background characteristics, and Mann-Whitney U-tests for the ordinal or interval variables.

In a similar way we investigated whether carers who showed substantial improvement after 7 months of participation in the support programme were different with respect to background characteristics from carers who did *not* change or who experienced more problems during this period.

RESULTS

There were no significant differences between the various meeting centres with regard to severity of dementia of the participants ($\chi^2 = 4.71$, df=7, p=0.70) or feeling of competence of the participating informal carers ($\chi^2 = 6.06$, df=7, p=0.53). However on neuropsychiatric symptoms we found a difference between the meeting centres ($\chi^2 = 15,5$, df=7, p=0.03): in two of the centres the frequency of neuropsychiatric symptoms of persons with dementia was lower than in the other centres. Because of the relatively small study sample we decided to treat the participants from the different meeting centres as one homogeneous group in the follow-up analyses.

Characteristics of the Carers and the Persons with Dementia

Table 1. Characteristics of carers (n=71)

Carer		
Gender		
male	12	(16.9%)
female	59	(83.1%)
Age	64.5	(sd 12.4)
Civil status		
married/cohabiting	66	(93.0%)
divorced/single	5	(7.0%)
Education		
primary education (including lower vocational)	33	(46.5%)
secondary education	28	(39.4%)
higher (vocational) education	10	(14.1%)
Gainfully employed		
yes	2	(16.9%)
no	59	(83.1%)
Relationship with person with dementia		
partner	46	(64.8)
daughter/son	19	(26.8)
other	6	(8.4)
Duration caregiving (in months)	28	(median)
Range	4-120	
Additional financial expenditures		
yes	34	(47.9%)
no	37	(52.1%)
Limited in activities by this:	4	(5.6%)
Coping (JCS: 0-180)	70.9	(sd 19.1)
Loneliness (Loneliness Scale: 0-11)	4.0	(sd 3.4)
Social support (SSL: 12-48)	28.7	(sd 6.1)
Use of services (Adapted use of services checklist: 0-14)	1.68	(sd 1.4)
Emotional impact of neuropsychiatric symptoms (NPI-D: 0-60)	12.7	(sd 7.4)

JCS= Jalowiec Coping Scale; SSL= Social Support List; NPI-D= Neuropsychiatric Inventory-Distress Scale.

The characteristics of informal carers and persons with dementia are represented in tables 1 and 2 respectively. The most common diagnoses are Alzheimer's disease (AD, 56%) or Vascular dementia (VD, 10%), or mixed AD and VD (11%). The severity of dementia varied from serious forgetfulness to severe dementia. For 90% of the respondents the diagnosis of dementia met the DSM-IV criteria or the Standard of the Dutch Society of General Practitioners according to GP or specialist. Seven percent did not meet the full diagnosis of dementia (they had severe memory problems or an amnestic syndrome) and for two persons (3%) it was unknown whether they met the diagnostic criteria because no information was received from the GP or attending specialist.

Table 2. Characteristics of persons with dementia (n=71)

Persons with dementia		
Gender		
male	41	(57.7%)
female	30	(42.3%)
Age	76.8	(sd 6.0)
Civil status		
married/cohabiting	50	(70.4%)
divorced/single	21	(29.6%)
Education		
primary education (including lower vocational)	34	(47.9%)
secondary education	27	(38.0%)
higher (vocational) education	10	(14.1%)
Diagnosis		
Alzheimer's disease (AD)	40	(56,3%)
Vascular Dementia (VD)	7	(9,9%)
AD/VD	8	(11,3%)
Dementia syndrom (NOS)	6	(8,5%)
Parkinson's disease with Dementia	1	(1.4%)
Korsakow Syndrome	1	(1.4%)
Frontal Lobe Dementia	1	(1.4%)
Severe memory complaints	4	(5.6%)
Amnestic syndrome	1	(1.4%)
Unknown	2	(2.8%)
Severity of dementia (GDS Stage)		
Severe forgetfulness	2	(2.8%)
Very mild cognitive decline	11	(15.5%)
Mild cognitive decline	21	(29.6%)
Moderate cognitive decline	21	(29.6%)
Moderately severe decline	14	(19.7%)
Severe cognitive decline	2	(2.8%)

GDS= Global Deterioration Scale.

Relation between Informal Carer Characteristics and Satisfaction with the Support Programme

The results regarding the evaluation of the support programme as a whole and the different support activities by the informal carers are represented in tables 3a, 3b, and 3c.

Table 3a. Satisfaction with the support programme (after 7 months participation)

	Total support programme	Discussion group	Informative meetings
Dissatisfied	--	2 (2.8%)	1 (1.4%)
Moderately satisfied	1 (1.4%)	1 (1.4%)	2 (2.8%)
Satisfied	36 (50.7%)	29 (40.9%)	36 (50.7%)
Very satisfied	29 (40.9%)	24 (33.8%)	19 (26.8%)
Unknown	5 (7.0%)	15 (21.1%)	13 (18.3%)

Table 3b. Evaluation of opening hours

	Opening hours meeting centre
Insufficient	10 (14.1%)
Sufficient	24 (33.8%)
Good	31 (43.7%)
Unknown	6 (8.4%)

Table 3c. Evaluation of consultation hour

Consultation hour:		
Made use of:	no	48 (67.6%)
	yes	19 (26.8%)
	unknown	4 (5.6%)
Feels it is:	not practical	13 (18.3%)
	practical	49 (69.0%)
	unknown	9 (12.7%)

The majority of carers were satisfied or very satisfied with the entire support programme and the different support activities (i.e. discussion groups, informative meetings and consultation hour).

Table 4 shows the results of the relation between carer characteristics and satisfaction with the entire support programme and the different support activities for carers. Carers who experienced a higher degree of social support from their own environment at the beginning of the support programme, proved to be very satisfied with the entire support offer more frequently ($U=-370,5$, $p=0.03$) compared to those who experienced a lower degree of social support from their own environment. We can observe a trend that people who take care of a relative for a longer period of time are more satisfied with respect to the total support programme ($U=363,5$, $p=0.06$).

A high degree of satisfaction about the discussion group turned out to coincide with a longer duration of taking care of a relative ($U=232,5$, $p=0.03$), and lower age of the informal carers ($U=234,0$, $p=0.03$). Furthermore, carers who felt more burdened at the beginning of participation in the MCSP seemed to be more satisfied with the discussion group ($U=252,5$, $p=0.06$).

None of the carer characteristics shows any relations with a high degree of satisfaction on the informative meetings. There also turned out to be no relationship between carer characteristics and the evaluation regarding opening hours of the meeting centres and use of the consultation hour. Some carer characteristics were related to the evaluation regarding the consultation hour: carers with higher levels of education ($U=203,5$, $p=0.03$), less emotional burden at the start of participation ($U=199,5$, $p=0.04$) and who felt less lonely ($U=203,5$, $p=0.05$) more frequently evaluated the consultation hour as practical.

**Table 4. Relation between carer characteristics and evaluation
of the programme after 7 months participation (n=71)**

Carer characteristics	Evaluation support programme		
	Very satisfied with total programme	Very satisfied with discussion group	Feels consultation hour is practical
Gender			
Higher age		-	
Higher level of education			+
Gainfully employed			
Partner of person with dementia			
Longer duration of informal care		+	
Additional financial expenditure			
More coping behaviour			
More loneliness			-
More social support	+		
More utilization of services			
More emotional impact of neuropsychiatric disorders			-

+ Positive and – negative significant correlation (p < 0.05).

Relation between Carer Characteristics and Positive Effects on Indicators of Burden

For a minority of the informal carers reliable changes were observed in two of the effect measures, i.e. *psychological and psychosomatic complaints* (21.1% of carers showed improvement; on the subscale "Anxiety and insomnia" 22.5% showed improvement) and *feeling of competence* (15.5% of the carers showed improvement).

When questioned about their *experienced burden* after 7 months participation as compared to before their participation in the MCSP, 29 carers (41%) answered they felt "much less burdened", 29 (41%) felt "somewhat less burdened", 8 carers (11%) felt "not less burdened", and for 5 carers (7%) the experienced burden was unspecified.

A final effect measure for the burden of informal carers was *admission into a nursing home* of persons with dementia within 7 months after the beginning of the support programme. Institutionalization was recorded for 92 person with dementia-carer dyads who enrolled in the study. Of these, 3 persons with dementia turned out to have been admitted into a nursing home *within* 7 months after the beginning of the support, after an average participation of 14 weeks (resp. after 5, 13 and 23 weeks).

**Table 5. Relation between carer characteristics and effects
of the support programme after 7 months participation (n=71)**

Carer characteristics	Improvement in effect measures								
	Psychological and psychosomatic complaints					Feeling of competence			
	A^1	B^1	C^1	D^1	Tot	A^2	B^2	C^2	Tot
Gender									
Higher age						−			
Higher level of education							+		
Gainfully employed									
Partner of person with dementia						−			
Longer duration of informal care				+					
Additional financial expenditure				+					
More coping behaviour									
More loneliness					+				
More social support									
More utilization of services						−			
More emotional impact of neuropsychiatric disorders									

+ Positive and − negative significant correlation (p ≤ 0.05)
A^1= Somatic symptoms, B^1= Anxiety and insomnia, C^1= Social dysfunction, D^1= (Severe) depression;
  A^2= Satisfaction with person with dementia as the cared for person, B^2= Satisfaction about oneself
as central carer, C^2= Consequences for private life of central carer .

Table 5 presents the results of the analyses of the relations between carer characteristics and improvements in the selected effect measures. With respect to the *psychological and psychosomatic complaints scale,* the carers who were more lonely at the beginning of participation in the support programme, more often experienced an improvement in psychological and psychosomatic complaints (U= 265,0, p= 0.03). Furthermore, the carers whose mood had improved after seven months, proved to have been taking care of the person with dementia over a longer period of time before the beginning of the support (U=54,50, p=0.05), and all had higher financial expenses in connection with the caregiving (χ^2 = 4,61, p= 0.03), compared to carers who did not show improvement in mood.

Although no relation was found between any of the carer characteristics and the total score on the Sense *of competence scale,* some relations were found with it's subscales. For example, carers who received less formal support before the support programme were more frequently satisfied about the person they cared for after seven months of participation in the MCSP compared to those who already received substantial formal support before joining the programme (U=98,0, p=0.04). Younger carers (U=72,0, p=0.04) and non-partners (χ^2=4,73, p=0.03) more often proved to be self-satisfied being the central carer than older carers and partners, and more highly-educated carers more often experienced a decrease in consequences of caring for the person with dementia for their private lives than low-educated carers (U=69,5, p=0.02).

None of the carer characteristics showed any significant relations with the reported *reduction of experienced burden* nor with *institutionalization* within 7 months after the support programme started.

Out of the other carer characteristics (gender, employment, emotional impact of neuropsychiatric disorders of the person with dementia, coping, and social support) that we investigated in this study, none were related to the observed improvements in the burden measures.

Finally, we investigated whether higher satisfaction and a positive evaluation by the carers of the support programme were related to an improvement in psychological and psychosomatic complaints, feeling of competence, and a reduction of experienced burden. A high degree of satisfaction about the informative meetings proved to be accompanied by lower improvements on the 'anxiety and insomnia' subscale (χ^2=4,28, p=0.04). Concerning the carers who indicated that they used the consultation hour, the feeling of competence increased more often as compared to those who did not use the consultation hour (χ^2=3,79, p=0.05). Also, over the course of the support period they more often felt that the impact of the care of the person with dementia on their private lives was diminished (χ^2=4,56, p=0.03).

We could not check the relation between satisfaction with the support programme and the effect measure 'time to admission into nursing home' because the evaluation of the support programme took place after 7 months, and thus persons who had been admitted into a nursing home within 7 months did not participate in this evaluation.

CONCLUSION

In this exploratory study we investigated how carer characteristics related to the evaluation and the effects of the MCSP. In general, informal carers of persons with mild to severe dementia who live at home proved to be very satisfied with the entire support programme and the different support activities offered to carers (informative meetings, discussion group, individual consultation hour), especially carers who at the beginning of their participation experienced more support from their social environment. It is possible that these people were more sensitive to support and were therefore more satisfied with the entire support programme. This is coherent with results of other research, that found a positive connection between social support and carer satisfaction with respite care [48]. The entire support programme was also more appreciated by those who had been taking care of their relative for a longer period of time. Duration of caregiving was also found to be related, as was younger age, to higher satisfaction about the discussion group. Furthermore, those carers who at the beginning of the support experienced more burden appeared to appreciate the discussion group more. The weekly consultation hour was appreciated as practical especially by the carers with higher levels of education and by those who at the start of the support felt less emotionally burdened and less lonely. This might be explained by the fact that higher educated carers appreciate individual counselling more than the lower educated carers and that the less burdened and less lonely carers found it less difficult to wait a few days before they could discuss their problems with the programme coordinator of the MCSP. However, for the majority a more flexible consultation opportunity was preferred to discuss their problems, reflected by the fact that many carers sought individual contact with the programme coordinator during the week, while only a quarter of the carers used the fixed weekly consultation hour.

Evaluation studies often find high degrees of satisfaction and this is partly due to a selection bias, because those who are not satisfied with the intervention have dropped out along the way [28]. However, in the current study reasons for drop-outs were not related to dissatisfaction with the support programme (see figure 1) and satisfaction therefore does not seem to be caused by selection bias.

With regard to the effects of participation in the support programme, on several indicators of experienced burden, the majority of the carers have shown neither improvement nor deterioration on psychological and psychosomatic complaints or feeling of competence during the research period. This outcome can be considered as positive, because during the study period an increase of behaviour problems in the persons with dementia was observed [18]. Moreover it has been documented that an increase in behavioural disorders is often accompanied by a *reduced* wellbeing of the carers [49-53]. The (sub)scales on which the participating informal carers most frequently improved on were: psychological and psychosomatic complaints, anxiety and insomnia, and feeling of competence. In addition, many carers indicated regarding the experienced burden question, retrospectively, feeling less burdened after seven months of participation in the support programme. We also considered quitting the support programme because of nursing home admission of the relative as an indication of carer burden. Only a very small percentage stopped participating in the programme within 7 months. All these results can be viewed as positive effects of participation in the support programme. The effects found confirm the results of other studies on combined support programmes for community dwelling persons with dementia and their caregivers, and in which positive outcomes were reported on variables such as delay in nursing home admission of the person with dementia, and burden and feelings of competence of carers [19,54-56].

Predictors were found for some of our effect measures of experienced burden. Carers who at the beginning of the support programme felt more lonely experienced a reduction in psychological and psychosomatic complaints more often than carers who felt less lonely. Earlier research has already shown that lonelier carers benefited more from the combined MCSP than from respite care only by means of regular psychogeriatric day treatment with regard to psychological and psychosomatic complaints [21]. This can be explained by the social contact and emotional support that the meeting centres offer carers. Predictors for a positive effect on mood were higher financial expenditure related to the caregiving and 'longer duration of caring for the persons with dementia'. The possibility of sharing the care task with professionals in the meeting centre and receiving advice on formal and financial support, might be especially beneficial for carers who have spent a lot on the caregiving and have cared for their relative already for a longer period of time.

We also found predictors for improvements on several dimensions of sense of competence. For example, receiving less formal support before participating in the MCSP predicted increased satisfaction with the person with dementia as the cared for person. This can be explained by the benefit of the psychoeducation offered in the MCSP, especially for carers who lacked this kind of support before participation in the programme. Younger age and not being the partner of the person with dementia were related to becoming more satisfied with oneself as a carer after participation in the MCSP. Children of people with dementia often have concomitant work and/or the care for their own family as well. This is a burdensome situation that easily leads to insufficiency feelings in regard of the different tasks. Sharing the caring with professionals in the meeting centre and discussing their feelings in the discussion group may be especially helpful for them. Finally, a higher level of education of the informal carer proved to be a predictor for a reduced impact of the caring on the carer's private life after participation in the MCSP. In other words, higher educated carers seem to have benefitted most of the psychoeducation offered in the support programme and actually learned to bring their care task into balance with their private life. In other research, contrary to what the researchers expected, a higher level of education was not related to a positive effect of a support programme [57].

One outcome that was striking in our study was that high emotional burden of the carer wasn't predictive for any of the outcome measures. Much research is being carried out on predictors of high risk of burden and distress [23,58-65], with the aim, among other things, to help to plan the correct support for carers [66]. However, it is not immediately obvious which type of support is most effective for the different subgroups of carers. It is therefore advisable to do more research in this complex field of effective support for different types of informal carers of persons with dementia in order to interpret our results.

A few critical remarks are in order. A large number of tests were carried out in a relatively small population, which increased the chances of finding significant results. Thus we must exercise caution when drawing conclusions about the effects found. A second remark is on the people that participated in the study: most people with dementia were male and most carers were partners. Naturally, this is not a representative sample of community dwelling persons with dementia and their informal carers, but an occasional sample in the meeting centres setting. Also, for some people with severe memory problems no detailed diagnostic data were obtained, and some others did not meet the criteria of a full dementia syndrome. We therefore have to be cautious generalizing the study outcomes as well.

Because of the relatively small study sample, we did not perform subgroup analyses. For instance, we did not differentiate between the meeting centres though there was some variation among the meeting centres with respect to the occurrence of neuropsychiatric symptoms of the participants with dementia at the start of the support programme. This might have influenced the burden of carers differently and possibly the effectiveness of the support programme. Neither did we make a distinction between carers of persons with different types of dementia, such as Alzheimer's disease and Vascular dementia, in our data analysis. However, we must be aware that it is possible that carers of persons with different types of dementia benefit differently from different types of support. Further research is needed to clarify this matter.

A fourth drawback is that the different types of informal care support were studied in a specific setting (i.e. in the meeting centres). Although this had the advantage that various carers could evaluate different types of support activities, the drawback is that we can no longer distinguish the effect of the separate types of support from the combined effects of support types. In addition, we should be aware that not all informal carers of people with dementia use all carer support activities offered in the meeting centres, and that we therefore studied a selective group that used the entire programme. Furthermore, Wettstein et al. [67] pointed out, that the lower socio-economic strata are underrepresented in psychosocial interventions. Although the distribution of educational level in our sample suggests this was not the case in our study, we do recommend further research into the evaluation of the different types of carer support.

This explorative study demonstrated that satisfaction with and effectiveness of the support offered is related to several characteristics of the carers, such as age, the period of time people provide care and the social support they receive. The carers who benefited most from the support they received were those who felt more lonely, had provided care for a longer period of time, had more financial burden because of the caregiving and received less formal support before they participated in the MCSP.

These kind of results should be accessible to referrers in order to facilitate a more efficient use of care facilities.

Future research should study what kind of support would better benefit carers with specific characteristics, such as being spouse, having advanced age and a lower educational level. This type of carers, at least in several Western countries, represent the most frequent carer category and they seem to benefit less than others of traditional support programmes and at the same time they experience high stress levels and psychosomatic disturbances. Furthermore, it should be investigated whether our results could also be found in larger samples and other settings, so that, eventually, a more efficient support for the growing numbers of informal carers of people with dementia can be achieved. Perhaps the results from this exploratory study may serve as a guide for such research.

ACKNOWLEDGMENTS

The province of Noord-Holland funded this research (no 2003-8132). There is no conflict of interest, the authors had full control of the research and all the data.

The authors confirm all participant/personal identifiers have been removed or disguised so the participants described are not identifiable and cannot be identified through the details of the story.

The researchers would like to thank every participant and the Meeting centres staff for their cooperation.

REFERENCES

[1]   Timmermans, JM. Mantelzorg. Over de hulp van en aan mantelzorgers. Den Haag: Sociaal en Cultureel Planbureau, 2003.

[2]   Health Council of the Netherlands. Dementia. The Hague: Health Council of the Netherlands, 2002.

[3]   Zarit, SM; Reever, KE; Bach-Peterson, J. Relatives of the impaired elderly: Correlates of feelings of burden. *Gerontologist* 1980;20:649-55.

[4]   Eagles, JM; Craig, A; Rawlinson, F; Restall, DB; Beattie, JA; Besson, JA. The psychological well-being of supporters of the demented elderly. *Br J Psychiatry* 1987;150:293-8.

[5]   Coope, B; Ballard, C; Saad, K; Patel, A; Bentham, P; Bannister, C; Graham, C; Wilcock, G. The prevalence of depression in the carers of dementia sufferers. *Int J Geriatr Psychiatry* 1995;10: 237-42.

[6]   Pot, AM. Caregivers' perspectives; a longitudinal study on the psychological distress of informal caregivers of demented elderly. Amsterdam: Vrije Universiteit, 1996.

[7]   Burns, A. The burden of Alzheimer's disease. *Int J Neuropsychopharmacol* 2000;3:31-8.

[8]   Meiland, FJ; Danse, JA; Wendte, JF; Klazinga, NS; Gunning-Schepers, LJ. Caring for relatives with dementia - caregiver experiences of relatives of patients on the waiting list for admission to a psychogeriatric nursing home in The Netherlands. *Scand J Public Health* 2001;29:113-21.

[9]   Vugt, ME de; Stevens, F; Aalten, P; Lousberg, R; Jaspers, N; Winkens, I; Jolles, J; Verhey, FR. Behavioural disturbances in dementia patients and quality of the marital relationship. *Int J Geriatr Psychiatry* 2003;18:149-54.

[10]   Greene, JG; Smith, R; Gardiner, M; Timbury, GC. Measuring behavioural disturbance of elderly demented patients in the community and its effects on relatives: a factor analytic study. *Age Ageing* 1982;11:121-6.

[11]   Teri, L. Behavior and caregiver burden: behavioral problems in patients with Alzheimer disease and its association with caregiver distress. Alzheimer Dis Assoc *Disord* 1997;11: S35-8.

[12]   Braekhus, A; Oksengard, AR; Engedal, K; Laake, K. Social and depressive stress suffered by spouses of patients with mild dementia. *Scand J Prim Health Care* 1998;16: 242-6.

[13]   Kaufer, DI; Cummings, JL; Christine, D; Bray, T; Castellon, S; Masterman, D; MacMillan, A; Ketchel, P; Dekosky ST. Assessing the impact of neuropsychiatric symptoms in Alzheimer's disease: the Neuropsychiatric Inventory Caregiver Distress Scale. *J Am Geriatr Soc* 1998;46:210-5.

[14]   Mirakhur, A; Craig, D; Hart, DJ; McLlroy, SP; Passmore, AP. Behavioural and psychological syndromes in Alzheimer's disease. *Int J Geriatr Psychiatry* 2004;19:1035-9.

[15]   Aalten, P. *Behavioral problems in dementia. Course and risk factors.* Maastricht: Maastricht University, 2004.

[16]   Vugt, M de. *Behavioral problems in dementia, caregiver issues.* Maastricht: Maastricht University, Department of Psychiatry and Neuropsychiatry, 2004.

[17]   Dröes, RM. In beweging: over psychosociale hulpverlening aan demente ouderen. Utrecht: De Tijdstroom, 1991.

[18]   Dröes, RM; Meiland, F; Schmitz, M; Tilburg; W van. Effect of combined support for people with dementia and carers versus regular day care on behaviour and mood of persons with dementia: results from a multi-centre implementation study. *Int J Geriatr Psychiatry* 2004;19: 673-84.

[19]   Vernooij-Dassen, M. Dementie en thuiszorg. Een onderzoek naar determinanten van het competentiegevoel van centrale verzorgers en het effect van professionele interventie. Amsterdam, Lisse: Swets & Zeitlinger, 1993.

[20]   Mittelman, MS; Ferris, SH; Shulman, E; Steinberg, G; Ambinder, A; Mackell, JA; Cohen, J. A comprehensive support program: effect on depression in spouse-caregivers of AD patients. *Gerontologist* 1995;35:792-802.

[21]   Droes, RM; Meiland, FJ; Schmitz, MJ; van Tilburg, W. Effect of the Meeting Centres Support Program on informal carers of people with dementia: Results from a multi-centre study. *Aging Ment Health* 2006;10:112-24.

[22]   Dröes, RM; Goffin, J; Breebaart, E; Rooij, E de; Vissers, H; Bleeker, C; Tilburg, W van. Support programmes for caregivers of people with dementia: A review of methods and effects. In Miesen B, Jones G (eds). Care-giving in dementia III. London: Routledge, 214-239, 2004.

[23]   Burns, A; Rabins, P. Carer burden dementia. Int J Geriatr Psychiatry 2000;15 Suppl 1: S9-13.

[24]   Mittelman, MS; Ferris, SH; Shulman, E. Steinberg G, Levin B. A family intervention to delay nursing home placement of patients with Alzheimer disease. A randomized controlled trial. *JAMA* 1996;276:1725-31.

[25]   Van der Roest, H. G; Meiland, F.J.M; Van Hout, H.P; Jonker, C; Dröes, R.M. What do community-dwelling people with dementia need? A survey of those who are known to care and welfare services. *Int Psychogeriatr* 2009, 21(5), 949-65.

[26]   Bruce, DG; Paterson, A. Barriers to community support for the dementia carer: a qualitative study. *Int J Geriatr Psychiatry* 2000;15:451-7.

[27]   Wright, SD; Lund, A; Pet, MA; Caserta, MS. The assessment of support group experiences by caregivers of dementia patients. *Clinical Gerontologist* 1987;6:35-59.

[28]   Brodaty, H; Gresham, M. Prescribing residential respite care for dementia - effects, side-effects, indications and dosage. *Int J Geriatr Psychiatry* 1992;7:357-62.

[29]   Cuijpers, P; Nies, H. Ondersteuning van familieleden van dementerende ouderen: de effecten. *Tijdschr Psychiatr* 1995;37: 790-800.

[30]   Thompson, C; Briggs, M. Support for carers of people with Alzheimer's type dementia. *Cochrane Database Syst Rev* 2000;2:CD000454.

[31]   Jeon, Y; Brodaty, H; Chesterson, J. Respite care for caregivers and people with severe mental illness: literature review. *J Adv Nurs* 2005;49:297-306.

[32]   Dröes, RM; Meiland, FJM; Lange, J de; Vernooij, MJFJ; Tilburg, W van. The Meeting Centres Support Programme: an effective way of supporting people with dementia who live at home and their carers. Dementia; *The international journal of social research and practice*, 2003;2:421-38.

[33]   Dröes, RM; Meiland, FJM; Vernooij, MJFJ; Lange, J de; Derksen, E; Boerema, I; Grol, RPTM; Tilburg, W van. Implementatie Model Ontmoetingscentra voor mensen met dementie en hun verzorgers. Amsterdam: VU Medisch centrum, *Afdeling Psychiatrie,* 2003.

[34]   Swanborn, PG. Methoden van sociaal-wetenschappelijk onderzoek. Meppel: Boom, 1987.

[35]   Cummings, JL; Mega, M; Gray, K; Rosenberg-Thompson, S; Carusi, DA; Gornbein, J. The Neuropsychiatric Inventory: comprehensive assessment of psychopathology in dementia. *Neurology* 1994;44:2308-14.

[36]   Kat, MG; de Jonghe, JF; Aalten, P; Kalisvaart, CJ; Dröes, RM; Verhey, FR. [Neuropsychiatric symptoms of dementia: psychometric aspects of the Dutch Neuropsychiatric Inventory (NPI)]. *Tijdschr Gerontol Geriatr* 2002;33:150-5.

[37]   Jalowiec, A. Jalowiec Coping Scale (Revised version of 1977) Chicago: Loyola University School of Nursing, 1987.

[38]   Jong-Gierveld, J de; Tilburg; T van. Manual of the loneliness scale. Amsterdam: Vrije Universiteit, 1990.

[39]   Schulz, C. Dementie onderzoek; een verkennende studie naar de verzorgers van dementerende bejaarden in Amsterdam. Amsterdam: PCA/Valeriuskliniek, 1991.

[40]   Eijk, LM van; Kempen, GIJM; Sonderen, FLP. Een korte schaal voor het meten van sociale steun bij ouderen: de SSL12-I. *Tijdschr Gerontol Geriatr* 1994;25:192-6.

[41]   Goldberg, DP; Hillier, VF. A scaled version of the General Health Questionnaire. *Psychol Med* 1979;9:139-45.

[42]   Teunisse, S; Haan, R de. Aanpassing van de competentielijst van Vernooij-Dassen (1993). Amsterdam: Academisch Medisch Centrum, *afdeling Neurologie*, 1994.

[43]   American Psychiatric Association. DSM-IV: Diagnostic and Statistical Manual of Mental Disorders. Fourth edition. Washington DC: American Psychiatric Association, 1994.

[44]   Nederlands Huisartsen Genootschap. Standaard Diagnostiek en behandeling dementie. Utrecht: Nederlands Huisartsen Genootschap, 1994.

[45]   Reisberg, B. The Brief Cognitive Rating Scale and Global Deterioration Scale. In Crook T, Ferris S, Bartus C (eds). Assessment in Geriatric psychopharmacology, New Canaan (Conn.): Mark Powley Ass. Inc., 1983.

[46]   Muskens, JB. Het beloop van dementie; een exploratief longitudinaal onderzoek in de huisartsenpraktijk. Nijmegen: Katholieke Universiteit, 1993.

[47]   Jacobson, NS; Follette, WC; Revensdorf, D. Psychotherapy outcome research: methods for reporting variability and evaluating clinical significance. *Behav Ther* 1984;15:336-52.

[48]   Nicoll, M; Ashworth, M; McNally, L; Newman, S. Satisfaction with respite care: a pilot study. *Health Social Care Community* 2002;10:479-84.

[49]   Zarit, SH; Todd, PA; Zarit, JM. Subjective burden of husbands and wives as caregivers: a longitudinal study. *Gerontologist* 1986;26:260-6.

[50]   Haley, WE; Pardo, KM. Relationship of severity of dementia to caregiving stressors. *Psychol Aging* 1989;4:389-92.

[51]   Wright, LK; Clipp, EC; George, LK. Health consequences of caregiver stress. *Med Exerc Nutr Health* 1993;181-95.

[52]   Schulz, R; O'Brien, AT; Bookwala, J; Fleissner, K. Psychiatric and physical morbidity effects of dementia caregiving: prevalence, correlates, and causes. Gerontologist 1995;35:771-91.

[53]   Acton, GJ; Wright, KB. Self-transcendence and family caregivers of adults with dementia. *J Holist Nurs* 2000;18: 143-58.

[54]   Smits, CH; de Lange, J; Dröes, RM; Meiland, F; Vernooij-Dassen, M; Pot, AM.Effects of combined intervention programmes for people with dementia living at home and their caregivers: a systematic review. *Int Psychogeriatr* 2007, 22: 1181-93, Epub 2007 Apr 24.

[55]   Graff, MJ; Adang, EM; Vernooij-Dassen, MJ; Dekker, J; Jöhnsson, L; Thijssen, M; Hoefnagels, WH; Rikkert, MG. Community occupational therapy for older patients with dementia and their care givers: cost effectiveness study. BMJ 2008, 336 (7636): 134-8.

[56]   Eloniemi-Sulkava, U; Saarenheimo, M; Laakkonen, ML; Pietilä, M; Savikko, N; Kautiainen, H; Tilvis, RS; Pitkälä, KH. Family Care as Collaboration: Effectiveness of a Multicomponent Support Program for Elderly Couples with Dementia. Randomized Controlled Intervention Study. JAGS, 2009, 57 (12): 2200-8

[57]   Brodaty, H; Roberts, K; Peters, K. Quasi-experimental evaluation of an educational model for dementia caregivers. *Int J Geriatr Psychiatry* 1994;9:195-204.

[58] Reis, MF; Gold, DP; Andres, D; Markiewicz, D; Gauthier, S. Personality traits as determinants of burden and health complaints in caregiving. *Int J Aging Hum Dev* 1994;39:257-71.

[59] Draper, BM; Poulos, CJ; Cole, AM; Ehrlich, F; Poulos, RG. Risk factors for stress in elderly caregivers. *Int J Geriatr Psychiatry* 1996;11:227-31.

[60] Bedard, M; Molloy, DW; Pedlar, D; Lever, JA; Stones, MJ. IPA/Bayer Research Awards in Psychogeriatrics. Associations between dysfunctional behaviors, gender, and burden in spousal caregivers of cognitively impaired older adults. *Int Psychogeriatr* 1997;9:277-90.

[61] Coen, RF; Swanwick, GR; O'Boyle, CA; Coakley, D. Behaviour disturbance and other predictors of carer burden in Alzheimer's disease. *Int J Geriatr Psychiatry* 1997;2:331-6.

[62] Pot, AM; Deeg, DJ; Dyck, R van; Jonker, C. Psychological distress of caregivers: the mediator effect of caregiving appraisal. *Patient Educ Couns* 1998;34:43-51.

[63] Dunkin, JJ; Anderson-Hanley, C. Dementia caregiver burden: a review of the literature and guidelines for assessment and intervention. *Neurology* 1998;51:S53-S60

[64] Donaldson, C; Tarrier, N; Burns, A. Determinants of carer stress in Alzheimer's disease. *Int J Geriatr Psychiatry* 1998;13:248-56.

[65] Freyne, A; Kidd, N; Coen, R; Lawlor, BA. Burden in carers of dementia patients: higher levels in carers of younger sufferers. *Int J Geriatr Psychiatry* 1999;14:784-8.

[66] Rinaldi, P; Spazzafumo, L; Mastriforti, R; Mattioli, P; Marvardi, M; Polidori, MC; Cherubini, A; Abate, G; Bartorelli, L; Bonaiuto, S; Capurso, A; Cucinotta, D; Gallucci, M; Giordano, M; Martorelli, M; Masaraki, G; Nieddu, A; Pettenati, C; Putzu, P; Tammaro, VA; Tomassini, PF; Vergani, C; Senin, U; Mecocci, P. Study Group on Brain Aging of the Italian Society of Gerontology and Geriatrics. Predictors of high level of burden and distress in caregivers of demented patients: results of an Italian multicenter study. *Int J Geriatr Psychiatry* 2005;20:168-74.

[67] Wettstein, A; Schmid, R; Konig, M. Who participates in psychosocial interventions for caregivers of patients with dementia? *Dement Geriatr Cogn Disord* 2004;18:80-6.

In: Dementia: Non-Pharmacological Therapies
Editor: Elisabetta Farina, pp. 259-273
ISBN: 978-1-61470-736-3
© 2012 Nova Science Publishers, Inc.

THE ABC GROUP FOR CAREGIVERS OF PERSONS LIVING WITH DEMENTIA: SELF-HELP BASED ON THE CONVERSATIONAL AND ENABLING APPROACH

*Pietro Vigorelli**

Gruppo Anchise (Milan, Italy)
Via Giovanni da Procida, 37. 20149; Milan, Italy.

ABSTRACT

Background. The ABC Group is different from other self-help groups, as well as from psycho-educational groups and the support groups usually organized by the parents associations of Alzheimer patients. The ABC Group is an original self–help group, led by a professional leader, addressed to caregivers of persons living with dementia, based on a new method developed in Italy, presented here for the first time in English: Conversational and Enabling Approach (CEA).

The ABC Group. The CEA is based on focusing the attention on the words exchanged between patient and caregiver during daily life and aims at favouring verbal expression in spite of the speech impairment and the deterioration of the communication function of speech, caused by dementia. In this way CEA aims at helping for the well-being (possible happiness) of both the caregiver and the patient.

The main components of CEA are here described: the Conversational Approach, the point of view of Multiple Identities and of Disidentity, The Elementary Competencies, and the Enabling Approach.

The ABC Group is based on the Twelve Steps proposal. They constitute the synthesis of CEA adapted to the caregiving practice.

A pilot study. This pilot study is carried out trough two ABC groups led following the CEA and a control group. Group A consists of 10 caregivers and 4 group sessions within a 6 weeks period, group B consists of 8 caregivers and 6 group sessions within 8 weeks, and the control group consists of 7 caregivers who have taken part to two informative sessions separated by 8 weeks.

The trial objective is the evaluation of the effectiveness of the ABC Group in modifying the Verbal Behavior of the caregivers, in the sense of greater adherence to the Twelve Steps. Furthermore the trial evaluates the changes of the Verbal Behavior of the patients and of the Caregiver Burden.

---

* Corresponding author: Telephone number 003902313301. E-mail: pietro.vigorelli@formalzheimer.it .
www.gruppoanchise.it

Conclusions. The results of this pilot study suggest the effectiveness of the ABC Group in modifying the Verbal Behavior of the caregivers, in the sense of greater adherence to the Twelve Steps. The Verbal Behavior of the patients and the Caregiver Burden of the caregivers appear unmodified.

Keywords: self–help group, ABC Group, Conversational Approach, Enabling Approach.

INTRODUCTION

The groups addressed to the relatives involved with the care of persons living with dementia are generally organized by the Alzheimer's Associations [1,2,3] and can be classified in three categories: *a*) Psycho - educational groups which give information about the illness and the strategies to cope with the Behavioral and Psychiatric Signs and Symptoms of Dementia (BPSD); *b*) Support groups with a professional leader, which want to give psychological help to caregivers; *c*) Self-help groups, with or without a professional leader.

These three categories of groups have the following objectives: *a*) the prevention of BPSD and the improvement of the care (in that case the aim is the well-being of the patients); *b*) e *c*) the comfort and mutual help between the participants (in that case the objective is the well-being of the caregivers).

Starting from this context the ABC Group is placed in a new position: the aim of the group is related primarily to the happiness of the caregiver (possible happiness) and secondarily to the happiness of the person living with dementia. The ABC Group intends to give to the caregiver the experience and the instruments needed to become an expert caregiver in the use of the speech. The satisfaction derived from the feeling of being an expert caregiver is the base on which the possible happiness of the caregivers is founded and secondarily also that of the patients.

The ABC Group is based on Conversational and Enabling Approach (CEA), an original method developed in Italy [4,5,6], freely extracted from distant cultural roots, such as Al-Anon and Alcoholic Anonymous self-help Groups [7], Michel Balint's Training Groups [8], Giampaolo Lai's *Conversazionalismo* (*Conversationalism*) [9,10,11,12].

It is however appropriate to remark that this method intersects a number of works of different Authors.

Tom Kitwood's (TK) *Malignant social psychology* highlights the environment pathogen power on the clinical evolution of the person living with dementia [13]. In a similar way CEA considers in particular the exchanged words as important elements of the environment that can affect the clinical presentation of the illness and the patient happiness.

Many non-pharmaceuticals treatments proposed for dementia are linked in various manners to Carl R. Rogers's (CRR) *Client-centered therapy* [14,15,16]. In a similar way CEA shifts the attention away from the illness towards the patient affected by dementia and the caregiver.

Naomi Feil's (NF) *Validation Therapy* highlights the relevance of emotive aspects in the relationship with the patient with dementia [17]. Similarly a CEA goal is to maintain the Elementary Competencies of the patient affected by dementia and among these the Emotional Competence.

The European Reminiscence Network (ERN) propose Reminiscence Therapy as method to improve the quality of life, of both the patient and the caregiver [18]. Similarly the ABC Group has the objective of improving the happiness of the caregiver and of the patient in each very instant and place of their mutual relationship.

The *Care Manual* of Alzheimer Europe (AE) aims at the harmonization of the person with dementia needs with the caregiver coping strategies [2]. Similarly the ABC Group assumes that one of the tallest challenges of the caregiver is to cope with the feeling of hopelessness before the illness and proposes the objective of meeting this challenge by becoming an expert therapist.

Kenneth Hepburn, Marsha Lewis, Jane Tornatore, Carey Wexler Sherman, Judy Dolloff - University of Minnesota - (KH, ML, JT, CWS, JD) in *The Savvy Caregiver Program* highlight how important is the self-care for the caregiver and the involvement and well-being of the patient [19]. In similar way the ABC Group has as objective the self-care of the caregiver and the possible happiness of the patient.

Amarthia Sen's (AS) *Capability Approach,* developed in a different field, finds many intersections with the ABC Group because of the relevance given to Multiple Identities and to the Contractual and Decision making Competence of the persons with dementia [20, 21,22].

SPECAL Approach (SPecialized Early Care for Alzheimer's) proposed initially by Penny Garner (PG) considers the well-being of the person with dementia as the top priority and concentrates on what a person with dementia can do, rather than what he cannot, in analogy with the ABC Group [23,24].

Moyra Jones's (MJ) *Gentlecare* highlights the importance of creating a prosthetic environment, where the persons with dementia can live 24 hours a day, rather than insisting on the value of the single rehabilitation session [25]. In similar way the ABC Group has the goal of creating a favourable environment throughout day life. CEA is a way of being and relating that everybody may learn and may be used in all contexts.

Traditional *Reality Orientation Therapy* (ROT) [26,27] has been the base from which Aimee Spector (AS) started *Cognitive Stimulation Therapy* (CST), an original program neatly differentiating from ROT and making the most not only of the proposed activities, but also of the relational behavior of the operator [28]. This evolution of ROT towards CST is another evident sign that presently many researchers are experimenting new techniques and pay great attention to the relational behaviour of the caregiver just as CEA does.

The environmental influence on the presentation of the illness (TK) and on the care results (MJ), the relevance of the relational behavior during care and rehabilitation (CRR), the need of considering the emotive world (NF) and of recognizing the free choice of functioning (AS) also for persons living with dementia, the possibility of choosing as objective the patient well-being (KH, ML, JT, CWS, JD; PG) as well as the caregiver's (AE; ERN), are all ideas which modify the approach to the care of the person living with dementia and that, considering the specific differences of expressions of each Author, still do intersect the CEA proposed here. This list, that is certainly incomplete, is reported to thank the previous Authors and to share with them the effort of finding instruments useful to improve the quality of life of persons living with dementia and their relatives.

The ABC Group

The ABC Group is based on the Twelve Steps proposal. They constitute the synthesis of CEA adapted to the caregiving practice [9, 10,11]. The main components of CEA are here described: the Conversational Approach, the point of view of Multiple Identities and of Disidentity, The Elementary Competencies, the Enabling Approach.

The Conversational Approach
Language disorders are a relevant component of the clinical picture of dementia, especially in Alzheimer's Disease, starting from the anomies of the initial phase to the lack of verbal communication of the advanced phase of the illness.

In these diseases the *communication function* of speech (which guaranties the ability of sending and recognizing messages linked to the meaning of words; in practice it allows the possibility of understanding and of being understood, and it is related to the semantic value of the verbal language) deteriorates earlier than the *conversational function* (which allows the exchange of words, in a more or less good manner, independently from the goal of producing information; eventually it makes possible a conversation without communication; that function is related to verbal fluency, independently of the semantic value of the words) As a result of that dissociation between the *communication function* and the *conversational function*, the patient and the caregiver tend to give up the use of speech when it would still be possible.

Starting from that observation, in Italy Lai has proposed a new approach to the care of persons living with dementia which makes the most of the verbal speech and which constitutes an application of the *Conversationalism* introduced by him in the eighties [9,10,11,12]. On these studies is based the Conversational Approach, the first of the two pillars of CEA. It should be noticed that in Italy the *Conversationalism* is developed later but independently of the Conversation analysis developed in the 70's by Sacks H., Schegloff E. and Jefferson G. [29].

The Conversational Approach wants to be a method to be used with the others rehabilitation treatments, a new method aiming at a new goal. The method originality consists in exploiting the *verbal language* instead that the *non-verbal*. It consists in keeping alive the use of speech when it is deteriorated but still possible, in the meantime giving up the recovery of the semantic value of words, when this is unattainable.

The two main techniques of Conversational Approach consist in two rules, *don't ask questions* and *give back the narrative motif* that is, re-expressing to the patient the minimum unit of meaning that the therapist detects from his words.

Multiple Identities and Disidentity
When dementia is diagnosed the ill person is considered by the caregiver only on the deteriorated aspects. The many features of the character, the long personal history, the capabilities still alive, are ignored.

Using Amarthia Sen's language [21], we can say that the ill person is deprived of his Multiple Identities (i.e. father, son, pensioner former teacher, music lover, dog owner…) and he is reduced to a mono-identity of 'affected by dementia'.

Using Lai's language [12], we can obtain an antidote to the reductive view of mono-identity with a different point of view, the Disidentity: "The Disidentity is a linguistic creation useful to solve a few practical problems: the concept of Disidentity gives us the possibility of accompanying the patient in all the possible worlds he inhabits".

The Disidentity, for example, allows the caregiver to relate to the patient as mother, when the patient acts as a daughter, as daughter when the patient acts as a mother.

In Lai's opinion, the Conversational method starts from the point of view of Disidentity and sees each interlocutor in the instantaneous '*I*' appearing in the pronounced sentence, a discontinuous and changeable '*I*'.

In other words, the Conversational Approach sees the dementia as an illness of identification, since the patient affected by dementia is not recognized in his/her Multiple Identities. The purpose of the ABC Group is to take care of the patient affected by dementia recognizing his/her Multiple Identities.

The Elementary Competencies

Considering the patient in his mono-identity of 'affected by dementia' triggers a series of phenomena aimed to eclipse the so called Elementary Competencies: the Emotive Competence, the Speech, Communication, Contractual and Decision making Competences [5,6].

The Emotive Competence consists in being aware of one's own emotions, to be able of feel, express and see them recognized.

The Speech Competence is shown with the use of verbal language, as it is possible in the different stages of the disease independently of the semantic value of the words.

The Communication Competence uses not only the verbal language, but also the non-verbal and near-verbal.

The Contractual Competence satisfies the need of participating to the choices regarding the everyday life.

The Decision making Competence is related to the choice criteria based on the system of values of patient, as he is able to conceive it.

The Enabling Approach

The Enabling Approach, the second of the two pillars of CEA, consists in creating the conditions where the person affected by dementia can perform the activities he is still able to do, as he can, without feeling of being in error.

The objective is to make, in the limits of possible, the person happy of performing what he does, as it is done, in the context of his environment.

The Enabling Approach is based on recognizing the Multiple Identities and the Elementary Competencies of the person living with dementia, it is not connected with the rightness of the action to be performed and it aims to the happiness of the patient.

This approach makes the most of the patient autonomy on the bases of an innovative concept.

Traditionally the autonomy is considered *the aim* of the rehabilitation intervention; the therapist works in order to increase the autonomy level of the patient.

Following the Enabling Approach, on the contrary, the autonomy is considered *the mean* to favor the possible happiness of the patient; the enabling therapist detects the autonomy whenever it appears, as it is shown or when it could have been shown but it is eclipsed. The task of the therapist becomes the favoring of the emerging of the Elementary Competencies to contract and to make decisions whenever he is interacting with the patient.

The Happiness as Objective

The CEA is a care method placed among the rehabilitation methods but which, due to his basic philosophy, is different from these methods. The CEA is not properly a rehabilitation method because it does not aim to recover the lost functions. The CEA final goal is the possible happiness of the person living with dementia, the happiness possible in the actual moment and in the given context.

The ABC Group

The ABC Group is based on a new, original, method inspired by Al-Anon and Alcoholic Anonymous Groups [7], by Balint Groups [8] and by Lai's *Conversationalism* [9,10,11,12].

A) The **Al**-Anon Groups address the alcoholic relatives and aim to objectives related to the relatives, not to the alcoholics. With the help of the group the relatives follow a path aimed to a personal improvement, convinced that, eventually, this will be useful also for the alcoholic. That path consists in Twelve Steps. The ABC Groups have a similar structure, leverage on strong group solidarity and propose a path with Twelve Steps, specifically designed, based on our last ten years experience.

B) The groups described by Michel Balint address doctors and nurses wanting to improve their interaction capacity with the patients and are focused on difficult situations experienced by the participants. Both the ABC and Balint Groups have a professional leader and are hetero-centric, that is they are based on accounts of facts happened outside the group, in particular on words exchanged between the caregiver and the patient.

C) The *Conversationalism* (see above)

The ABC Group is addressed to caregivers of person living with dementia and offers them a direct CEA experience during group sessions, in order to better adopt the approach in the daily life with the person living with dementia.

It contributes to build around the patient an environment where the CEA would be the base of the interaction 24 hours a day, not only during the sessions with the therapist.

As we consider the patient happiness the goal of our activities with the patient, so we consider the caregiver happiness the aim of our activities with him during group sessions.

The ABC Group intends to give to the caregiver the experience (within the group) and the instruments (Twelve Steps) needed to become an expert caregiver.

The Expert Caregiver

Both the CEA taking care of persons living with dementia and the ABC Group for caregivers, focus their attention on the exchanged words.

In CEA the therapist focuses on the words exchanged with the patient whenever they emerge, in ABC Group the leader focuses on two levels, the level of the words exchanged during the working sessions and the level of the words exchanged daily between the caregiver and the patient.

In conducting the group, the goal is the caregiver happiness; we will now explain how we intend to reach this goal.

It is known that the caregiver suffering is in part due to the feeling of being impotent in front to the relentless evolution of the illness, in spite of the continuous end heavy effort put into the care.

To overcome this sense of impotence and frustration, the ABC Group proposes to the participants to become expert caregivers as a way out from the impotence tunnel.

In this way we modify the care-giving objective, shifting the attention from the patient to the caregiver. Specifically, the caregiver should become expert in the use of the language instead of looking for a non-realistic improvement of the functionality and autonomy of the patient. The ABC Group meetings and the Twelve Steps are the instruments which allow the caregiver to achieve the objective. The improvement in the patient Speech Competence and other Elementary Competencies is considered a good but secondary result. In our opinion, the primary objective of the work with the caregivers must be placed at the caregivers own level, not at a different one, like that of the patient.

The Twelve Steps

The Twelve Steps are a synthesis of CEA made suitable for caregivers and are used as guidelines to become a caregiver expert in the use of the speech with relatives living with dementia (see Table 1). They aren't strict rules; everyone should follow them as far as it is possible, keeping in mind that their main objective is, in first instance, to favor the caregiver happiness, and in second instance the patient's.

The first five Steps refer to Conversational Approach and are used to keep alive the Speech and Communicating Competencies. The first step in particular makes this approach different from others rehabilitation approaches.

Questions like *Which day is today? Who am I? What have you had for lunch?* are considered obstacles to the flux of everyday's conversation and are avoided. The 5th Step consists in accompanying the patient in his possible world, adjusting to his space-time, using specific techniques as *Give back the narrative motif, Echoing response* and *Supplying fragments of autobiography,* which means allowing personal involvement, enriching the conversation with personal memories related to the patient's narrative motif.

Table 1. The Twelve Steps

1.	Don't ask questions
2.	Don't correct
3.	Don't interrupt
4.	Listening, respecting the silence and the slowness
5.	Accompany with the words
6.	Answer the questions
7.	Communicate also through non verbal language
8.	Recognize the emotions
9.	Answer the requests
10.	Accept whatever the patient does
11.	Accept the illness
12.	Taking care of one's own well being

The next five Steps refer to Enabling Approach. The 8th Step is meant to keep alert the Emotional Competence and consists in recognizing the patient's emotion (so like is expressed), in identifying it and giving it back with a verbal acknowledgement. The 9th and 10th Steps are meant to keep alert the Contractual and Decision making Competencies and to help the active participation to everyday's life choices.

The 11th and 12th Steps help the caregiver to overcome his own feelings of guilt and inadequacy and are important to reach a sufficient happiness (the possible happiness).

The ABC Group Creation

The ABC Group is made by a small number of caregivers (6-12) meeting for two hours every 2-4 weeks. The participants are seated in circle. The leader is a psychotherapist expert in CEA, trained in conducting ABC Groups. In selected cases can be a different professional (occupational therapist, speech therapist, pedagogue...) with the right training.

Leadership of the ABC Group

The leadership of the group is directive and hetero-centric. The group leader with his comments wants to prompt the direct participation of all the members of the group.

At the opening of the meeting he addresses the group inviting whoever wishes to report about a difficult, unsatisfactory or unintelligible conversation held with the sick relative. While the speaker reports, everyone else is invited to listen while keeping quiet, without interrupting.

When the speaker is through with his contribution, the group leader invites the participants to identify a critical moment in the conversation, helping to focus attention on words exchanged.

Anybody can report analogous conversations occurred to him, or possible *ways out*, alternative to that used by the speaker, in terms of words used.

The group leader listens to all reports then takes the floor to point out what happens, in the conversations reported, when the words uttered agree or disagree with one of the Twelve Steps.

For instance, if a caregiver tells that when asked questions, the patient replies he does not remember or interrupts the conversation, getting irritated, the group leader focuses attention on this fact and asks the group whether other words (different from those of the question) could be used in a similar situation, to help carrying on with a fluent conversation.

During the meeting, discussions are avoided. Everyone is free to tell his own experience, and to listen to the experience of others and to take home those ideas and suggestions that might be more valuable for him.

A PILOT STUDY

Starting from 2008 the ABC Groups have spread in different italian regions (Lombardy, Liguria, Trentino, Emilia, Tuscany, Marche, Sicily, Sardinia) through group leaders trained by the "Associazione Gruppo Anchise" (www.gruppoanchise.it). The present study is meant to start the process of evaluation of the effectiveness of the method.

AIMS

The study assesses first the changes in Verbal Behavior of the caregivers in applying the Twelve Steps; secondly the changes in Verbal Behavior of the patients and the changes of the Caregiver Burden.

Materials and Methods

The study is concerned with two ABC Groups, carried out in different centers, Group A structured in four meetings with 10 caregivers, Group B structured in six meetings with 8 caregivers, held within 6 and 10 weeks respectively. As a control group we consider 7 caregivers taking part to two informative meetings, one on the dementia diseases and another, after an 8 weeks gap, on the pharmacological treatment. All the participants are caregivers of dementia patients who live at home and are usually followed in a specialized health center. All patients, already under treatment with anticholinesterasic drugs, have continued the treatment during the period of the study.

The participants to the non random control group have been recruited immediataly after the conclusion of the two ABC Groups.

The characteristics of the participants are summarized in Table 2.

Two questionnaires are presented to all participants (ABC Groups and Control Group), for self-evaluation of Verbal Behavior and Caregiver Burden, before and after the intervention (*ante/post*). The Verbal Behavior of patient and caregiver is evaluated by an original Questionnaire prepared for the present research: 9 items of the Questionnaire refer to the caregiver Verbal Behavior (Table 5) and 9 to the Verbal Behavior of the persons with dementia [On the whole, how do you judge his/her way of speaking? Does he/she start speaking on his own initiative? Does he use well built sentences (subject, verb and possible object)? Does he/she use only mono-syllables (yes, no,…)? Does he/she use very short and stereotyped answers (I don't know, let me be, I'm tired,…)? Does he/she tend to jam or interrupt? Does he/she seem to be happy when speaking to you? How much does he/she speak, compared with the situation before the illness? Comparing with the situation before the ABC Group how much time do you spend talking with him/her?].

The answers to the Questionnaire *ante* refer to the situation of the week preceding the start of the ABC Group; the answers to the Questionnaire *post* refer to the situation of the week preceding the last meeting of the ABC Group. Low scores indicate a higher closeness to the Twelve Steps.

The Caregiver Burden is measured by the Caregiver Burden Inventory (CBI) [30] .

The person responsible of the evaluation of the results (Antonio Guaita, Geriatric Institute Camillo Golgi, Abbiategrasso, Italy) is not involved in the running of the groups activity and in the data collection.

Table 2. Characteristics of the participants

Group	A	B	A e B	Control
Location	Don Gnocchi[1]	Segesta[2]		Don Gnocchi[1]
Sex				
Males	2	3	5	1
Females	8	5	13	6
Relationship				
Spouse	3	1	4	2
Children	3	5	8	2
Daughter/Son- in-law	2	2	4	0
Other	2	0	2	3
Total	10	8	18	7

[1] S. Maria Nascente Clinical Research Centre, Don Gnocchi Foundation, Milan, Italy.
[2] Saccardo Residences of Segesta Group, Milan, Italy.

Results

The data related to the Verbal Behavior are considered separately from those related to the Caregiver Burden. Only 15 caregivers out of 18 have handed in the Questionnaire *post* related to the Verbal Behaviour, and 13 the Questionnaire *post* related to the Caregiver Burden.

The Verbal Behavior of Caregivers and of Persons with Dementia

A comparison has been made between the results *ante/post* and also the *cases/controls* have been compared.

As already mentioned, 9 items of the Questionnaire refer to the Verbal Behavior of caregivers and 9 to the Verbal Behavior of persons with dementia. Two summarizing variables, called "Verbal Behavior of caregivers" and "Verbal Behavior of persons with dementia" have been built using the sum of the results of the two groups of 9 answers: the so built variables have a good internal consistency, measured with Cronbach's alfa and however greater than 0,70. The *ante/post* differences have been analyzed using Student's "t" for data pairs. The *cases/controls* differences have been analyzed using Student's "t" for independent samples.

The results related to the two summarizing variables (Table 3) show that the caregiver's Verbal Behavior improves significantly within the *cases* and not within the *controls*; the Verbal Behavior of persons with dementia doesn't change significantly within the *cases,* instead it changes significantly (p 0,049) within the *controls*.

A specific analysis of the answers on the Verbal Behavior of persons with dementia shows only one answer significantly different comparing *ante/post* (Table 4). The *post* lower values indicate that the caregivers, after attending the ABC group, spend more time talking with the patient.

A specific analysis of the answers on the Verbal Behavior of Caregivers of ABC Group (see Table 5) shows that 5 have significantly improved, 2 are close to a significant improvement, 2 result stable.

The Control Group answers do not show any significant improvement and 4 show no significant worsening.

Table 3. Summarizing variables "Verbal Behavior of caregivers" and "Verbal Behavior of persons with dementia"

ABC Group		average	sd	p	Control Group	average	sd	p
Verbal Behavior of persons with dementia	ante	23,00	7,34	0,143	Verbal Behavior of persons with dementia	23,29	7,32	**0,049**
	post	20,93	4,62			18,43	6,19	
Verbal Behavior of caregivers	ante	24,47	4,02	**0,036**	Verbal Behavior of caregivers	23,29	7,32	0,818
	post	21,07	5,18			23,71	4,50	

Table 4. The Verbal Behavior of persons with dementia evaluated by caregivers

Caregivers of ABC groups		average	sd	p	Caregivers of Control Group	average	sd	p
Comparing with the situation before how much time do you spend talking with him/her?	ante	3,93	1,163	**0,006**	Comparing with the situation before how much time do you spend talking with him/her?	3,57	0,976	**0,030**
	post	2,93	0,961			3,00	0,577	

Correlation between the Summarizing Variables "Verbal Behavior of Caregivers" and "Verbal Behavior of Persons with Dementia"

It is interesting to notice the correlation between the considerations about the Verbal Behavior of the patients and their own Verbal Behavior for the participants to the ABC Group (Table 6). Before starting the Group the two behaviors are not correlated, afterword they become correlated with a negative sign.

To explain this, *the more the patient Verbal Behavior is compromised, the more the Caregiver Verbal Behavior, after participating to the ABC Group, is close to the Twelve Steps.*

Indeed, if instead of referring to the absolute values, the relationship between the increase of the scores of the patients and those of the caregivers (i.e. the two differences *ante* and *post)* is analyzed, these increases are positively correlated, at the limit of significance ($p = 0,054$) (analysis made using Pearson's "r").

Caregiver Burden

The Caregiver Burden has been evaluated using the *Caregiver Burden Inventory* (CBI) [30]. No difference *ante/post* has been found for the global scale value (Table 7), and none for the single items inside the *cases* and the *controls*.

It should be noted that the initial average Burden shown by the controls has resulted significantly lighter ($p = 0.039$).

Table 5. Verbal Behavior of Caregivers of ABC Group

		media	n.	sd	p
When speaking to him, do you pose any question? (i.e.: do you remember what you had for lunch?)	ante	3,60	15	1,183	**0,060**
	post	2,73	15	1,486	
When he finds difficult starting speaking, do you try to help him with some questions or suggesting the answer?	ante	3,40	15	0,986	**0,004**
	post	2,47	15	1,187	
When he has started speaking, it happens to you to interrupt?	ante	2,33	15	1,113	**0,013**
	post	1,53	15	0,834	
When he makes errors when speaking, do you correct him?	ante	3,20	15	1,014	**0,022**
	post	2,33	15	1,113	
When he speaks in a sufficiently understandable way, do you try to follow his speech?	ante	1,33	15	0,488	0,110
	post	1,80	15	0,862	
When speaking to you he doesn't find a word, do you suggest the missing word or complete the sentence?	ante	3,47	15	0,990	**0,022**
	post	2,60	15	1,242	
When his speech is not enough understandable, however do you try to follow what he is saying?	ante	1,47	15	0,640	**0,010**
	post	2,33	15	0,900	
When speaking to him, it happens to tell him something about you or your life?	ante	2,93	15	0,884	1
	post	2,93	15	0,799	
Thinking back to your conversations, how do you globally judge your speaking ability?	ante	2,73	15	0,799	**0,052**
	post	2,33	15	0,617	

Table 6. Correlation between "Verbal Behavior of caregivers" and "Verbal Behavior of persons with dementia" before and after the ABC Group

		Verbal Behaviour of caregivers *ante*	Verbal Behaviour of caregivers *post*
Verbal Behavior of persons with dementia *ante*	"r" Pearson	0,383	-0,545
	p	0,159	0,035
Verbal Behavior of persons with dementia *post*	"r" Pearson	0,175	-0,579
	p	0,533	0,024

Table 7. Caregiver Burden *Comparison for data pairs ante and post for Caregivers of ABC Groups (cases) and Caregivers of Control Group (controls)*

	Cases averages	sd	n	*Controls* averages	n*	sd
Caregiver Burden *ante*	24,46	17,28	13	12,17	6	4,26
Caregiver Burden *post*	25,62	19,27	13	10,33	6	7,71
"p"	ns			ns		

*An "outliner" has been eliminated for those variables.

CONCLUSION

The present pilot study has shown that the caregivers' Verbal Behavior improves significantly in the *cases* and not in the *controls* (Table 3) and the Verbal Behavior of patients with dementia is not significantly modified in the *case's* while it is modified significantly in the *controls* (p 0,049).

This latter result probably is brought both by the effect of the two questionnaires, that have focused attention on the subject , and by the informative course based more on the patient and the illness than on the caregiver.

The detailed analysis of the answers on the Verbal Behavior of people with dementia shows that significantly different *ante/post* results (table 4) are given only by the amount of speech, a measure that involves both the Verbal Behavior of the dementia patient and that of the caregiver.

Also in the *controls* this is the only answer that gives a significant *ante/post* difference. It should be noted that although both meaningful, the "score" value is about double for the caregivers that have taken part to ABC Groups, compared with the *controls* (Also the "t" Student distribution, not shown in Table 4, gives 3,24 *versus* 2,83).

The detailed analysis of the answers on the Verbal Behavior of caregivers (Table 5) shows that what improves is especially the ability of "not interfering" negatively and that approach mistakes in the conversation are reduced (the caregivers have learnt not to suggest the answer, not to interrupt, not to correct, not to complete sentences).

Less evident, down to the significant level, is the improvement of the ability to reduce the questions, both in giving a positive appraisal of them and of the ability of speaking.

Finally for the two questions whose answers don't change, one has positive answers from the start (*ante*) that remain so (*post*) (When he speaks in a sufficiently understandable way, do you try to follow his speech?), the other has negative answers from the start (*ante*) that remain so (*post*) (When speaking to him, it happens to tell him something about you or your life?).

The single items analysis, that mainly highlighted the improvement of the "relational" behaviours, is supported also by the described correlation between verbal behaviour of the caregivers and of the patients, gained only after the ABC training.

For what concerns the answers of the control Group no significant improvement has been detected.

For what concerns the Caregiver Burden, measured using CBI, it doesn't show any significant change.

Our opinion is that CBI has proved to be an unsuitable tool for evaluating the results of this type of training path.

Indeed the caregivers attending the Groups gain awareness on what happens in everyday life and on their own specific role. However the resulting greater perception of the Caregiver Burden is not directly correlated with the Caregiver well being level.

Furthermore CBI considers the care relationship just as a burden and values it only through negative situations.

Whoever follows closely the complex relationship between patient and caregiver, knows that there are also positive aspects linked to the care activity, i.e. the affection of the patient and the rewards coming from the caring role. Therefore the negative drawbacks (*burden*) of the care giving task could be at least partially balanced by other positive aspects not detected by CBI.

This Pilot Study has highlighted that the participation to the ABC Group is followed by a change in the caregivers Verbal Behavior, which become closer to the Twelve Steps, without significantly modifying the patients' Verbal Behavior and the Caregiver Burden, measured using CBI. The perception by the caregivers of the changing in their own Verbal Behavior is stronger when the patient Verbal Behavior is more compromised. This study has been limited to the measurement of short term effects of the intervention with ABC method. Further studies are needed to assess long term effects, both for caregivers and for the persons with dementia.

REFERENCES

[1]   http://www.alzheimer.it (Federazione Alzheimer Italia)
[2]   http://www.alzheimer-europe.org (Alzheimer-Europe)
[3]   http://www.alz.org (Alzheimer's Association)
[4]   Vigorelli P. (2004). La conversazione possibile con il malato Alzheimer. Milano: Franco Angeli.
[5]   Vigorelli P. (2008). Alzheimer senza paura. Perché parlare, come parlare. Milano: Rizzoli.
[6]   Vigorelli P. (2010). Il Gruppo ABC. Un metodo di autoaiuto per i familiari di malati Alzheimer. Milano: Franco Angeli.
[7]   http://www.aa.org *(Alcoholic Anonymous)*
[8]   Balint M. (1956). The Doctor, his Patient and the Illness. London: Pitman Medical Publishing.
[9]   Lai G. (1985). La conversazione felice. Milano: Il Saggiatore.
[10]   Lai G. (1993). Conversazionalismo. Torino: Bollati Boringhieri.
[11]   Lai G. (1995). La conversazione immateriale. Torino: Bollati Boringhieri.
[12]   Lai G. (1999). Disidentità. Milano: Franco Angeli.
[13]   Kitwood T. (1997). Dementia reconsidered: the person comes first. Open University Press.
[14]   Rogers C. R. (1951*). Client-Centered Therapy*. London: Constable.
[15]   Cooper M., O'Hara M., Schmid P F. and Wyatt G. (2007). *The handbook of person-centered psychotherapy and counseling*. Palgrave Macmillan.
[16]   Brooker D. (2004). What is person-centered care for people with dementia? *Clinical Gerontology,* 13 (3).
[17]   Vicki de Klerk-Rubin V. (2007). *Validation Techniques for Dementia Care: The Family Guide to Improving Communication*. Edward Feil Productions.
[18]   Schweitzer P. and Bruce E. (2008). Remembering Yesterday, Caring Today. Reminiscence in Dementia Care: A Guide to Good Practice. Jessica Kingsley Publishers.
[19]   Hepburn K., Lewis M., Tornatore J., Sherman C. W. and Dolloff J. (2002). The Savvy Caregiver. A Caregiver Manual. Kenneth Hepburn
[20]   Sen A. (1992): Inequality reexamined. Oxford University Press.
[21]   Sen A. (1999). *Development as Freedom*. New York: Knopf, and Oxford: Oxford University Press.
[22]   Sen A. (2006). *Identity and Violence. The Illusion of Destiny*. New York – London: W.W. Norton & Company.
[23]   Garner P. (1995) SPECAL (Specialized Early Care for Alzheimer's) Project Report, Burford.

[24] *James O. (2008).* Contented Dementia. Publicher *Vermilion.*

[25] Jones M. (1999). *Gentlecare.* Changing the experience of Alzheimer's disease in a positive way. Moyra Jones Resources Ltd.

[26] Folsom J. C. (1966). Reality Orientation for the elderly mental Patient. Read at 122th annual meeting of American Psychiatric Association, May 1966.

[27] Spector A., Davies S., Woods B. and Orrell M. (2000): Reality Orientation for Dementia. A Systematic Review of the Evidence of Effectiveness from Randomized Controlled Trials. *Gerontologist* 40:206-212.

[28] Spector A. and Orrell M. (2006). A review of the use of Cognitive Stimulation Therapy in dementia management. *British Journal of Neuroscience Nursing,* 2 (8), 381-387.

[29] Sacks H., Schegloff E. and Jefferson G. (1974). A simplest systematics for the organization of turn-taking for conversation. *Language* 50: 696-735.

[30] Novak M. and Guest C. (1989). Application of a multidimensional Caregiver Burden Inventory. *Gerontologist* 29:798-803.

INDEX

N

O

T